Joe Rosales Jr. 1982

Joe Rosales Jr. 1982

HUMAN CHLAMYDIAL INFECTIONS

Julius Schachter, Ph.D.
Chandler R. Dawson, M.D.

PSG Publishing Company, Inc.
Littleton, Massachusetts

Library of Congress Cataloging in Publication Data

Schachter, Julius.
    Human chlamydial infections.

    Bibliography: p.
    Includes index.
    1. Chlamydia infections.   I.   Dawson, Chandler R.,
joint author.   II.   Title.
RC124.5.S3   616.9'22   75-12032
ISBN 0-88416-043-2

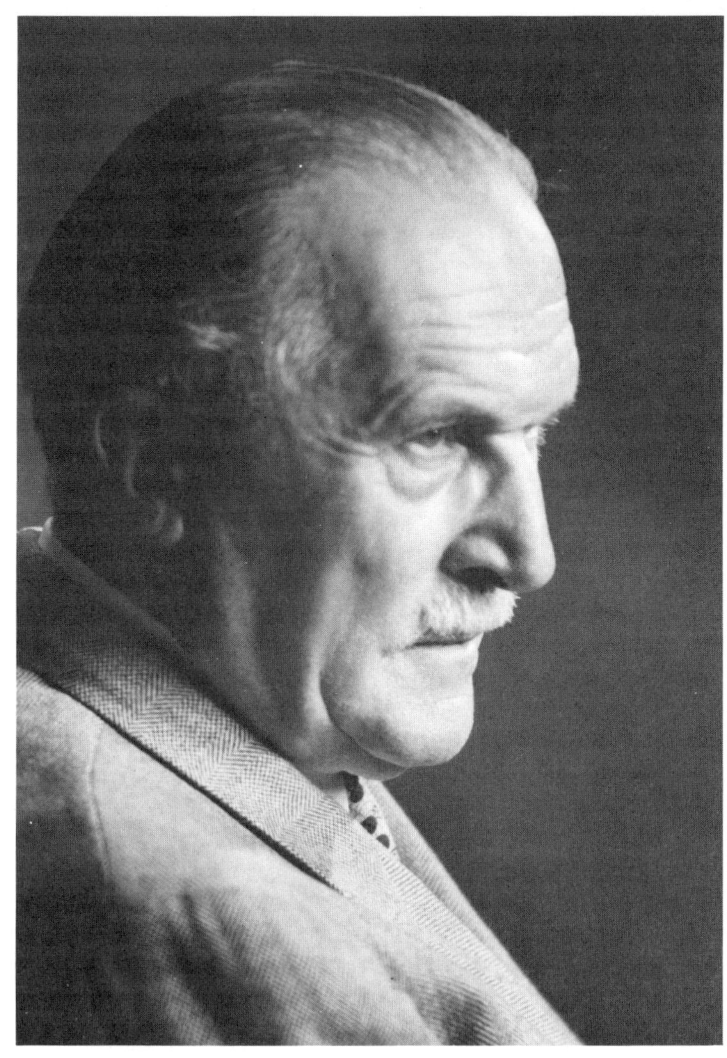

This book is dedicated to the memory of Karl F. Meyer (1884–1974).
He led us here.

The Authors

Julius Schachter, Ph.D.

Professor of Epidemiology
Acting Director of the George Williams Hooper
    Foundation for Medical Research
Codirector of the World Health Organization
    Collaborating Centre for Reference and Research
    on Trachoma and Other Chlamydial Infections
University of California
San Francisco, California

Chandler R. Dawson, M.D.

Professor of Ophthalmology
Associate Director of the Francis I. Proctor
    Foundation for Research in Ophthalmology
Codirector of the World Health Organization
    Collaborating Centre for Reference and Research
    on Trachoma and Other Chlamydial Infections
University of California
San Francisco, California

CONTENTS

1 Introduction   1
   Taxonomy
   Chlamydia and *Neorickettsia*

2 Psittacosis   9
   Historical Aspects
   Prevalence
   Clinical Picture
   Laboratory Diagnosis and Specimens
   Differential Diagnosis
   Treatment
   Immunity
   Pathology
   Epidemiology
   Latency in Psittacosis
   Natural History in Birds
   Diagnosis of Infection in the Avian Contact
   Experimental Host Range
   Public Health Considerations
   Perspectives

3 Lymphogranuloma Venereum   45
   Historical Aspects
   Clinical Manifestations
   Serologic Abnormalities
   Differential Diagnosis
   Chemotherapy
   LGV and Cancer
   Diagnostic Methods

4 Trachoma   63
   Historical Aspects
   Clinical Description
   Epidemiology
   Differential Diagnosis
   Laboratory Diagnosis
   Immunization
   Treatment and Control

5 Adult Inclusion Conjunctivitis   97
   Historical Aspects
   Epidemiology
   Clinical Disease
   Differential Diagnosis

vi

      Laboratory Tests
      Treatment

6 **Inclusion Conjunctivitis of the Newborn and Chlamydial Pneumonia in Infants**   **111**
      Historical Aspects
      Epidemiology
      Clinical Disease
      Differential Diagnosis
      Laboratory Tests
      Treatment
      Pneumonia in Infants

7 **Genital Tract Infections**   **121**
      Historical Aspects
      Nongonococcal Urethritis in Males
      Diagnosis of Nongonococcal Urethritis
      Cervical Infection with Chlamydiae
      Postgonococcal Urethritis
      Treatment
      Discussion

8 **Reiter's Syndrome**   **141**
      Historical Aspects
      Clinical Description
      Evidence for Chlamydial Involvement
      Studies at the University of California,
        San Francisco
      Isolation Attempts
      Cytologic Studies
      Studies Performed in Other Laboratories
      Immunologic Response to Chlamydiae in Reiter's
        Syndrome
      Experimental Studies
      Diagnosis of Reiter's Syndrome
      The Role of Chlamydiae in Reiter's Syndrome

9 **The Role of Chlamydiae Derived from Lower Mammals in Human Disease**   **153**
      Proven Human Infections
      Cat-Scratch Disease

10 **Microbiology of the Chlamydia**   **157**
      Morphologic Characteristics
      Bacterial Nature
      Developmental Cycle
      Effect of Penicillins
      Chemical Composition

Nutritional Requirements
Metabolism
Protein Synthesis
DNA Synthesis
DNA Homology
Lipid Synthesis
Synthesis of Polysaccharides
Growth in Cell Culture
Latent Infections in Vitro
Stability of Chlamydiae
Chlamydial Antigens
Specific Antigens
Hemagglutination Reactions
Cross-reactions with Other Organisms

11 **Laboratory Diagnosis   181**
Cytologic Techniques
Serologic Diagnosis
Isolation of Chlamydiae

Bibliography   221

Index   265

AHC	acute hemorrhagic conjunctivitis
AVU	arbitrary vaccine units
CF	complement-fixing (fixation)
CSD	cat-scratch disease
EB	elementary body
EKC	epidemic kerato-conjunctivitis
FA	fluorescent antibody
GC	gonorrhea
IC	inclusion conjunctivitis
ICN	inclusion conjunctivitis of the newborn (inclusion blennorrhea)
IDU (IUDR)	5-iodo 2-deoxyuridine
IgA, IgG, IgM	immunoglobulin classes
HSV	herpes simplex virus *(Herpesvirus hominis)*
LGV	lymphogranuloma venereum
Micro-IF	microimmunofluorescence
MRC	Medical Research Council
NAMRU	Naval Medical Research Unit
NDV	Newcastle disease virus
NGU	nongonococcal urethritis
PBS	phosphate buffered saline
PCF	pharyngoconjunctival fever
PEB	purified elementary body
PGU	postgonococcal urethritis
PID	pelvic inflammatory disease
PMN	polymorphonuclear neutrophil
RS	Reiter's syndrome
TPK	TRIC agent punctate keratoconjunctivitis
TRIC	trachoma–inclusion conjunctivitis
VD	venereal disease
WHO	World Health Organization
YS	yolk sac

ACKNOWLEDGMENTS

We would like to thank our colleagues, Drs. S. Darougar, E.M.C. Dunlop, A.W. Hoke, A. Kaufman, G.P. Manire, J. Swanson, G. Wachendörfer, and S.-P. Wang for supplying some of the illustrations used in this volume. Permission to reproduce illustrations has been graciously granted by the journals cited in the text.

Original work of the authors has been generously supported by funds from the National Institutes of Health, Dr. Schachter, CC-00553, AI-07439, AI-10193, AI-11881, CA-14427; Dr. Dawson, 2 RO1 EY00427, 5 RO1 EY01198, 2 RO1 EY00186, NO1 AI-22520, 2 PO1 EY00310, 1-KS NB-31,781, PL.480 07-075, PL.480 03-024. The World Health Organization has also provided support.

We would like to acknowledge the help we have had in preparing this volume. Our thanks to Ms. Janette Reseco and Ms. Joan Williamson for typing the manuscript, Ms. Carol Fegte for editorial assistance, and Ms. Joanne Zidek for putting it together.

Julius Schachter, Ph.D.
Chandler R. Dawson, M.D.

1 Introduction

In this volume the authors cannot make any claim to performing a complete survey of the literature. Because of the ubiquitous nature of chlamydial parasites and the significance of the human diseases they cause, the list of references could easily number many thousands.

It should be obvious that each of the chapters in this book could well be the subject of its own volume. It was not our purpose to write an "Encyclopedia of the Chlamydiae" — nor would we be suitable authors in some areas. However, we have long felt the need for a single volume reviewing certain aspects of chlamydiae and their role in human disease. Therefore, our goal has been the preparation of a relatively concise review of our knowledge in this area to 1977. To keep the volume within manageable size, we have tried to discuss most of the major issues but have refrained from in-depth analysis of individual points. We leave this to those who may focus on single chlamydial diseases.

The book is designed to cover points of interest to clinicians, epidemiologists, and public health and laboratory workers. Because the emphasis is on human disease, microbiology and laboratory diagnosis are discussed later. Realizing we must compete for the reader's time, we have written the text so that each chapter can be read independently; this is a reflection of the clinical spectrum of human chlamydial diseases. Obviously the ophthalmologist's major interest will be in the chapters dealing with eye disease, and the venereologist may be most interested in the chapters on lymphogranuloma venereum and other chlamydial infections of the genital tract; neither may be concerned with psittacosis. Therefore we must apologize to the person who has the interest and patience to read the whole book for the slight redundancy this has caused. The diagnostic procedures, discussed under specific diseases, are presented in the chapter on laboratory diagnosis in sufficient detail to allow the interested worker to implement the methods. Interpretation of results is also discussed; thus we hope the reader may benefit from our experience.

We feel that perhaps one of the most important things we can do is suggest additional reading for those students who may wish to delve further into selected aspects of chlamydial biology. Some of the references suggested here are presented because they cover areas beyond the scope of this particular volume; others are given because they represent the most complete, up-to-date reviews available. We have also included a number of papers published many years ago, because some of these observations are as significant today as they were when originally made. It is doubtful, for example, that there will be another psittacosis pandemic such as occurred in 1929 and 1930, but this does not diminish the value of the epidemiologic and pathologic studies done at that time. And, although trachoma is rapidly disappearing from some parts of the world, the disease still remains as the most important cause of preventable blindness in other regions.

For the historical aspects of psittacosis, the authors suggest the following: Bedson's Harben lectures (1959); and the recapitulation of the pandemic of 1929 and 1930 in England (Sturdee and Scott, 1930), in the United States (Armstrong, 1930), and in Europe and Argentina (Elkeles and Barros, 1931; Pfaffenberg, 1936; Barros, 1940). We recommend the monograph by Lillie (1933) for studies of the pathology of psittacosis. The Public Health Reports, Reprint No. 2580, reviewing the study of an epidemic outbreak of human psittacosis in Louisiana, is recommended as a complement to the studies of the 1929–1930 pandemic. For reviews of the physiology of chlamydiae we suggest the series of publications from Moulder: the two books *The Psittacosis Group as Bacteria* (1964) and *The Biochemistry of Intracellular Parasitism* (1962a); and the reviews "The Relation of the Psittacosis Group (Chlamydiae) to Bacteria and Viruses" (1966) and "A Model for Studying the Biology of Parasitism" (1969). Weiss (1968) has also reviewed the physiology of these organisms, and Becker (1974) has written specifically on the biology of the trachoma agent. For a review of chlamydial infections with an emphasis on diseases in lower mammals, see Storz's *Chlamydia and Chlamydia-Induced Diseases* (1971); for reviews of the biology of the chlamydiae causing avian diseases, refer to the chapters by Meyer in the 1965 edition of *Diseases of Poultry* and by Page in the 1972 edition. For review of chemotherapy for chlamydial infections in general, see Jawetz (1969), and in the field of trachoma (Tarizzo and Nataf, 1970); this is, however, an area which needs much greater knowledge. For review of trachoma, the volumes by MacCallan (1936); by Bietti, Freyche, and Vozza (1962); and by Bietti and Werner (1967) are recommended. The field of chlamydial genital tract infections is not presented in any single book, but the most recent review is by Grayston and Wang (1975); the authors suggest that the interested reader refer to the 1964 and 1972 volumes of *The British Journal of Venereal Diseases* for a series of original articles, mainly by English workers, that review and present the then current status of chlamydial genital tract infections. Lymphogranuloma venereum (LGV) was reviewed by Sigel (1962).

For an interesting perspective on the evolution of research approaches to trachoma and oculogenital chlamydial infections, we recommend the three proceedings that have resulted from the international symposia held on these subjects in 1960, 1966, and 1970:

The biology of the trachoma agent. Proceedings of a conference, May 26–27, 1961. F.B. Gordon (ed.). *Ann. N.Y. Acad. Sci.* 98:382, 1962.

Trachoma and allied diseases. Proceedings of a conference, August 25–31, 1966. Sponsored by the Francis I. Proctor Foundation for Research in Ophthalmology and the Harvard School of Public Health. *Am. J. Ophthalmol.* 63:631, 1967.

Trachoma and related disorders caused by chlamydial agents. Proceedings of a symposium, August 17–20, 1970. R.L. Nichols (ed.). *Excerpta Medica,* International Congress Series No. 223, 586 pp., Amsterdam, 1971.

TAXONOMY

In recent years the chlamydiae have been known by a variety of names. Most important among these various epithets are *Bedsonia*

4

and *Miyagawanella*. The confusion was largely resolved by Page (1966), who reviewed the classification of this group of agents and suggested that the genus *Chlamydia* be used for all members of the psittacosis-lymphogranuloma venereum-trachoma group. He pointed out that this term had taxonomic validity over the various other proposals. The adoption of a single genus served to unite these organisms which have common antigenic and biological properties, and stressed their similarities rather than their differences. The name *Chlamydia* may be traced back to the original description by Halberstaedter and von Prowazek (1907a,b), who thought they were dealing with protozoan parasites and proposed the term *Chlamydozoaceae* for these "mantled animals" (von Prowazek, 1907). Unfortunately this is a misnomer (there is no mantle), and the derivative term is one which must be accepted because of priority in conformity with the systematics of bacterial nomenclature.

Differences in biological properties of various isolates within this genus had long been recognized. However, the first functional segregation was by Gordon and Quan (1965a), who studied 27 chlamydial isolates and divided them into two groups on the basis of inclusion morphology and the presence or absence of glycogen in the inclusion. The tight, compact inclusions containing glycogen were designated as group A, while diffuse inclusions which did not stain for glycogen (iodine stain) were designated group B. Lin and Moulder (1966) extended this grouping to include inhibition of growth by sulfadiazine, with all subgroup A strains being sensitive to the action of sulfadiazine and most (excepting only the psittacosis, 6 BC isolate) B strains being resistant. These authors also found that sensitivity to cycloserine was associated with group A isolates to a greater degree than with group B.

The morphologic criteria are not particularly useful, but the association of iodine-staining inclusions (glycogen) and sensitivity to sulfadiazine appear to be useful taxonomic tools. Sensitivity to sulfa alone will not give perfect discrimination between species because, in addition to the 6 BC strain, the Gleason strain and several recent chlamydial isolates have been shown to be sensitive to sulfadiazine, although they are clearly psittacosis strains and have glycogen negative inclusions. Thus, it would appear that the most useful distinction between these two groups is the ability to stain the inclusion with iodine in order to detect glycogen.

Page (1968) proposed that two species be recognized within the genus, and he utilized the terms *C. trachomatis* and *C. psittaci* to represent Gordon and Quan's groups A and B, respectively.

The following description of these species is taken from the eighth edition of *Bergey's Manual of Determinative Bacteriology* (Page, 1974) under the general heading "The Rickettsias":

Order II.   Chlamydiales Storz and Page, 1971

Chla.my.di.a′les. M.L. n. *Chlamydia* type genus of the order; *-ales* ending to denote an order; M.L. fem. pl. n. *Chlamydiales* the *Chlamydia*.

Coccoid microorganisms whose obligately intracellular mode of multiplication is characterized by change of the small, rigid-walled infectious form of the organism (elementary body) into a larger, thin-walled, non-infectious form (initial body) that divides by fission. The developmental cycle is complete when daughter cells reorganize and condense to become elementary bodies which survive extracellularly to infect other host cells. Metabolically limited, Gram-negative parasites of vertebrates in which they may cause various diseases. Occasionally found in arthropods.

Family I.   Chlamydiaceae Rake, 1957

Chla.my.di.a′ce.ae. M.L. fem. n. *Chlamydia* type genus of the family; *-aceae* ending to denote a family; M.L. fem. pl. n. *Chlamydiaceae* the *Chlamydia* family.

Coccoid microorganisms, 0.2–1.5 μm in diameter, which multiply only within the cytoplasm of host cells by a developmental cycle characterized by change of a small elementary body into a larger initial body that divides by fission. The cycle is complete when daughter cells reorganize and condense to become elementary bodies which survive extracellularly to infect other host cells. Elementary bodies contain compactly arranged nuclear material and ribosomes and are bounded by a rigid, trilaminar cell wall that is chemically similar to that of Gram-negative bacteria. Initial bodies contain amorphous nuclear material less electron-dense than that of elementary bodies, have thin, fragile cell walls and apparently are non-infectious. Metabolically limited, Gram-negative parasites of vertebrates in which they may cause various diseases. Occasionally found in arthropods. Cultivatable in yolk sac of chicken embryos. Sensitive to tetracycline antibiotics. Stain with aniline dyes.

Genus I.   Chlamydia Jones, Rake and Stearns, 1945

Chla.my′di.a. Gr. fem. n. *chlamys, chlamydis* a cloak, M.L. fem. dim. n. *Chlamydia* a cloak.

Only two species are recognized. Type species: *Chlamydia trachomatis* (Busacca) Rake, 1957.

Key to the species of genus Chlamydia:
 I. Forms compact microcolonies within cytoplasmic vesicles. Produces iodine-staining compounds within vesicle. Growth in the yolk sac of chicken embryos is inhibited by sodium sulfadiazine (1 mg/embryo).
1.   *Chlamydia trachomatis*
 II. Forms microcolonies within cytoplasmic vesicles which tend to rupture early in microcolony development, and the organisms in various stages of growth become distributed throughout the host cell cytoplasm. Does not produce iodine-staining compounds in vesicles. Growth in the yolk

sac of chicken embryos is not inhibited by sodium sulfadiazine (1 mg/embryo).

2. *Chlamydia psittaci*

Page's proposal has the merit of dividing the chlamydiae into two groups which can be differentiated by relatively simple biochemical tests. It suffers because organisms possessing a great diversity of biological and antigenic properties have been somewhat awkwardly compressed into each of these species. Easier methods of differentiating the agents will have to be developed before new species can be proposed. The current data suggest that there are differences readily demonstrable within either species, with the greatest diversity of biological properties in the species *C. psittaci*. Most members of the species *C. trachomatis* appear to present a spectrum of antigenic relationships and biological properties (with the singular exception of the markedly different mouse pneumonitis strain). That is, the lymphogranuloma venereum and trachoma-inclusion conjunctivitis strains are clearly very closely related. In spite of its drawbacks, this general system of nomenclature will be utilized here, largely because it has the general acceptance of the scientific community.

The chlamydiae for many years were included in the order Rickettsiales. Weiss (1968) showed that there are significant differences in the metabolic reactions of rickettsiae and chlamydiae. Among these differences are the metabolic independence of the rickettsiae with aerobic metabolic cycles resulting in energy production and including complete cytochrome systems; the chlamydiae, on the other hand, are essentially anaerobic, have no cytochrome system, do not produce ATP, and do not preferentially utilize glutamate as do the rickettsiae. Moulder (1964) had emphasized the unique nature of the chlamydial developmental cycle. Storz (1971) pointed out that this difference was probably sufficient to justify removing the chlamydiae from the Rickettsiales, and this proposal to establish a separate order Chlamydiales was formalized by Storz and Page (1971).

CHLAMYDIA AND NEORICKETTSIA

There is much literature, primarily French, on human and animal diseases associated with what are called neorickettsiae. Giroud (1969), who has been responsible for much of the original work in this area, has stated that he feels the terms neorickettsiae and bedsoniae (now chlamydiae) are essentially synonymous, and that these strains have the same biological properties. It is clear that at least some neorickettsial strains are chlamydiae, but it is not clear that all of them are. At any rate, it has been very difficult to determine from the literature and simple strain designations which neorickettsiae really are chlamydiae and which might be rickettsiae that have not been identified properly on the basis of serologic or other reactions. Because of this difficulty, we have chosen not to consider the neorickettsiae in this review.

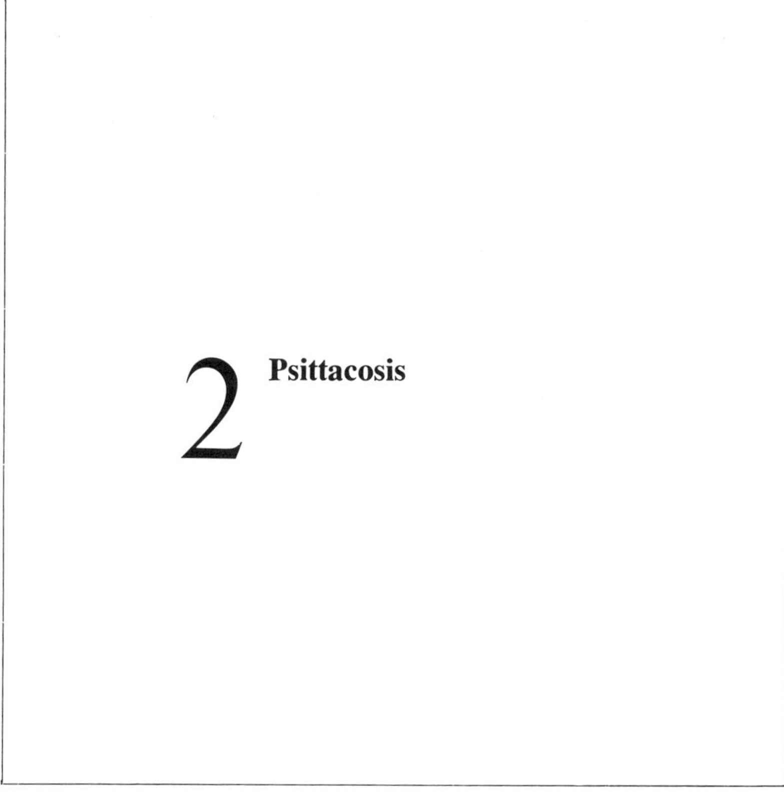

Psittacosis is a chlamydial infection contracted by humans through exposure to infected avian species. The term psittacosis is also applied to chlamydial infection of psittacine species (parrots and related birds), while the term ornithosis is used for chlamydial infection of other avian species (such as turkeys, pigeons, and egrets).

HISTORICAL ASPECTS

Human psittacosis often causes an atypical pneumonia, and it may have been described in this form by Jüergensen as early as 1874. However, the first recognition of psittacosis is generally attributed to Ritter, who reported an outbreak of pneumotyphus in Switzerland in 1879 (Ritter, 1880). The disease was typified as a severe pneumonia with stupor (hence the descriptive term) and a scattering of rose spots. An association of human disease with exposure to exotic pet birds was observed in the Swiss outbreaks; this association was confirmed in a series of outbreaks in France in the 1890s. Morange, describing some of these cases in 1895, coined the term psittacosis, derived from the Greek word for parrot.

A number of these outbreaks in the late nineteenth century foreshadowed the events that occurred in the larger outbreaks of the 1930s. For example, in the Paris outbreaks in 1892 and 1893, unscrupulous pet bird dealers made every effort to sell diseased parrots before they died; in the United States in the 1930s, bird dealers, to obtain some use for their dying merchandise, gave away sick birds as prizes at state fairs in Wisconsin and Minnesota. In 1897, cases of psittacosis in Italy were traced to diseased parrots shipped from Argentina. This outbreak was controlled when quarantine measures were instituted and importation of parrots was banned.

Psittacosis was first described in the United States in 1904 (Vickery and Richardson, 1904), and there were a number of relatively small outbreaks after that, the most notable being traced to infected birds on sale in a department store in Wilkes Barre, Pennsylvania (McClintock, 1925). However, psittacosis remained a relatively uncommon disease, with only scattered case reports in the scientific literature until the great pandemic of 1929–1930.

This pandemic, ultimately involving at the very least 700 to 800 cases, started in Argentina in July 1929 when Barros (1930) observed an unusual form of pneumonia, occurring in Cordoba and other provinces, which seemed to be associated with exposure to parrots. The disease soon spread to Europe and North America and, by November 1930, major epidemics had occurred in England, Germany, and the United States, with well over 100 cases in each of these countries. Most recognized cases were severe and in each country where the pandemic struck the outbreaks received considerable publicity. There were thousands of references in the newspapers and many hundreds in the scientific literature. There were many small outbreaks. For example, in the United States in a five-month period there were 169 cases with 74 different foci (Armstrong, 1930). Seamen working on the ships that transported the infected birds from the Argentine were also exposed and became ill. The mortality rate was relatively high — up to 40% in certain outbreaks. The near panic associated with the disease was increased when many laboratory workers attempting to define the disease's etiology contracted laboratory infections, resulting in a number of fatalities (Hasseltine, 1932). Some laboratories were completely closed down due to aerosol type infections, where researchers in adjacent laboratories, not even working on this problem, became victims.

The interest and the concern of public health officials were obviously great, and many researchers sought the cause of the disease. The timing of this outbreak on a world-wide basis was so acute that the morphologic descriptions of the causative agent appeared almost simultaneously in Germany, the United States, and England. Levinthal on April 5, Lillie on April 11, and Coles on May 10 of 1930, each described the characteristic coccoid forms and inclusions found in the tissues of infected birds or humans. The agent causing the disease was isolated by Bedson and Western in 1930 by inoculation of human and avian material into budgerigars (parakeets). Krumwiede and associates (1930) in the United States and Gordon (1930a,b) in England made the observation that the agent of psittacosis was transmissible to mice. This provided a convenient laboratory system for isolation and assay of the organism and led to the development of useful screening methods. Bedson and Western (1930) demonstrated a complement-fixing antibody response to the organism which ultimately led to the development of serologic tests for diagnosis (Bedson, 1935). (It should be noted here that these studies were initially clouded by a previous report by Nocard [1893] of isolation of the causative bacteria. Much of the early work emphasized attempts to confirm Nocard's studies, and were virtually complete failures. Unfortunately, there were occasional successes in recovering the organism, which was then called *Bacterium psittacosis* or *B. aerytrycke*. This organism is now known as *Salmonella typhimurium* and is recognized to be a common contaminant or pathogen in avian species.)

The major public health measure to control the epidemic was embargo. Many countries refused to accept birds from Argentina or instituted a complete ban on importation of psittacine species. This was markedly successful in some countries. In England there were no new cases for many months following the ban on importation. In the United States, however, although the incidence decreased, there continued to be sporadic outbreaks of psittacosis. Meyer and Eddie (1933b), following up on the Grass Valley, California, epidemic, discovered the reservoir of what they called "endemic psittacosis"; the locally bred psittacine bird, the parakeet, was infected. Within a few years there were approximately 145 cases of human psittacosis traced to these birds (Meyer, 1935). Essentially all these cases derived from California breeding establishments (Hoge, 1934). This led to a ban on interstate transport of parakeets, which stopped the outbreak. Because of the economic importance of the pet bird industry, Meyer and Eddie developed methods of testing breeding flocks for infection levels, and this led to the development of certified clean breeding establishments (Meyer, 1942).

Up to 1938 it was thought that all human psittacosis cases were associated with psittacine species, but then an atypical pneumonia which occurred in epidemic form in the Faroe Islands was traced by Haagen and Mauer to infected fulmars. Thus, passerine species were

12

shown to be infected with a chlamydial agent. The disease was quite severe, with a relatively high fatality rate, 23.1% (42 deaths/182 cases). Vaag (1950) has emphasized that the mortality rate was exceptionally high (78%) in pregnant women, with 11 of the 14 cases succumbing. Among the other cases, both mild and severe infections were observed. The general pattern was similar to previous outbreaks of respiratory disease among the Faroe Islanders that had always been considered to be influenza.

The awareness of what came to be known as ornithosis (a term used to indicate that species other than psittacine birds could be reservoirs) was soon followed by the recovery of a chlamydial agent from pigeons placed under stress by a thiamine-deficient diet (Pinkerton and Swank, 1940). Shortly thereafter, Meyer (1941b) diagnosed a human infection resulting from exposure to pigeons. This was followed by demonstration that chickens could be a source of human infection (Karrer, Eddie, and Schmid, 1950). Then, in 1951, in Texas, the first mass outbreak of human chlamydial infections associated with turkey ranching was proved (Irons, Denley, and Sullivan, 1955; Irons, Sullivan, and Rowen, 1951; Meyer and Eddie, 1953). Here many of the infections were associated with the processing of the birds, with high infection rates in eviscerators and pickers. These Texas outbreaks were followed by epidemics associated with turkeys in the mid-1950s in Oregon, Washington, and California (Meyer, 1965). In 1952 it was discovered that ducks could be a significant source of human infection (Korns, 1955). Thus, in the 25 years after the isolation of the psittacosis agent, the potential reservoirs of human psittacosis were recognized not to be restricted to exotic birds but to include many avian species.

By the mid-1950s effective methods for treating human psittacosis had been developed and improved diagnostic techniques were available. Until the late 1960s importation of birds still represented a potential threat, but then Arnstein, Eddie, and Meyer (1968) developed methods of treating psittacine birds with medicated feed which theoretically promised to control the infections. Similar methods are possible in the poultry industry, but problems concerning the long-term effect and advisability of adding tetracycline to feed are still unsolved.

The Louisiana Outbreak

There have been a number of outbreaks of human psittacosis where the source of infection has never been positively identified. It seems worthwhile to briefly recount one of the more dramatic of these outbreaks. In 1943 and 1944, in the bayou region of Louisiana, 19 cases of psittacosis resulted in 8 deaths (Olson and Treuting, 1944). There was no documented history of avian contacts. This epidemic is particularly noteworthy for the frequency of secondary infections, as there were only 5 primary cases. The secondary cases occurred exclusively in individuals who came in close proximity to fatal cases within 48 hours before death. In one instance, 3 of the 7 individuals attending a fatally ill patient expired.

In most patients the onset was mild and appeared to have an incubation period ranging from 6 to 19 days (Treuting and Olson, 1944). Patients developed fevers that reached 103° to 105° F 4 to 7 days after the onset. The pulse and respiration in these cases tended to rise (which is not typical for psittacosis). A productive cough developed in many of the patients approximately 7 to 14 days after onset of symptoms, and cyanosis occurred in 14 of the 19 individuals. The pulse fluctuated and circulatory collapse was common. In general, the clinical findings indicated a process much more severe than the patients' illness appeared to be upon gross examination. The later cases, when tested, readily yielded isolates (3 of the 4 so tested) of a highly virulent chlamydial strain (Olson and Larson, 1944). Death, when it occurred, was usually between 7 and 14 days after onset. In the patients coming to autopsy, marked focal consolidation of the lung was observed, with very sharp demarcation from the adjacent normal tissue. Spleens were enlarged, with infiltrated pulp, and degeneration of the rectus muscle was common (Binford and Hauser, 1944). Historical reconstruction, together with the isolation of virulent chlamydial strains from egrets (Rubin et al., 1951) in the area, suggests that the egrets, with the possibility of a further zoonotic complication from egret-muskrat interaction, may have been the source of the infecting organism.

Although this is certainly one of the most dramatic instances of an outbreak of this nature, it is not unique, since similar outbreaks have occurred in Illinois, San Francisco, and elsewhere. Neither the high case fatality rates nor the high rate of man-to-man transmission demonstrated in the Louisiana outbreak are common features of human psittacosis. But both have been observed in selected outbreaks, and some man-to-man transmission has been noted in a number of other instances where fatal disease was not involved.

PREVALENCE

In the decade after the epidemic years of 1929 and 1930 there were relatively few cases of psittacosis reported annually in the United

States. From 1931 to 1940 virtually all human cases were associated with parakeets. With the recognition of ornithosis, human infections in the 1940s were occasionally associated with chickens (Meyer and Eddie, 1942), or more often with pigeons (Meyer, 1959). As is shown in Figure 1, the increases in the number of reported cases could be associated with each relaxation of quarantine or restriction placed on interstate commerce or importation of exotic birds (Drachman, 1953; Steele and Scruggs, 1958). The number of cases increased dramatically in 1952 and for several years thereafter, largely as a result of recognition of the domestic turkey reservoir (Irons, Denley, and Sullivan, 1955; Meyer, 1965). By this time, at least in the United States, the epidemiologic profile of psittacosis had changed from that of a household disease in humans, with occasional outbreaks in employees of pet shops or in bird breeders, to an occupational hazard involving individuals exposed to birds in poultry processing plants. However, by the 1960s and early 1970s, the number of reported cases had again dropped dramatically, so that fewer than 50 cases were being recognized each year. The 1974 outbreaks in Texas, Missouri, and Nebraska served as a reminder of the ever present threat of psittacosis in the turkey industry (Durfee et al., 1975).

It must be recognized that the diagnosis of psittacosis is not readily obtained in all cases. In many cases of psittacosis, it is likely that this diagnosis is not even considered. The disease, of course, is now recognized to have a broad clinical spectrum and is not nearly as severe as it was in the 1930s when the case fatality rates were so high. It is characteristic in any disease that earlier recognized cases represent the more severe forms and later studies demonstrate the presence of a milder form of infection.

Serologic studies on individuals at risk have demonstrated that subclinical infections are not uncommon (Meyer, 1965; Fransén, 1969). Many veterinarians, individuals involved in raising or handling exotic birds, and employees in poultry industries have antibody titers (Meyer and Eddie, 1939; Graber and Pomeroy, 1958; Meyer and Eddie, 1962). These high seropositive rates are often associated with previous histories of minor respiratory disease or influenza-like symptoms which in some cases probably represent mild psittacosis infections. It is likely that the true incidence of psittacosis is much higher than that reflected by the cases reported. For example, Germany, with approximately one-quarter the population of the United States, regularly

Fig. 1. Reported psittacosis cases in the United States, pertinent regulations, and recognition of reservoirs. (From National Communicable Disease Center, with permission.)

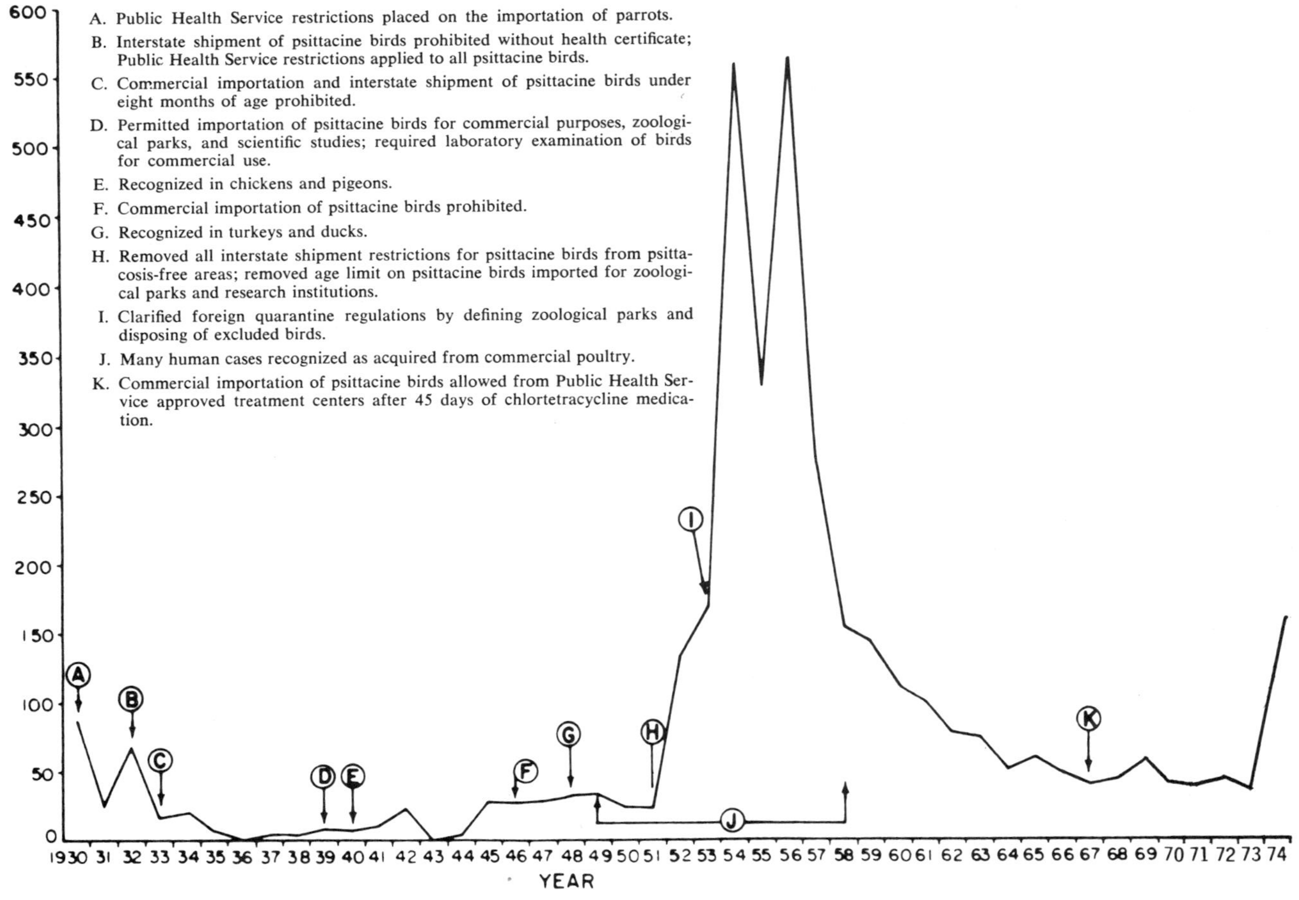

CASES
A. Public Health Service restrictions placed on the importation of parrots.
B. Interstate shipment of psittacine birds prohibited without health certificate; Public Health Service restrictions applied to all psittacine birds.
C. Commercial importation and interstate shipment of psittacine birds under eight months of age prohibited.
D. Permitted importation of psittacine birds for commercial purposes, zoological parks, and scientific studies; required laboratory examination of birds for commercial use.
E. Recognized in chickens and pigeons.
F. Commercial importation of psittacine birds prohibited.
G. Recognized in turkeys and ducks.
H. Removed all interstate shipment restrictions for psittacine birds from psittacosis-free areas; removed age limit on psittacine birds imported for zoological parks and research institutions.
I. Clarified foreign quarantine regulations by defining zoological parks and disposing of excluded birds.
J. Many human cases recognized as acquired from commercial poultry.
K. Commercial importation of psittacine birds allowed from Public Health Service approved treatment centers after 45 days of chlortetracycline medication.
1930 31 32 33 34 35 36 37 38 39 40 41 42 43 44 45 46 47 48 49 50 51 52 53 54 55 56 57 58 59 60 61 62 63 64 65 66 67 68 69 70 71 72 73 74
YEAR

records more human psittacosis cases (Fig. 2). The higher rate probably reflects slight epidemiologic differences together with somewhat greater surveillance.

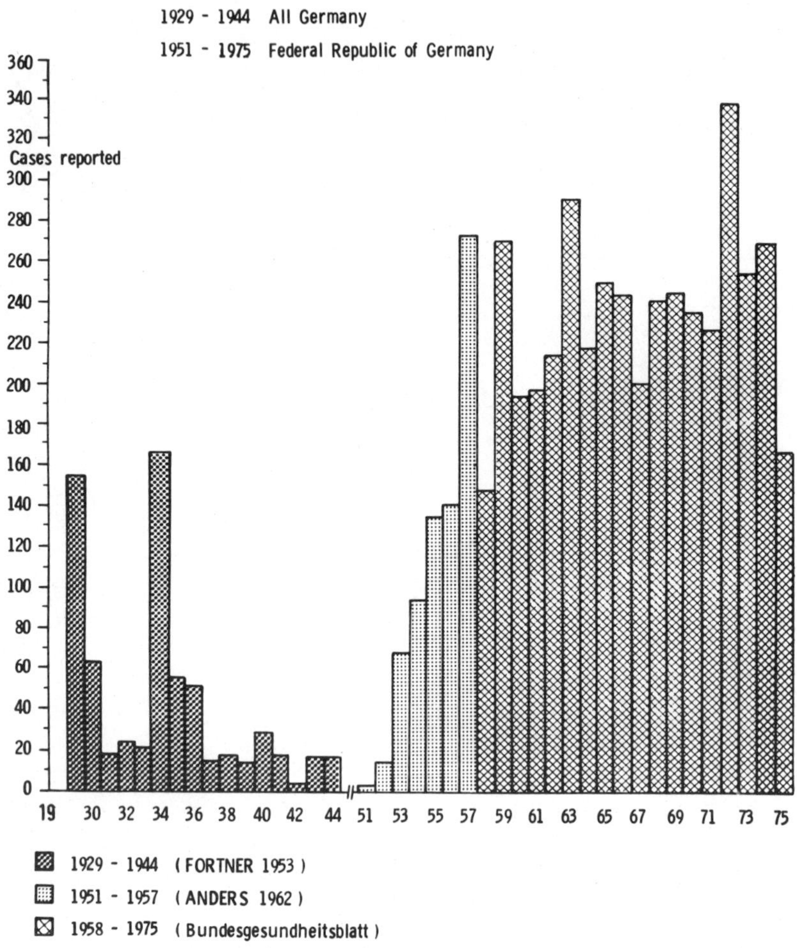

Fig. 2. Incidence of psittacosis and ornithosis in humans in Germany. (Courtesy of Dr. J.G. Wachendörfer)

The significance of psittacosis in atypical pneumonia is difficult to determine. Originally, prior to the identification of *Mycoplasma pneumoniae* and the introduction of specific serologic tests, it was thought that psittacosis might be a major cause of atypical pneumonia (Eaton, Beck, and Pearson, 1941; Smadel, 1943). After the introduction and widespread use of the complement fixation test and use of cold agglutinins to differentiate the two, a number of studies based on these methods indicated that psittacosis might be responsible for as many as 20% to 25% of human cases of atypical pneumonia. For example, Smadel (1943), in a small series, found that 10 out of 45 cases of atypical pneumonia were, in fact, psittacosis, probably associated with pigeons. As late as 1961, Goto et al., in Japan, tested 160 patients with atypical pneumonia and found that 33 of them could be shown by serologic methods to have had psittacosis. On the other hand, a number of large serologic surveys on respiratory diseases have shown that psittacosis is a very minor problem. Most of these studies were performed in North America and Europe, but similar results have been obtained in surveys of respiratory disease among children in the tropics (Chanock et al., 1967; Mufson et al., 1967).

CLINICAL PICTURE

Clinical Description of Untreated Psittacosis

It should be noted that the clinical conditions and progression described here are generally those of untreated psittacosis, based on descriptions culled from the literature of the early 1930s together with the results from some very carefully studied laboratory infections and more recent small outbreaks (Sturdee and Scott, 1930; Armstrong, 1930; Treuting and Olson, 1944). The advent of chemotherapy obviously removed the necessity of following this disease through its course.

The incubation period is often difficult to ascertain because exposure to the infected bird or to infected premises may be either fleeting or constant. In general, the incubation period is considered to be between 6 and 15 days (Sturdee and Scott, 1930; Armstrong, 1930) although periods of up to 39 days have been proven.

The disease may have either an acute or insidious onset. There are usually two forms of the disease: The first, a pneumonitis or atypical pneumonia, is more common and is the one in which the diagnosis is most often made. It has clinical features somewhat similar to both influenza and typhoid, although it lacks the man-to-man transmission common to both these other conditions. The second general form of human psittacosis is associated with a toxic or almost septic condition where pneumonic findings and symptoms are not prominent. In either instance, fever is virtually always present. Temperatures as high as 100° to 103° F are common in the first week of the disease, and temperatures as high as 103° to 105° F are often reached in the second week. Chills often accompany the fever. Many, if not most, patients become constipated, although 10% to 12%

develop diarrhea. There is often a dry, hacking, nonproductive cough associated with the pneumonic process.

Two features of psittacosis that may help in the diagnosis are a pulse rate much slower than expected in view of the accompanying high fever, and pneumonic symptoms that are mild considering the extensive lung involvement shown by roentgenogram. Often there are radiologic findings of considerable pneumonitis in the total absence of any signs of respiratory distress.

The leukocyte count is usually normal or slightly low; leukopenia is marked in about 25% of cases, and late onset leukocytosis is often attributed to secondary bacterial infections.

Muscle aches and pains are common. Muscle involvement has recently been shown to be documentable by measurement of enzyme and creatine levels (Sullivan and Brewin, 1974). Occasionally, rose spots, similar to typhoidal rash, have been observed. The spleen is often involved and hepatitis has occasionally been clinically prominent and pathologically confirmed (Yow et al., 1959; Reinicke and Søndergaard, 1969). Hepatosplenomegaly is not rare, although it

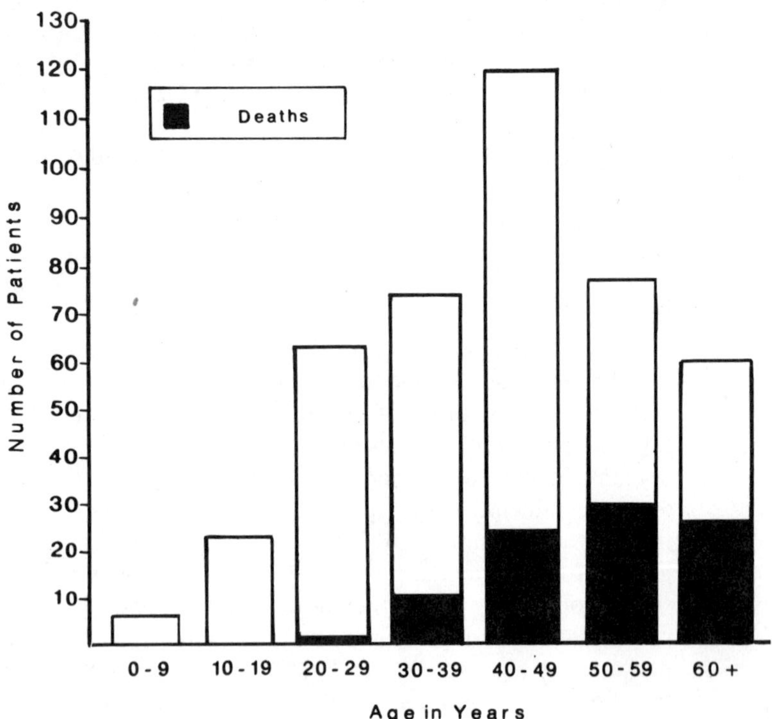

Fig. 3. Age distribution of cases and deaths in untreated human psittacosis.

appears to be variable depending on the series studied. Some authors found the spleen palpable in most cases, with tenderness and apparent extension of the liver border (Schaffner et al., 1967). Photophobia may occur but there is no conjunctivitis. Confusion and delirium are not rare and meningitis has been reported.

The temperature usually declines gradually (not by crisis) in the second week, although it may continue longer, and has been shown in some cases to persist for as long as 82 days (Jørgenson and Steffensen, 1956). Case fatality rates are shown in the accompanying figures which are a synthesis of several large series reported in the early 1930s together with records of untreated cases from the Hooper Foundation files (Figs. 3, 4). Case fatality rates have often been quite significant, varying between 20% and 40% in untreated, clinically ill patients. Serologic studies have detected clinically inapparent infections and mild influenzal forms. Cases generally occur in adults and are more severe in older patients, with most fatalities occurring in patients over 50 years of age. It is uncommon for children to contract the disease, although fatal infections have been reported (Berman et al., 1955). There is no definite prognosticator, even though some observers have felt that an increasing pulse means a poor prognosis (Sturdee and Scott, 1930).

The recovery is often prolonged, even after effective chemotherapy (Schaffner et al., 1967; Anderson and Bridgwater, 1968;

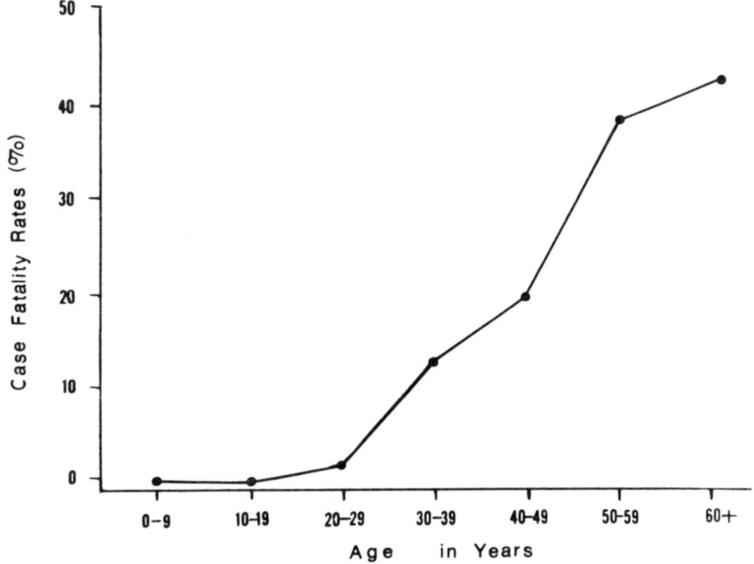

Fig. 4. Age-specific case fatality rates in untreated human psittacosis.

Jørgenson and Steffensen, 1956; Strauss, 1967). Relapses are not uncommon and may follow inadequate therapy. In general, complications are rare, although femoral vein thrombosis has been reported and may have led to fatal outcome in some relapsing cases. Myocarditis has been observed as a complication and is occasionally the only finding. The possible role of chlamydial infections in human cardiac disease is discussed later in this chapter.

It may be useful to review the symptoms associated with 22 confirmed psittacosis infections among workers at the Hooper Foundation during the past two decades. There were 17 individuals involved (3 relapses and 2 reinfections). One infection was limited to the conjunctiva. Of the 21 systemic infections, 20 were febrile. Severe headache was a common feature (16 cases) and often the major complaint. Chills were noted in 12 episodes. The disease was termed "flulike" in 10 instances. Although only 2 patients had pneumonia, 5 of the 10 patients X-rayed had evidence of lung involvement. Two of the patients had diarrhea and 1 was disoriented. Three required hospitalization. Tetracycline (250 mg q.i.d. for 21 days) was the prescribed treatment and generally achieved good results. In three instances the tetracycline was taken for less than a week because the acute symptoms had disappeared; in each instance relapse occurred (three to five weeks later). Among the successfully treated cases, 5 complained of marked fatigue well into convalescence.

Persistent infection may occur in humans. In one classic case cf a laboratory infection prior to adequate methods of treatment, the patient yielded the agent from sputum and blood for 10 years after the initial episode (Meyer and Eddie, 1951). Shorter-term post-convalescent shedding is recognized.

Clinical Spectrum in Sporadic Cases

The clinical variation of psittacosis has led to several publications describing apparently atypical clinical findings in a limited number of patients seen at major medical centers in the United States. The cases were not very similar in nature. It must be recognized that there is a wide range in the severity of the disease; also, the availability of accurate diagnosis, supportive therapy, and effective chemotherapy influences the clinical course. Part of the variation inherent here can be shown by considering two types of studies. The first type reflects cumulative experience at major medical centers. One by Seibert, Jordan, and Dingle (1956), reporting on 13 cases of psittacosis seen in Cleveland during an approximate five-year period, showed all patients with some degree of lung involvement, ranging from minimal to quite severe. Small series in Denver and Nashville are generally similar (Fitz, Meiklejohn, and Baum, 1955; Schaffner et al., 1967). In contrast, in the large outbreak associated with turkeys in Texas in 1952, the 22 of the 92 exposed workers who developed the disease had illnesses of varying severity, but without pneumonic involvement (Dickerson, 1962). Clearly, the current diagnosis of psittacosis reflects the index of suspicion of the attending physicians. At the major medical centers, it is likely that psittacosis was considered in the differential diagnosis of patients with pneumonias, either on epidemiologic grounds or after other causes had been excluded. In the Texas epidemic, there was a point source outbreak of a disease with many cases studied and diagnosed in a short period. In the latter type of series it is easier to identify unexpected differences in a syndrome.

It is obvious that psittacosis could well be considered in the differential diagnosis of any undiagnosed pneumonic process or any obscure febrile disease. The experiences of Kukowka, Stephan, and Krebs (1960) in Czechoslovakia may be of interest here. In a small outbreak involving 10 cases occurring in workers at a duck farm, the first 2 cases had an admitting diagnosis of bronchial pneumonia. The next 5 cases were considered to have typhoid fever on clinical grounds. In retrospect a diagnosis of psittacosis was made on serologic tests and the next 3 cases (quite similar, in fact, to some of the prior 7) were admitted with a diagnosis of psittacosis. The clear lesson here is that it is virtually impossible to diagnose human psittacosis on clinical grounds and that the physician should seek laboratory assistance in establishing the diagnosis as soon as possible.

Chlamydiae (Psittacosis) and Cardiac Involvement

Cardiac involvement has been well documented during systemic chlamydial infections of humans. In experimental animals it is characteristic, and pericarditis is a very significant part of the clinical response to chlamydial infection in avians. When autopsies are performed on birds presumed to have psittacosis or ornithosis, pericarditis and pericardial adhesions are among the lesions sought. This is particularly true in turkeys, where pericarditis may be the only major finding (Davis and Delaplane, 1958; Page, Derieux, and Cutlip, 1975).

Among the hundreds of case reports resulting from the pandemic of 1929–1930, there were occasional mentions of human psittacosis cases complicated by cardiac involvement. In the years since, there have continued to be a number of reports on myocarditis and, rarely, endocarditis. Occasionally inclusions have been shown in the macrophages in the myocardium (Jannach, 1958) or in the vegetations, in endocarditis. Levison et al. (1971) described two cases of fatal endocarditis where the diagnosis of chlamydial infection seemed reasonably certain (based on serology); in one case they demonstrated typical inclusions in impression smears and sections from valvular vegetations. Pericarditis (Schoenemann and Glasel, 1965) has also been reported. Grist and McLean (1964) consider cardiac involvement a common feature of psittacosis.

In the great majority of cases there has been a pneumonitis, either as a major complication of the cardiac involvement, or as the primary reason for presentation which was then followed by cardiac involvement. The patients appear to develop typical, but severe, pneumonia, with systemic spread of the agent and cardiac involvement, and often signs of encephalitis. For example, Schiraldi and Pesce (1965) described cases of pleuro-pericarditis. Similar observations have come from many countries (Valero, 1953; Kemmerer et al., 1956).

Many of the cases have been fatal — Jannach's case was fatal; Vosti and Roffwarg's (1961) patient with pneumonitis, encephalitis, and myocarditis died. The two cases described by Levison and colleagues were fatal. Yow et al. (1959) also described cardiac involvement in fatal psittacosis. Thus, most of these diagnosed cases have been severe. However, Coll and Horner (1967) reported a case of serologically proved psittacosis myocarditis which resulted in spontaneous remission, the patient becoming completely asymptomatic without any specific treatment.

Sutton in Chicago has attempted a systematic study of myocardial disease. In 1964 he reported one case of psittacosis complicated by myopericarditis (Sutton et al., 1964). Because of this observation, Sutton's group studied 599 patients suspected of having acute pericarditis or myocarditis (Sutton et al., 1967). Nine cases showed fourfold or greater increases in complement-fixing antibodies, and three had good response to tetracycline, as well as previous exposure to parakeets. Sutton et al. (1971) expanded their previous studies to focus on patients with primary myocardial disease and serologic evidence of exposure to chlamydiae. The rate of chlamydial seroreactors was greater than serologic reactions observed in control populations. Patients with coronary disease of known etiology were used as controls and did not show reactivity to chlamydiae. There was no apparent clinical difference between chlamydia-seropositive and chlamydia-seronegative patients with primary myocardial disease. A major finding in this study was that these seropositive patients usually did not have clinically evident psittacosis. It was thus suggested that otherwise inapparent chlamydial infections might cause a proportion of the primary myocardial disease seen at a time when there was a sudden increase in diagnosed chlamydial infections in Illinois. Some of their patients appeared to have alcoholic and postpartum "myocardial" involvement. Since the group-specific CF test was used, it is possible that chlamydial genital tract infections with TRIC agents might be involved in the primary coronary involvement. By inference, one could assume that chlamydiae present in the cervix might become bloodborne following delivery. (Parenthetically, one may note that we have observed rising CF titers after the infected women have come to term.) LGV would be another potential cause of this disease and, of course, the lymphogranuloma venereum agent has been recovered from autopsy tissue collected from a patient with hilar lymphadenopathy and pericarditis (Sheldon et al., 1948).

However, in a later study, 19 of Sutton's 40 patients had proven exposure to psittacosis reservoirs (Sutton et al., 1971). These cases occurred in a temporal cluster, at a time when the rate of positive CF reactions detected at the Illinois viral laboratories also peaked. It should be noted that the common nature of avian chlamydial infections had at this time only recently become clear, but effective chemotherapy for pet birds was not yet readily available. An obvious interpretation of these data is that the clinical spectrum of mild human psittacosis may include cardiac involvement.

Most case reports of cardiac involvement associated with psittacosis describe the condition as rare. Since psittacosis is itself not a common diagnosis, it is obvious that cardiac involvement, which appears to be an infrequent complication of psittacosis, could not be a common disease. However, rare diseases only stay rare when the diagnosis is not often sought. There is a consistent background of reports dealing with chlamydial infection and cardiac involvement. It is obvious that psittacosis is not often sought as a diagnosis in most cases of respiratory disease where it could be considered; certainly, it is not considered in the differential diagnosis of myocardial disease. Considering the number of reports together with the rarity of the disease, one may speculate that chlamydial infections may indeed be a definite, albeit minor, cause of coronary involvement, and that this area deserves further study.

LABORATORY DIAGNOSIS
AND SPECIMENS

The laboratory diagnosis of psittacosis is most conveniently established by serologic means. In general, cytologic examination of human material is unrewarding. The complement fixation test is quite effective, although early effective treatment with tetracycline may abolish an antibody response (Meyer and Eddie, 1956). A fourfold increase with paired acute and convalescent sera is usually considered necessary for a diagnosis. If an acute serum specimen is not obtained, single titers of 1:64 to 1:256 or higher are supportive of the diagnosis of ornithosis. It must be emphasized that the antibody response measured in the complement fixation test is group-specific and could indicate exposure to any chlamydiae. Low-level titers, particularly unchanging ones, may reflect exposure to the very common genital tract chlamydial infections and do not support a diagnosis of psittacosis.

The causative agent may be isolated in the yolk sac of the embryonated hen's egg, in the mouse, or in tissue culture systems. In the patient with a pneumonic process, sputum is most likely to yield chlamydiae, can be positive for weeks in untreated cases, and is usually chlamydia-positive between the fifth and eleventh day of disease (Rivers and Berry, 1932). An expectorant should be given if needed to produce sputum, and the collected material should be held in a liquid medium (e.g., balanced saline solution, nutrient broth) containing antibiotics. Streptomycin is the major component of the many antibiotic mixtures that have been specifically designed for collection of chlamydial specimens. Whole blood (heparinized or citrated), serum, or plasma may also be tested, and in the untreated case the agent may be recovered for several weeks (Bedson, Western, and Levy, 1930). The sterile citrated or heparinized blood should be collected and submitted to the laboratory. If it cannot be processed within 24 hours after collection, it should be frozen at $-60°$ C. It may be helpful to test a number of specimens because the agent is not consistently present in either sputum or blood. Although many animals have been shown to be susceptible to infection with psittacosis or ornithosis isolates, the useful host systems are restricted to those mentioned above.

Diagnostic methods are presented in detail in the last chapter. Although the techniques are not particularly difficult, the hazard of laboratory infection is so great that isolation attempts are best left to specially equipped laboratories.

DIFFERENTIAL DIAGNOSIS

Clinically, psittacosis must be differentiated from a variety of pneumonic processes. Viral pneumonias should be eliminated by appropriate serologic tests, as should primary atypical pneumonia and Q fever, which can be clinically quite similar. Protracted influenza is the virus infection most likely to be a source of confusion. Typhoid fever and brucellosis may also occasionally appear similar to psittacosis.

From the previous descriptions, it is obvious that human psittacosis may have many clinical manifestations. It would not be useful to recommend the routine consideration of psittacosis (an uncommon disease) in all cases of hepatitis or myocarditis. The diagnosis would be worth considering when the usual tests are negative, or when there is persistent fever or other indications. It may be reasonable to consider psittacosis in the diagnosis of persistent fevers of unknown origin, a persistent influenzal disease, or the unresolved pneumonia that might follow an influenzal illness (Anderson, 1973). Typhoid-like conditions with negative routine tests would also be candidates. If the patient has an unresolved condition, the test for serologic diagnosis would simply be a complement fixation test; many diagnostic laboratories and certainly all public health laboratories perform this test. A history of avian contact is obviously a paramount indicator of psittacosis, and questions about a patient's possible exposure should be asked as early as possible. Lack of contact with birds does not rule out a diagnosis of psittacosis, since at least 25% of proven infections have no such history; clearly, however, the index of suspicion is higher when there is close avian contact.

There is no place in the diagnosis of psittacosis for "therapeutic trials." The response to chemotherapy is too variable. If there is a good response, in the absence of accurate diagnosis, the course of therapy is liable to be too short, thus risking relapse. Cases have been reported where inadequate tetracycline therapy (not uncommon in treating patients with fevers of unknown origin) may result in a persistent psittacosis infection. In one such case the organism was recovered as late as the 97th day of the disease (Irons, Sullivan, and Rowen, 1951). We have observed one case of six months' duration. Antibiotics should be given only for a specific diagnosis where treatment should be decisive.

TREATMENT

The only treatment that can be readily recommended is tetracycline at a minimum dose of 250 mg four times a day for 21 days. A recommendation often given is that treatment should be continued for 7 days after temperature has returned to normal. We feel this may be inadequate because occasionally there is a very dramatic clinical response to tetracycline, with temperatures returning to normal in

24 to 48 hours (Fitz et al., 1955; Seibert, Jordan, and Dingle, 1956). In some such cases the shorter course of tetracycline has resulted in a relapse. We prefer to recommend the 21-day course. It should be noted that response is not always dramatic (Schaffner et al., 1967; Anderson, 1973). Recovery, even during and after successful therapy, may be protracted. The acute symptoms — chills, fever, headache — tend to disappear, but the patient may be debilitated for months (Anderson and Bridgwater, 1968; Strauss, 1957, 1967).

In years gone by there were therapeutic claims for penicillin. It is probable that many patients were treated with this drug as their psittacosis infection was naturally resolving. Also, the penicillin therapy was actually effective against secondary bacterial infections, which may be common, rather than against the chlamydial infection itself. It is extremely unlikely that penicillin would have any dramatic effect on the course of the psittacosis case unless it were given in very high doses (20 million units a day). Relapses often followed apparent improvement after penicillin therapy, and many workers have observed penicillin treatment failures (Fitz et al., 1955; Goto et al., 1961; Grist and McLean, 1964). The occasional claims for a therapeutic response to sulfa drugs may be explained by the observation that some psittacosis strains are sensitive to sulfonamide drugs. These include a strain isolated in 1941 (6 BC) from a parakeet, a strain isolated in 1943 from human lung (strain Gleason), and a strain recovered in 1969 from parakeets in Maryland, as well as others (Meiklejohn, Wagner, and Beveridge, 1946; Schachter, unpublished). However, the great majority of psittacosis isolates are completely unaffected by sulfas.

Chloramphenicol has some therapeutic effect, but is not highly effective and has other obvious drawbacks. Erythromycin may be effective (Timberger and Armstrong, 1969), and is the recommended alternative to tetracycline. Aminoglycosides have no demonstrable activity.

IMMUNITY

For many years workers in the field have hoped to develop an effective vaccine for the protection of individuals at high risk of contracting psittacosis. Obviously, a very real degree of self-interest is present in this approach, since many laboratory workers have been infected with psittacosis in the course of their work. During the 1930s there were a disconcerting number of fatalities among researchers (55 cases, 8 deaths). In a series of experiments, Rivers and Schwentker (1934) developed a vaccine that proved somewhat protective in monkeys and in man. Low levels of neutralizing antibody were shown to follow immunization and infection (Rivers and Schwentker, 1934), but their role in natural infection is not clear. In the 1930s there were many efforts at treating patients with immune sera from previously recovered individuals, but there was no appreciable success. The ability of hyperimmune or convalescent sera to neutralize small infectious doses has been shown in a number of studies (Meyer and Eddie, 1962). Resistance to challenge has also been demonstrated in immunized laboratory animals. However, this resistance has always been relative and often a function of the route of challenge as well as of the inoculum size. In many instances where the challenged animals survived, they showed neither resistance to, nor enhanced clearance of, infection. They remained alive but became persistent carriers of the organism.

There is no convincing evidence of a persistent immune response to psittacosis (Meyer and Eddie, 1962). Second infections and attacks of clinical diseases are well documented even in patients with high titers of complement-fixing antibodies. In the outbreaks in turkey processing plants, workers with high CF titers developed psittacosis. Strauss (1957, 1967), in his study of the outbreaks among workers on the duck farms in Czechoslovakia, showed that the secondary infection rate, in cases where consistent exposure to highly infected birds was maintained, was essentially the same as the primary infection rate. He felt the occupational reinfection could be as high as 66%.

Even the natural host does not appear to develop solid immunity to chlamydiae. Resistance in avian species appears largely to reflect persistent infection; in fact, it would appear that birds (or laboratory animals) resist superinfection and do not possess a solid immunity (Meyer and Eddie, 1962; Fortner, 1936). If an infected bird is treated with tetracycline, it becomes highly susceptible again.

In mammalian chlamydial infections there is conflicting evidence about development of immunity in virtually any system. Many of the positive reports have not been confirmed by other researchers, or have only led to small-scale successes followed by large-scale failures (Storz, 1971; Page, 1973). It is clear that there is little hope for development of effective vaccines, and prevention of human disease and infections depends upon minimizing exposure to the organism.

It is likely that efforts at developing vaccines have been premature. Certainly we know very little about the pathogenesis of psittacosis and the biological roles of the various antibodies produced after infection. Meyer (1941a) has presented evidence suggesting that cellular response to infection is paramount, but this lead has not been exploited. Many studies have shown that a true immunity of limited effectiveness may be acquired. But there is no evidence to suggest that immunity may be the basis for psittacosis prevention.

PATHOLOGY

Pathology in Human Psittacosis

In man virtually all cases coming to autopsy exhibit extensive pulmonary involvement (Sturdee and Scott, 1930; Lillie, 1933; Binford and Hauser, 1944). The pneumonia is usually a focal or lobar consolidation. It may be confluent, although the bronchioles are virtually never involved. The alveoli may be completely filled with an exudate containing fibrinous red cells and polymorphonuclear cells, as well as epithelial cells, in the early stages. In later stages this serofibrinous exudate may diminish with increasing evidence of hemorrhage; large mononuclear cells are very common. There is alveolar septal cell hyperplasia which may be quite marked. Phagocytic activity is high. Persistence of polymorphonuclear cells usually indicates secondary bacterial infection.

The spleen is usually enlarged and normal architecture may be obliterated by the congestion caused by infiltration of lymphoid tissues. There appears to be marked increase in mononuclear phagocytic cells. In the liver, focal necrosis is quite common, often with marked phagocytic activity of the Kupffer cells. Noncaseating granulomas have been observed.

The central nervous system may be involved, with congestion and edema of the brain and spinal cord often noted. There may be slight meningeal hemorrhaging. In frank meningitis, inclusions have been found superficially.

Pleural effusion is unusual, although pleural involvement is common. Often a large part of the pleura may be covered by thin layers of fibrin that detach readily. Involvement of the rectus muscles is not uncommon. The lesions are usually hemorrhagic with some degeneration.

Generally the genital tract, gastrointestinal tract, and thyroid are not involved. Lack of involvement of the gastrointestinal tract is perhaps surprising in view of the constipation or diarrhea reported in psittacosis. The kidneys and the adrenals may show some degeneration.

Sequential Pathology in Monkeys

Most of the pathologic studies or surveys reporting histopathologic findings in man have been based on terminal cases or on postmortem findings. Obviously, there is little opportunity for sequential studies. There has been one study with serial clinical and pathologic observations in rhesus monkeys following aerosol infection (McGavran et al., 1962). The subhuman primate is not a particularly suitable model since the disease is relatively mild (even with the most virulent psittacosis isolates), with clinically inapparent infections and rapid clearance rather than the occasionally severe disease observed in man. In monkeys exposed by aerosol route, the organism could be recovered from the lungs for periods ranging from 2 to 23 days after infection; the regional (tracheobronchial) lymph node yielded the organism between 7 and 20 days, and the blood was positive from 8 to 10 days following infection. Interestingly, the liver was infected almost as soon as the lung and remained positive for approximately 3 weeks. The spleen was the site at which the organism persisted for the greatest length of time, being recoverable for 6 to 29 days after inoculation. Histopathologic findings were most marked in the lung, with minimal changes observed (small clusters of monocytes and scattered polymorphonuclear leukocytes in the bronchial walls) during the first week of infection. By the 10th day the lesions were grossly visible and reached a peak 14 to 16 days postinfection. In the early lesions, alveoli were filled with fibrinous exudate (primarily mononuclear cells with some neutrophils and occasional red blood cells). At the edges of the lesion, septal cell hyperplasia and hypertrophy were obvious. At the reaction peak (14 to 16 days) the consolidation increased and the exudate began to organize and involved the respiratory bronchioles. As is typical in human disease, the radiologic findings were more severe with microscopic resolution initiated before radiologic evidence of improvement was noted. Between days 16 and 20 the foci of lobular pneumonia were still active at their periphery, and appeared consolidated; however, clearing was apparent in the central portion of the lesion. Macrophages became predominant later. Some hepatocellular necrosis and small granulomas in the liver were observed in a few monkeys. Inclusions were rarely seen and were only found in the lungs.

EPIDEMIOLOGY

For all practical purposes, it can be said that human psittacosis is contracted by exposure to infected avian species. The disease may be considered an occupational hazard to those people engaged in the pet bird or poultry industries. The individuals working in poultry processing plants, particularly those involved in cleaning and processing carcasses, are at greatest risk. One can consider all avian species as potential reservoirs. Meyer in 1967 reviewed the host range of chlamydiae and tabulated approximately 130 species of birds known to harbor chlamydiae. In fact, the omission of mention of a species probably represents lack of adequate research rather than lack of infection in that species.

Man-to-man transmission, although known to occur, is quite rare except in unusual circumstances. Most documented cases have occurred in individuals exposed to severely ill patients with productive coughs and in individuals attending fatally ill patients. It should be noted that there have been cases of human psittacosis, proven by agent isolation, where there was no known avian exposure, but where man-to-man transmission had been proven. In the Louisiana outbreak the assumption that an avian species — the egret — was the ultimate source was inferred retrospectively, based on the similarity of biologic characteristics of the (Borg) agent recovered from humans and that recovered from egrets in the area of the outbreak (Rubin, 1954; Meyer and Eddie, 1952). However, in San Francisco, one outbreak of psittacosis, with several fatal cases and man-to-man transmission (Eaton, Beck, and Pearson, 1941), was associated with a chlamydial agent having biological characteristics unlike those of any known avian chlamydiae.

Human infection has followed casual exposure to birds or to premises where an infected avian species has lived. Infection is transmitted by the aerosol route from dried feces, infected bird droppings being the common source. The birds do not have to be ill, and many outbreaks have been associated with exposure to healthy carriers.

The avian source of infection is not conclusively known to play a major role in the severity of the human disease. In the past it was assumed that agents recovered from psittacine species were more virulent for humans than those associated with passerine species or poultry (Meyer, 1958). This, however, is very difficult to prove, because the recognition of non-psittacine sources of infection tended to occur at a time when antibiotic therapy was available and when improved diagnosis led to identification of mild and subclinical infection. This was not the case during the psittacine-associated cases of the 1929–1930 pandemic.

Although many domestic and other lower mammals are known to be infected with chlamydiae, agents in these species do not seem to play a significant role in producing human disease. The only two documented systemic infections with chlamydiae recovered from domestic mammals have occurred in the laboratory. Chlamydiae recovered from sheep or cattle may be capable of infecting turkeys (Pierce, Carroll, and Moore, 1964), and it is possible that these organisms may play a role in causing psittacosis-like disease in man, but this has not yet been described. These organisms are suspected of causing other human infections (discussed in Chapter 9).

Psittacine Species as Sources of Human Infections

As mentioned previously, most human psittacosis cases have been traced to exposure to parrots and parakeets. These birds tend to be sources of sporadic cases or small household outbreaks, although somewhat larger outbreaks have been traced to exposure to these birds in department stores (Badger, 1930; McClintock, 1925; Drachman, 1953). In Meyer's (1965) tabulation of human cases, 60% of the more than 5,000 reported cases involved psittacine contact.

Poultry as Sources of Human Infections

As discussed earlier, turkeys have been a major source of human infections. Meyer (1965) has estimated that 25% of all human cases were from turkey exposure. The major danger is industrial, and there is no evidence of any threat to the consumer. Cooking kills the chlamydiae, and no cases have been traced to the handling of infected visceral organs packaged with the carcasses.

Chickens may harbor chlamydiae capable of causing human infections, but there has been little disease attributed to this host.

Ducks (Korns, 1955) may be the source of human infection. Workers in eastern Europe, particularly Czechoslovakia, East Germany, and Hungary, have emphasized the importance of ducks as a reservoir (Strauss, 1967; Dömök, 1963; Ortel, 1964). The mortality associated with human infections here seems to be quite low; however, the morbidity is extensive, with prolonged hospitalization, protracted recuperation, and high incidence of clinical relapse. The disease among these workers is an occupational hazard of considerable concern and considerable economical import.

Pigeons as a Source of Human Infection

Although the chlamydial infections in pigeons were demonstrated in 1941, and their potential as sources for human infections was demonstrated shortly thereafter by Meyer, these birds have not been significant reservoirs for human disease. It seems most likely that these organisms are not highly virulent for man although a number of infections have been documented in breeders, bird fanciers, and racers. We have documented a small outbreak at the San Francisco campus of the University of California, traced to pigeons that spend much time on office window sills. The workers in these offices contracted clinical chlamydial infections. It is tempting to postulate that many, if not most, of the human psittacosis cases with no avian contact

32

probably result from exposure to infected pigeon droppings. Certainly these birds are ubiquitous, and in some surveys the infection has been found to be almost universal among them. For example, the review by Page and Erickson showed that only 2 of 50 flocks that were tested were serologically negative (1969). Although pigeons in many countries around the world have been shown to carry chlamydiae, with infection rates as high as 25% (Meyer, 1965), relatively few (only 1% of proven cases) of the reported human cases have been due to pigeon exposure. Meyer (1955) has speculated that "New York dressed" squabs (birds packaged with intact visceral organs) may present a potential source of infection to anyone preparing them for consumption.

Wild Birds as Sources of Human Infections

Fulmars were shown to be the reservoir for the Faroe Islands outbreak, and egrets were suspected in the Louisiana outbreak. Many species of wild birds have yielded chlamydiae. Sporadic human cases have been seen in hunters, people studying birds (though most outbreaks in zoological gardens have been traced to psittacine species), or people trying to help sick birds. We have diagnosed a psittacosis infection in an arbovirus researcher who was bleeding cormorants in the field and in a research worker studying vultures. It must be reiterated — any avian species must be considered a potential source of chlamydial infection.

Man-to-Man Transmission

As mentioned above, man-to-man transmission of psittacosis has been most convincingly demonstrated in series where contacts have had very close exposure to fatal cases in the last 48 hours of illness. This was the case in the Louisiana and San Francisco outbreaks (Olson and Treuting, 1944; Eaton, Beck, and Pearson, 1941). There have been a number of other instances where individuals coming into contact with psittacosis patients developed clear-cut cases of psittacosis. This has been shown in many countries around the world: England (Bedson, Western, and Levy Simpson, 1930), Germany (Günther, 1930; Hegler, 1934), Switzerland (Schmid, 1931), Argentina (Garcia, 1940), and others. At least 30 nurses have been infected by patients in their care. In Buenos Aires, Barros (1940) observed an outbreak in a hospital where patients in the ward were exposed to the index case.

However, Gerlach's (1936) observations in Vienna were quite different from those above: in this instance sequential infection in a hospital ward occurred in the absence of symptoms in the contacts. The index case was symptomatic; his two bed neighbors and three other patients in the ward developed asymptomatic infections proven by isolation of the organism from sputum. A potential rationale for Gerlach's findings would be that even the most virulent psittacosis agents may cause clinically inapparent infections in man. This has been suspected on the basis of serologic reactions found in high-risk individuals with no clinical history consistent with psittacosis. Meyer and Eddie (1951) documented one case where, following laboratory infection, an individual yielded a psittacosis-like agent for 10 years after the initial attack. Isolation of the agent from this patient was irregular with positive results from blood and sputum 10 days after the initial attack, followed by a sporadic history of clinical exacerbation and remission. The agent was recovered from the sputum intermittently throughout this decade. It is of interest that neither this carrier nor the one studied by Dekking and Ruys (1951) was a source of other human infections. Further evidence for the chronic carrier is supported by the fact that prior to the introduction of chemotherapy the organism could be recovered for at least five weeks postonset from sputum specimens of many patients. There are a number of other histories which suggest long-term infection with late onset. The possibility, of course, that there is occasionally a very long incubation period may explain the lack of avian contact in at least some of the human psittacosis cases.

Gordon (1958) has speculated that the inoculum size may be an important variable in the evolution of the clinical picture in human psittacosis. Since sputum contains highly variable amounts of organism, it is also possible that Gerlach's patients had exposure to very few infectious particles.

Psittacosis as an Occupational Disease

It is clear that individuals involved in the pet bird industry, whether in breeding, shipping, or direct consumer sales, run a high risk of developing psittacosis. There is abundant evidence in the United States and elsewhere that such individuals have much higher rates of CF antibodies than comparable control populations (Meyer, 1965; Meyer and Eddie, 1962). Many of the infections are inapparent, with only a minor history of respiratory disease being elicited from many of the seropositive patients. However, severe clinical disease was not rare in the past and still occurs. For instance, in the statistics published by the U.S. Public Health Service in recent years, many of the individuals with proven psittacosis have known avian contact due to their occupations.

In the poultry industry, psittacosis is an occupational hazard of greater potential for large outbreaks than in the pet bird business. It is clear, from previous experience, that there are two epidemiologic patterns of human psittacosis in poultry processors. Although there is an obvious threat to turkey ranchers (for turkeys are usually the avian reservoir in the United States, although ducks and geese have been implicated in Europe), it appears that the highest risk is in the poultry processing plant. Studies in Texas (Irons, Denley, and Sullivan, 1955) and in Wisconsin (Graber and Pomeroy, 1958) and other parts of the United States (Meyer, 1965) have shown that pickers and eviscerators are at highest risk, although infections may occur via the aerosol route in any area of the plant. Of the two major types of outbreak, the point source outbreak has usually reflected exposure to the highly virulent turkey strains that have been producing epizootics in birds, with a concomitant increase in condemned carcasses. Often, in fact, morbidity and mortality have been observed on the turkey ranch, and efforts have been made to butcher the whole flock before the disease progressed further. The continuing-exposure type of outbreak has resulted from infections of the turkeys with low-virulence strains. In this type of outbreak there is no excess mortality in the turkey flocks, and little or no increased condemnation of carcasses for gross lesions. The isolates recovered from these two types of situations have differed markedly in their virulence for laboratory animals (mainly the mouse), and have shown different pathogenicity indices.

The continuous exposure situation was documented by a series of surveys performed at the same processing plants in Wisconsin (Graber and Pomeroy, 1958). In 1955, approximately 18% of the turkey flocks surveyed had antichlamydial antibodies with the absence of overt clinical findings and little pathology at autopsy. No chlamydiae were recovered. After many negative efforts, the first of the low-virulence chlamydial strains were recovered from the turkeys. In 1956 a follow-up serologic study indicated that there had been approximately a 40% increase in seroreactors among workers at the turkey processing plant (from 11.6% to 16.1%). During this period of approximately 19 months, there had been 10 clinically compatible and serologically confirmed cases of psittacosis in the employees of the plants, and 9 inapparent but serologically confirmed infections. The cases occurred over a 4½-month period during which no birds had been condemned. This was in marked contrast to the previous outbreaks in New Jersey and Texas (and, in fact, to the later outbreak in Texas in 1974), where the onset had been explosive and where there had been an attack rate of up to 44% in potentially exposed employees with a 13% fatality rate (Steele and Scruggs, 1958). In Wisconsin, the decreased fatality rate in man could not actually be credited to early and effective chemotherapy; there is a real suspicion that there were human virulence differences in the infecting agents. It is clear from these studies, however, that the so-called high- and low-virulence strains are both highly contagious to man, and that it is very hard to differentiate the clinical diseases they cause in humans. We know nothing about the size of the inoculum, and extrapolations concerning human virulence are at best conjectural.

LATENCY IN PSITTACOSIS

The evidence clearly shows that apparently healthy birds may be sources of human infections. A major characteristic of virtually all chlamydial infection is latency. The natural history of the infection in parakeets may well be a model for other psittacine, and perhaps most avian, species. Parakeets were shown to be major reservoirs for psittacosis following the bans on importation of more exotic psittacine birds after the pandemic of 1929–1930. Exhaustive inquiries were made into the natural history of the infection in these birds. It was recognized quite early that the birds could be latently infected (Meyer and Eddie, 1933b,c). In the Grass Valley, California, outbreak, exposure to two parakeets was the common source for the infected individuals. One bird had died by the time the outbreak was investigated; the other appeared to be perfectly healthy. However, Meyer and Eddie, after confirming the diagnosis in the patients and examining the recovered body of the dead bird, brought the healthy-appearing bird to the laboratory and introduced an uninfected cage mate. This sentinel bird quickly developed psittacosis and died. A series of sentinels were exposed to this carrier; virtually all of them contracted the infection and died. In the parakeet breeding establishments, infections were contracted by the young birds who developed symptoms, were weak (crawlers), and often died. The resistance of the birds increased with age. The older birds could appear to be perfectly healthy parakeets but, when stressed by crowding or other conditions, would shed increasing amounts of the organisms and occasionally become symptomatic and die. The infections were spread by both nasal and fecal discharges. The judicious use of sentinel birds, particularly the rice bird, was instrumental in elucidating the healthy-carrier stage (Meyer and Eddie, 1933b; Meyer, 1942, 1965). Studies were also conducted with mice in California and Germany (Meyer and Eddie, 1933a; Fortner and Pfaffenberg, 1934), and it was shown that a persistent carrier state could be produced in the mouse.

NATURAL HISTORY IN BIRDS

One can assume that in their natural state, the chlamydiae and their avian hosts live in a delicate balance. The infected birds may appear to be healthy, but will develop clinical symptoms and overt disease when stressed or when some outside factor upsets the equilibrium (Meyer, 1942). The general consideration is that the natural infection rate tends to be relatively low (Doherty et al., 1961). The shedding adults (whether healthy carriers or symptomatic) infect the nestlings. The stress of egg laying and the activities involved in rearing the young bird seem to precipitate both symptomatology and shedding of the chlamydiae. Nasal secretions and feces are both highly infectious. The nestlings, while more susceptible to development of overt disease, seem to handle the infections reasonably well and the survivors grow up with chronic infections, and reach maturity to continue the cycle. Some researchers have speculated that this persistence of the organism at a low level maintains an immunity to superinfection.

Although Meyer and Eddie had shown that parakeets were infected in California early in the 1930s, the infection in Australia was not recognized until approximately 1934–1935. Burnet (1935, 1936), following reports by Meyer of psittacosis in a shipment of parakeets, investigated the situation and discovered that the infection existed in Australia (where parakeets are native). He found infected wild budgerigars and Australian parrots, and within a few years epizootics were recognized. However, it was later shown that the birds trapped in the wild and transported quickly and under good conditions had a very low rate of seroreactors or of infections when tested by serologic or isolation techniques (Doherty et al., 1961).

It was demonstrated that poor shipping or holding of the birds in crowded conditions increased the spread of the agent and resulted in a much greater infection rate, with a parallel increase in symptoms and shedding of chlamydiae. Thus, naturally low infection rates were amplified by the treatment the birds received between the time of trapping and the time of marketing. One may expect any large accumulation of birds to be a potential source of environmental contamination and human infection. The brief description above is generally consistent with our knowledge of infection chains in parrots, parakeets, other psittacine species, and pigeons.

In turkeys another problem exists in that there appear to be at least two well-differentiated groups of chlamydial parasites. The first isolates characterized were of high virulence with infection resulting in extensive morbidity and mortality in the turkeys (Meyer and Eddie, 1953). Later, isolates of lower virulence were recovered (Gale, Pomeroy, and Sanger, 1959; Page, 1959a). These turkeys had no apparent signs of infection until they were autopsied or inspected in processing plants. Some apparently healthy birds had all the gross anatomic signs consistent with chlamydial infection; this, of course, resulted in many of these birds being declared unfit for human consumption. Outbreaks of psittacosis have occurred in workers at rendering plants where some condemned carcasses had been sent for disposal (Meyer, 1965). In Wisconsin, an outbreak of psittacosis in processing plant workers was shown to be due to exposure to infected turkeys that were not only clinically healthy, but had no gross lesions (Graber and Pomeroy, 1958).

The natural chain of chlamydial infections in turkeys is not clear. With virulent strains the younger birds are more susceptible (Davis and Delaplane, 1958) and perhaps in a natural breeding situation the transmission of chlamydiae might be similar to transmission among psittacine species. However, the industry today depends upon rearing a large cohort of incubator-hatched poults to a simultaneous harvest. Thus there is no opportunity for "nest" infection. In fact, it is difficult to understand how chlamydiae persist on a turkey ranch with such cyclical harvests. It has been postulated that the chlamydiae of different biological characteristics have different survival (persistence) advantages in various ranching techniques. Persistence of viable chlamydiae in litter or in feather mites represents environmental contamination that might allow the agent to infect the next flock to be introduced (Eddie et al., 1962). Interspecies transfer of chlamydiae has also been postulated as an explanation of both continuing infections in turkey flocks and the diversity of isolates recovered.

There has been considerable research on this latter speculation (Page, 1966b, 1967; Page and Erickson, 1969) and it has been shown that sheep and turkeys may exchange chlamydiae (Pierce, Carroll, and Moore, 1964). Obviously infected feral birds are a potential reservoir.

DIAGNOSIS OF INFECTION
IN THE AVIAN CONTACT

The birds involved as the source of infection may be either healthy or diseased. The diseased birds often appear emaciated ("gone light") — having ruffled feathers, conjunctivitis occasionally, and usually showing evidence of diarrhea (Meyer, 1965). Latent and subclinical infections are not uncommon. In the diseased bird, psittacosis or ornithosis is essentially a disease of the reticuloendothelial system and of the digestive tract. At necropsy, characteristic lesions may be observed. Often the spleen is grossly enlarged and boggy. The liver may have focal necrosis, which can be quite marked. Air sacculitis, appearing almost purulent in nature, may exist, and there may be a pericarditis. Any of the involved organs may be covered with the so-called plastic exudate. Impression smears from cut specimens or touch preparations (particularly in the presence of the fibrinous or plastic exudate) may be stained by Giemsa, Macchiavello, or Giminez methods to demonstrate the chlamydiae. Although the lesions described above are characteristic, they are not pathognomonic, and chlamydiae may be recovered from grossly normal tissues (Weyer, 1964). Serologic tests may be performed on birds, but indirect complement fixation tests must be utilized for domestic fowl whose sera will not fix guinea pig complement (Karrer, Meyer, and Eddie, 1950). Isolation of the organisms may be attempted from spleen, liver, pericardial fluid, lung, involved air sacs, intestine, and cloacal specimens (Meyer, Eddie, and Schachter, 1969; Hanna, Schachter, and Jawetz, 1974).

EXPERIMENTAL HOST RANGE

All psittacosis and ornithosis isolates appear to grow well in cell culture systems. They can be isolated in these systems, and inclusions may be demonstrated readily. The agents are cytopathogenic and may form plaques (Piraino and Abel, 1964; Banks et al., 1970a). Limited serotyping is available by plaque reduction methods (Banks et al., 1970b).

Mice and embryonated hens' eggs are the usual host systems for isolation (Meyer, Eddie, and Schachter, 1969; Hanna, Schachter, and Jawetz, 1974). Virtually all psittacosis strains are virulent for mice by intracerebral, intranasal, and intraperitoneal routes. Highly virulent (so-called toxigenic) ornithosis strains have the same pathogenicity pattern, although the ornithosis isolates of lessened virulence (from turkeys, pigeons, chickens, ducks) have less pathogenicity by the intraperitoneal route than by the intracerebral route. Many of these isolates do not kill mice after intraperitoneal inoculation, although they may produce ascitic fluid extremely rich in agent. Therefore, for isolation of chlamydiae from turkeys, intracerebral inoculation of mice has been found to be as sensitive as yolk sac isolation, but the intraperitoneal route is less sensitive (Fagan, 1958).

Pathogenicity indices (i.e., the relationship of LD_{50} by the intracerebral route to the LD_{50} by the intraperitoneal route) have been used to characterize some of these isolates (Page, 1959a). The virulent organisms are highly lethal to guinea pigs and hamsters, but rabbits tend to be refractory to infection except by the intratracheal route. Psittacine birds are generally quite susceptible to infection, and the finch or rice bird has often been used in sentinel cage mate experiments to detect shedding by healthy carriers.

PUBLIC HEALTH CONSIDERATIONS

The student of human psittacosis becomes aware that the incidence of these infections has, in large part, been dictated by governmental and administrative action. For example, the pandemic of 1929–1930 was essentially stopped by bans on the importation of psittacine birds. The bans effectively removed most of the reservoir, because the majority of psittacine birds sought by fanciers cannot be bred in captivity or in temperate climates and therefore must be trapped and shipped from the tropics. The awareness of the parakeet as a reservoir led to the ban on interstate shipment of parakeets in the United States. This ban was particularly aimed at California, where most of the breeding establishments were located. It succeeded in effectively minimizing the residuum of cases occurring in the early 1930s. Meyer and Eddie developed a systematic and painstaking method for removing psittacosis-infected parakeet flocks from routine breeding by selection for normal birds and sacrificing infected birds. The resultant clean flocks were certified, and, following continued surveillance, shipment of parakeets was again allowed.

Unfortunately, there have always been a few individuals who attempt to circumvent the rules. Many abuses of the certification process took place, leading to increased infections when the birds were shipped. Birds have been smuggled to avoid quarantine stations in more recent years. Moreover, every time there is a relaxation of a ban, there has been an increase in infections. The graphs of annual cases of psittacosis show a very marked increase in the early 1950s (Fig. 1). There is usually a footnote appended to such graphs which states that the increases are more apparent than real, and simply reflect the discovery of infections due to turkeys, as well as the awareness of ornithosis and psittacosis as occupational hazards in poultry processing plants. This unfortunately is not wholly true; and Steele and Scruggs (1958) have very clearly pointed out that 125 human cases in 1952 were due to parakeets, and that those 125 cases represented a major increase in the incidence from previous years. Thus, the domestically bred parakeet has continued to be a source of human infections.

It would seem safe to say that the system of overseas quarantine centers has failed. Its demise was due to the cumulative effects of poor supervision, inadequately treated birds, smuggling, and contamination of susceptible birds during shipment from quarantine centers. The failure of the overseas quarantine center has led to the establishment of the in-country designated treatment center. In theory, all psittacine birds imported into the United States pass through these treatment centers, are treated under government agency supervision, and are then shipped out as psittacosis-free birds suitable for commerce. This system is almost certainly doomed to failure, for a number of reasons. There is the ever present problem of smuggled birds (occasionally a very major problem). But more important is the fact that this system is based on the erroneous assumption that having birds and tetracycline together on the same premises assures that the birds are adequately treated. The experience in Germany (Wachendörfer, 1973) has clearly shown that many of the birds in unmonitored treatment centers never receive therapeutic doses of tetracycline, and that more stringent surveillance is required. Standard doses of drugs in standard preparation form should be given to the birds in all treatment centers, and routine monitoring for tetracycline blood levels should be performed on a proportion of the birds to guarantee their acceptance of the food and chemotherapy. The increase in charges or cost for this procedure would be minimal, and could certainly be absorbed by instituting either a tax or a standard charge for this service. Inadequate surveillance and inadequate supervision are the seeding grounds for more psittacosis outbreaks.

Parakeets are bred in the United States and have provided a persistent (albeit minor) reservoir for human psittacosis. This situation should not be tolerated. An effective means for controlling psittacosis in parakeets is commercially available. The product, a chlortetracycline-impregnated seed (Meyer et al., 1958) quickly produces adequate blood levels and will eradicate psittacosis infection after a 30-day course of treatment. Unfortunately, in practice, the product tends to be misused because the bird breeders often receive poor advice. There appears to be a plethora of old wives' tales associated with the use of tetracyclines ("they cause permanent sterility," "interfere with feathering," among others). Although unfounded, these concerns have led to such practices as mixing medicated feed with other bird feed (resulting in inadequate blood levels) or short-term treatment (inadequate duration).

An effort must be made to educate the parakeet breeders in the proper use of the medicated seed. A full 30-day course of medicated seed, as a sole food source, will eradicate psittacosis infection in the breeding stock. Maintenance of a closed premises (no untreated birds introduced into the aviary) will prevent reinfection with chlamydiae. Self interest should dictate the breeders' desire to maintain a clean premises — after all, confirmation of psittacosis may result in quarantine and significant financial loss.

Realistically, one could assume that many of the parakeet breeding establishments in the country have a background level of psittacosis infections that is suppressed by tetracycline in subtherapeutic levels and that these birds, once shipped from the breeder to the pet store, may well begin shedding the organism, whether or not they become clinically ill. The imported birds coming out of the treatment centers, even if effectively treated, are highly susceptible and will certainly have a high risk of exposure to the infected parakeets.

Some research is needed to develop a well-accepted long-term tetracycline treatment which could be used when the birds are being shipped and while they are held in retail establishments. The birds need not be maintained on tetracycline after they have been purchased. In an effectively treated and infection-free bird, there is minimal chance of re-exposure once the bird is in the household. Therefore, what we must have as a goal is the adequate treatment of birds in the treatment center and the prevention of new infections or reinfections of the birds while in transit or in the store. The possibility that the birds may suffer from enteritis, aspergillosis, yeast infections, or the other types of infections often associated with prolonged tetracycline consumption is not an insolvable problem. Work at the Hooper Foundation and in Germany has shown that much of the enteritis in these birds can be prevented by providing them with a multivitamin supplement in their drinking water. The tetracycline and the vitamin supplement are inexpensive additives. Certainly it is a very small price to pay to minimize psittacosis as a public health problem. It is obvious that if no effort is made to implement a system like the one discussed here, there is an excellent chance that another round of increased incidence of psittacosis will be initiated, together with the increased administrative problems associated with control of such epidemics. It seems obvious that we should seek stability and not allow the evolution of situations that we will be forced to correct in the future.

PERSPECTIVES

It must be recognized that psittacosis is not a major public health problem in terms of national priorities. The number of cases reported per year has decreased (Fig. 1) from the peak of 500 to under 50 per year in the United States. Obviously, this disease is largely under-reported and under-diagnosed, but even if it were diagnosed properly and all cases reported, it is highly unlikely that it would be a major health problem. It is a significant problem as an occupational disease; the large outbreaks associated with turkey processing in midwestern states again in 1974 were a reminder of this dilemma. There have been many administrative procedures (generally involving, first, banning of shipments, then quarantines, and, finally, required treatment with tetracycline) which have proven effective to varying degrees in controlling psittacosis. With each relaxation or change in these procedures there have been small increases in human cases noted.

There is today adequate technology to remove psittacosis in psittacine species as a threat to human health. However, current national policies and implementation of the program are inadequate. The current program involves quarantine of imported psittacines in treatment centers in the United States. In these centers the birds are placed on a specifically prescribed chlortetracycline-containing mash for a period of approximately 30 days.

The major problem as we see it in the current system is that there is no monitoring for efficacy of treatment in the centers. In addition, the requirement for treatment following importation appears to be applied inadequately, as many birds are imported by individuals allowed — apparently illegally, due to a communication failure with customs officials — to bring single birds into the country without treatment. Occasionally bird dealers will promise to treat the birds under the supervision of a veterinarian, but often such treatment can be quite expensive and feed containing antibiotics is not commercially available. These birds generally represent little danger to the community at large, being a greater risk to their owners and their contacts.

The birds coming from treatment centers do represent a potential danger to the community because these birds will be housed in pet stores, department stores, etc., with a possibility of point source infections. We do not regularly test birds, but we occasionally receive avian specimens for screening for a chlamydial infection. We have isolated chlamydiae from a number of birds recently released from treatment centers. We do not know how long the birds had been held in treatment, but no traces of tetracycline were found in their bone marrow. Some of the birds have caused human infections. Occasionally we cannot trace the histories of the birds. There is no requirement for banding imported birds. (In California, there is a requirement for leg banding parakeets, which makes it easy to trace a bird's origin.)

This is a ridiculous situation if one considers the economics of the pet bird industry. Healthy birds command a premium price. Under any circumstances price is not a major consideration with exotic birds commanding exorbitant prices. We have seen relatively common gray parrots sell at retail for $300 to $400 — then be submitted to us shortly after purchase to determine cause of death, psittacosis. It would be reasonable to add a small tax per bird to assure adequate monitoring of efficacy of treatment in the treatment centers. This can be done by testing a sample of each group of birds for antibiotic levels. Arnstein, Eddie, and Meyer (1968) have shown that adequate levels (> 1 μg/ml) are readily achieved and easily measured. This procedure is followed in West Germany where Wachendörfer (1973) has shown it to be highly effective. After certification each bird would receive a coded leg band. It would be highly advantageous to both the industry and the public to see that such measures are instituted.

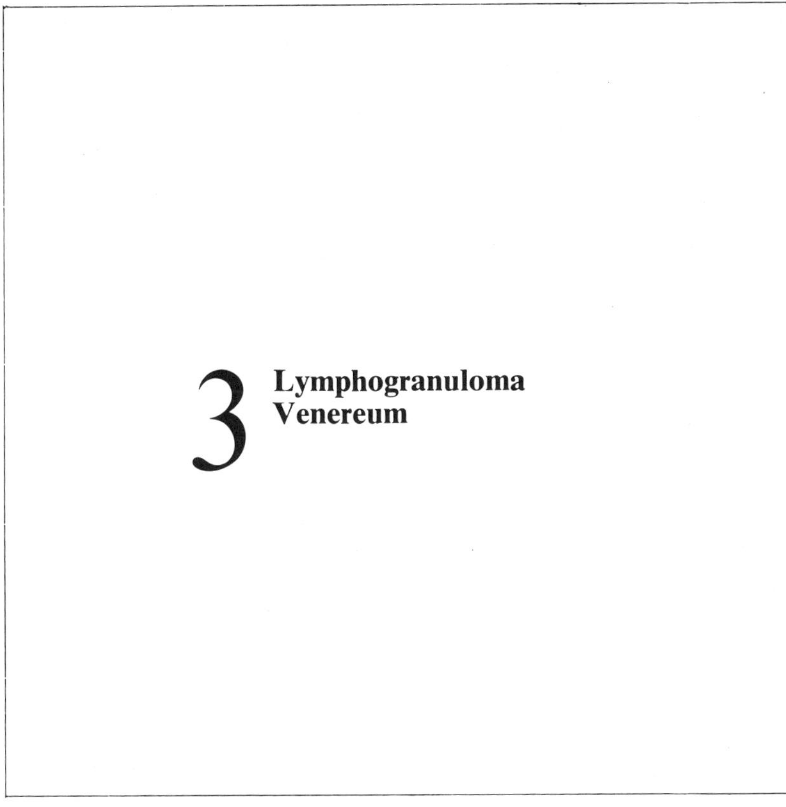

3 Lymphogranuloma Venereum

HISTORICAL ASPECTS

Lymphogranuloma venereum (LGV), a systemic disease transmitted almost exclusively by sexual contact, was probably first described in 1786 by John Hunter. It has been known by a variety of different terms, including malady of Durand, Nicolas, and Favre; lymphopathia venereum; climatic bubo; venereal bubo; lymphogranuloma inguinale; and, numerically, the third through the sixth venereal disease. Early in this century it was named lymphogranuloma by Durand, Nicolas, and Favre (1913), who noted its histologic similarity to lymphadenomas. A major advance in the diagnosis of LGV was made in 1925 when Frei introduced a specific skin test. Shortly thereafter, Hellerström (1929) succeeded in transmitting the disease by intraurethral inoculation of a man; later, with Wassén (1930), he transmitted the infection to monkeys by the intracerebral route. In a series of studies where he infected mice intracerebrally, Findlay showed similarities between the developmental cycle of the lymphogranuloma venereum agent and that previously described for the psittacosis agent

45

(1933). Final identification of the agent as a member of the *Chlamydia* was made in the 1940s when Rake, Eaton, and Shaffer (1941) demonstrated antigenic similarities, first between the LGV agent and psittacosis agents and then between LGV and trachoma-inclusion conjunctivitis (TRIC) agents (Rake, Shaffer, and Thygeson, 1942).

LGV was once more common, and its prevalence seems to have declined due to improving standards of living rather than as a reflection of specific control measures. The disease is found worldwide, although it is apparently more prevalent in warmer climates. Infectivity is unknown but is probably low, and it is possible that broad use of chemotherapeutic agents may have suppressed chlamydial levels sufficiently to reduce incidence.

The causative agents of LGV and the TRIC agents are now placed in the same species, *Chlamydia trachomatis*. Although closely related, LGV and TRIC agents are readily differentiated in the laboratory. There are three LGV serotypes (Grayston and Wang, 1975).

Widespread screening tests indicate the high prevalence of either asymptomatic LGV or previous exposure to the LGV agent in sexually active populations. The asymptomatic female is probably the major reservoir of the agent, and Caminopetros (1935) claimed to have recovered the agent from cervical and urethral cultures of apparently healthy prostitutes. However, the serologic tests were performed before our current state of knowledge enabled finer distinctions between chlamydiae-causing LGV and the closely related TRIC agents that cause oculogenital infections. Thus, the many papers that refer to positive CF reactor rates of 10%, 20%, or 30% in studies conducted in various VD clinics or among sexually active populations must be reinterpreted. The same holds true for results gained by using the Frei test. For example, King, Barwell, and Catterall (1956) found 18.4% (206/1119) of their patients at a VD clinic had positive skin tests and 2% (24) had high CF titers, but only 10 had clinical signs of LGV. Most of their positive reactions probably do not reflect LGV infection, but are most likely the result of infection with the chlamydiae that cause nongonococcal urethritis and cervicitis, since these two conditions are certainly prevalent in VD clinic populations.

At various times in the past, much has been made of the so-called racial predisposition to LGV (Gray et al., 1936), once erroneously considered a disease of blacks in the southeastern United States. The prevalence of LGV in a specific population probably reflects sexual activity and socioeconomic class. In a controlled comparative study, Luger and Cheatham (1950) found that the LGV rates in black college students were much lower than in black factory workers, the same as in the white population. Invariably, in reports of this nature, the differences in LGV rates represent the tendency of lower socio-economic classes to use public health facilities where reporting of venereal diseases is usually more accurate. LGV has been found to be common in other areas of the United States besides the southeast (Haim and Mathewson, 1937), as well as in European countries such as Finland, where blacks comprise a small proportion of the population (Sonck, 1972).

Grace (1941, 1943) and Greaves (1963) have pointed out that LGV is probably a relatively common venereal disease among homosexuals and probably represents a significant proportion of the proctitis seen in VD clinics. In fact, it has been suggested that male patients appearing with rectal LGV were probably homosexual. Recent experience has been inadequate to corroborate this association, but, since primary implantation of the agent in this site will probably cause this syndrome, there appears to be no reason to question it. Thus, it would seem reasonable to perform Frei and CF tests routinely on homosexuals with proctitis. In addition, the possibility of homosexual contacts in patients presenting with rectal LGV should be considered since the approach to their medical care and epidemiologic studies might be modified.

CLINICAL MANIFESTATIONS

The clinical course of LGV may be divided into three stages: primary, involving the initial infection and early lesions; secondary, involving the regional lymph nodes; and tertiary, with late sequelae.

The Primary Lesion

Following an incubation period that may be extremely variable (ranging from 3 to 30 days), a primary genital lesion may develop. In males, the lesion is commonly on the penis, often on the glans (Fig. 1, Plate 1); in women it is often on the vaginal wall or on the labia, and occasionally on the cervix. The primary lesion is usually transient and often imperceptible. It is painless and may take one of four forms: a papule, a shallow ulcer or erosion, a herpetiform lesion, or a nongonococcal urethritis (possibly due to an intraurethral primary lesion). Occasionally primary lesions are found on extragenital sites, which indicate the primary site of infection — for example, lesions have been described on the fingers and the tongue.

Histopathologically, no specific finding is associated with the primary lesion. In the ulcerated form, there is often a complete loss of epithelial cells with a relatively nonspecific inflammatory response in the surrounding tissue. However, the primary lesion may heal quite rapidly; in some cases scars may be found only after careful examination of the genital area. It should be noted that in recent times the primary lesion has usually not been found. For example, Alergant (1957) elicited a history of primary lesions in only 24% (13/55) of his cases in Liverpool, and Sigel (1962) in 26% (39/147), while Abrams (1968) saw lesions in 40% (8/20) of his patients in San Francisco. Only two of Alergant's patients had primary lesions at their initial examination; similarly, Erskine (1958) found only 4 out of 61 patients with a primary lesion. Obviously, the primary lesion, if present, is not considered serious enough by the patient to require medical attention. It may have completely healed before the sequential development of the disease brings the patient to the physician.

The Secondary Lesions, Lymphadenitis or Lymphadenopathy

Most patients who are subsequently diagnosed as having LGV come to venereal disease clinics seeking medical attention because of their enlarging buboes (Figs. 1, 2, Plate 1). Some complain of pain (although the bubo can be painless).

Lymphadenopathy, which is unilateral in two-thirds of patients, follows the primary lesion by a period of a few days to weeks. Since the primary lesion is not observed in many cases, those attempting to establish an incubation period have usually relied on the patient's recollection of the time of the presumed infecting sexual contact. Most patients develop lymphadenopathy in two to six weeks after the presumed infection, although incubation periods have ranged from a few days up to six months or longer.

Many series of lymphadenopathy show a 9:1 or greater ratio of males to females. This does not mean that lymphadenopathy actually occurs at this ratio, but it does reflect a possible sex difference in anatomic sites of lymph node involvement. One (not wholly satisfactory) explanation is based on the difference in distribution of pelvic lymphatics in the male and the female. This theory presumes that a primary penile lesion in male patients or an external primary lesion in female patients, drained by inguinal lymph nodes, will result in inguinal lymphadenopathy; however, women whose primary lesions are intravaginal will have posterior drainage of the lesion, thus involving the retroperitoneal lymph nodes.

In the bubonic form, the involved lymph nodes are usually inguinal, although several lymph node systems may be involved. When both inguinal and femoral lymph nodes are involved, they may be separated by the so-called groove sign, which consists of the separation of these two lymph node systems by the inguinal ligament. The groove sign is considered pathognomonic of LGV (Greenblatt et al., 1964), but only occurs in 15% to 20% of the cases. In instances where primary lesions are extragenital, other sites of lymph node involvement (such as axillary or submaxillary) may be seen.

Early in the secondary stage, a single lymph node may be involved, but inflammation may extend to an entire chain that then becomes matted with considerable periadenitis. Epithelioid and endothelial cells proliferate; clusters of large mononuclear cells and small abscesses are found in the lymph nodes (Sheldon and Heyman, 1947). The abscesses expand to become necrotic foci, which may progress to suppuration in some nodes, or the nodes may become fluctuant and then harden. The course of lymph node involvement is highly variable. An acute lymphadenopathy in some patients is followed by spontaneous remission; others undergo spontaneous rupture of the suppurative lymph node and develop draining fistulae. In a relatively small percentage of patients (approximately 5%), this lesion becomes a chronic lymphadenopathy, which may persist for many years. Occasionally patients with buboes progress, in approximately 5 to 10 years, to the tertiary stage of LGV.

If deep iliac lymph nodes are involved, an initial presumptive diagnosis of appendicitis may be made (Law, 1943), although in our experience a more common misdiagnosis is inguinal hernia. We have tested specimens from four patients whose buboes were recognized during surgery for hernia repair. This diagnostic confusion probably reflects the lack of clinical experience with LGV in recent years.

Fluctuant buboes may be aspirated in order to reduce risk of spontaneous rupture(Fig. 3, Plate 1), but incision of nodes is contraindicated.

In the acutely ill patient, fever, headache, and myalgia are common (Abrams, 1968; Annamunthodo, 1962). White cell counts are often normal, although occasionally mild leukocytosis with normal differential is seen.

The Tertiary Stage
or the Genito-Ano-Rectal Syndrome

The term "tertiary" is slightly misleading because this chronic LGV manifestation is usually not preceded by lymphadenopathy. The tertiary stage covers a variety of conditions, generally resulting from progressive spread of the disease, with destruction of tissue in the involved areas. This condition occurs most frequently in women, perhaps reflecting the involvement of retroperitoneal lymphatics as well as the proximity of the rectal and vaginal tissue. A variety of rectal strictures are found, involving small areas just above the rectum, or occasionally involving extensive areas of the lower intestinal tract. Proctitis without strictures, which may occur early, is probably the first objective sign in the anorectal syndrome, and usually persists as strictures develop (Grace, 1941).

Strictures may be considered in two forms, one due to chronic inflammatory reaction and granulation tissue, the other from late scarring. Strictures are generally annular or funnel shaped and are usually found 3 to 10 cm from the anal margin. Patients with this condition are usually seen in hospitals, not in venereal disease clinics. They may complain of constipation; they may be suffering from bloody, mucoid discharges and, occasionally, obstruction. Grossly, involved areas show thickening of the wall with ulcerated mucosa and fistulas in the chronic form of LGV; in the male, they are penile fistulas (Hopsu-Havu and Sonck, 1973) and in the female they are rectal or rectovaginal. Histologically the rectal lesions will show complete loss of the mucosal epithelium with replacement by granulation tissue, and plasma cell infiltration in the surrounding tissue.

Esthiomene (Greek, "eating away") is the misnomer applied to the hypertrophic, chronic granulomatous condition of the vulva occurring in LGV where the organ is quite swollen and disfigured, often with associated fistulae and ulcers. Elephantiasis may occur in both the male and the female.

Systemic Complications and Extragenital Infection

There are a number of secondary complications of LGV, as well as extragenital infections. These include a conjunctival infection causing blocked lymphatics and regional adenopathy that may mimic Parinaud's oculoglandular syndrome. Buboes may form in lymph nodes draining any primary site of infection, such as axillary buboes following infection of the fingers (Cole, 1933) and submaxillary buboes following oral infection (Buschke and Curth, 1931).

In addition to involvement of the lymphoid tissue, LGV may affect the central nervous system. The agent has been recovered from cerebrospinal fluid in several meningitis cases (Sabin and Aring, 1942); in some instances (before the organism was cultured) cerebrospinal fluid from cases was shown to be a potent Frei antigen. There have been a few cases of salpingitis presumably due to infection by the LGV agent, the abscess fluid being a potent Frei-type antigen. Erythema nodosum, erythema multiforme, and other cutaneous manifestations have been reported (Hickam, 1945). Arthritis has been observed in a number of LGV cases (Koteen, 1945; Dawson and Boots, 1939; Grace, 1941); synovial effusion in some cases has been shown to contain LGV antigen (Coutts, 1936). Cardiac involvement has been observed clinically and in cases coming to autopsy (Sheldon et al., 1948), and cases of pneumonia have also been attributed to LGV infection (Wood and Felson, 1946).

We have observed some of these complications in a series of 63 patients presumed to have LGV. However, only in one case, that of a febrile woman with pneumonitis from whose blood we isolated an LGV agent, did we feel secure in attributing the "complication" to LGV infection. In the past, when more LGV cases were seen, there was greater opportunity to observe the uncommon complications. This is particularly true of the tertiary stage, which is rarely reported today. Most of the LGV cases in our experience are young men (early twenties, 15:1 sex ratio) who contracted the infection in Southeast Asia or Central America and were usually seeking medical attention for their inguinal lymphadenopathy. Many of the proven LGV cases had constitutional symptoms (e.g., fever and chills, headache, myalgias).

The pneumonitis case mentioned above, and a male patient recently brought to our attention by Dr. Lawrence Drew of San Francisco, are of particular interest. The woman became febrile and developed pneumonia. Her chlamydial CF titers in paired sera were 1:16 and 1:256 and we isolated an LGV agent (Type L-2) from her blood. The other patient presented initially with painless superficial ulceration on the shaft of the penis. In the absence of bubo formation the lesions progressed, resulting in extensive necrosis requiring debridement of the penis, scrotum, and inguinal areas, followed by skin grafts. There were numerous complications, including urethral stricture and periurethral abscess. This patient's CF titers on paired sera were 1:16 and 1:1024. Isolation attempts were not performed.

Although the clinical presentations are unusual, what is especially remarkable about these two patients is their histories. She was 77 years old and he was 72. Both denied recent sexual activity — she for 25 years and he for several. But their serologic results are suggestive of recent infection. Since we do not know of an extra-human reservoir or nonvenereal mechanism for transmission of the LGV agent, another explanation must be sought. The most likely one is that these cases represent the LGV agent manifesting a characteristic of all chlamydiae — latency. Subclinical and chronic LGV infections are recognized. It is probable that these two patients had contracted the infection years before their symptoms developed. They probably carried the infection until, with advancing age, there was some decrease in a defense or immune mechanism, allowing the infection to develop and produce disease. It will be interesting to see whether other similar infections are recognized as a result of the combined effect of improved diagnostic techniques and expanded use of immunosuppressive agents.

We must strongly caution against over-attribution of clinical findings to LGV based on positive CF or Frei tests. Our current confirmation of the nonspecificity of these tests due to the prevalence of genital tract chlamydial infections in sexually active individuals necessitates a more critical analysis of some previous reports based on these tests.

SEROLOGIC ABNORMALITIES

Patients with LGV often show abnormal serum protein concentrations (Williams and Gutman, 1936). Reversal of the albumin-globulin ratio may occur (Saad et al., 1961). This abnormality is most marked in the chronic infection. Shaffer and Rake (1947) found that hypergammaglobulinemia caused the shift and that the increase in gamma globulin was proportional to increases in CF titers. Abrams (1968) observed serum protein electrophoresis patterns to be abnormal in 8 of 20 patients. Although different immunoglobulin classes may be elevated, the most consistent elevation is of IgA; Lassus et al. (1970) found IgA elevated in 6 out of 8 of their patients. Using the Mancini method we have observed IgA elevation in 5 of 10 patients from whom LGV agent has been isolated. Cryoglobulins were found in serum from 8 of 14 LGV patients by Lassus et al. (1970). Abnormal serum proteins may persist, even in old treated LGV cases (Sonck et al., 1972).

DIFFERENTIAL DIAGNOSIS

The first consideration in differential diagnosis of LGV is the possibility that the patient may have another venereal disease with similar clinical symptomatology. But over and above the problem of a specific diagnosis, is the consideration that many patients with lymphogranuloma venereum do have other venereal diseases as well; thus, proper clinical work-up should include, at the very least, tests for gonorrhea and syphilis as well as for LGV. Patients with positive syphilis serology may have a relatively high rate of seroreactions to LGV, and vice-versa. There is a very real question as to whether these so-called nonspecific reactions are, in fact, nonspecific (Simpson, 1954). It is obvious that sexually active individuals might have been exposed to many venereally transmitted pathogens. Gonorrhea has been diagnosed in a significant proportion of LGV patients, and in some studies up to one-third of the patients with LGV had syphilis. In Alergant's series, 11 of 55 patients had other venereal diseases in addition to LGV, and Sonck (1972) recorded 192 of 810 cases with two or more venereal diseases.

Syphilis can present a problem in differential diagnosis, not only because it has so many clinical forms, but also because much of the classic symptomatology of syphilis is similar to some of the findings in LGV. For example, inguinal lymphadenopathy commonly occurs in syphilis and a healed syphilitic chancre looks somewhat like a primary lesion in LGV. However, the hard lymph nodes of syphilis are different from the matted lymph nodes of LGV.

It cannot be emphasized too strongly that any patient being examined for LGV should have an examination for syphilis. There are numerous reports of the occurrence of biological false-positive syphilis reactions in patients with LGV. The reasons for this are still unclear. Possibly the serum abnormalities observed in LGV result in reaction with reagin antigens.

Herpes genitalis may also mimic LGV, particularly in an initial infection. The primary lesion of patients with this disease may be a healing herpetic vesicle with the appearance of a shallow ulcer, similar to the appearance of the healed primary lesion of LGV. In addition, regional (inguinal) lymphadenopathy is not uncommon, accompanied by systemic manifestations such as low-grade fever. In general, this disease follows a much shorter course than does untreated LGV, although specific diagnosis must be made by either serology or culture. Herpesvirus may be isolated from the vesicular lesion, but if the patient's ulcer has healed, it is probably too late to recover the virus.

Granuloma inguinale and chancroid are often considered in the differential diagnosis, but the similarities between these diseases and LGV are more apparent than real. A true bubo is not formed. In granuloma inguinale there is usually a beefy exuberant granulomatous response in superficial tissue, with lymph nodes being involved, often as a result of secondary infection. With chancroid there is usually a characteristic active primary ulcer of the genitalia, with either constant or sharp pain in the lymph nodes. Specific diagnosis may be made by deep scraping of the chancroid lesion and demonstration of the characteristic *Haemophilus ducreyi,* which may be shown by cytology or culture (Young, 1974). In addition, diagnosis can be made by the Ito-Reenstierna skin test, if available. The Donovan bodies (*Calymmatobacterium granulomatosis*) of granuloma inguinale may also be demonstrated in a similar manner by deep scraping and Giemsa or Wright staining of the smear (Kellogg, 1974).

Cat scratch disease may also be confused with LGV, although most patients with this syndrome are prepubescent. Lymphadenopathy commonly occurs in these patients following trauma associated with either a cat bite or scratch on an extremity. If it is on the leg, inguinal lymph nodes may be involved. Occasionally these patients will have high CF titers to chlamydial antigen, further confusing the picture. Such a syndrome appearing in a sexually active individual may readily be confused with LGV. Cat scratch disease does not respond to chemotherapy.

Tests for bacterial lymphadenitis should be done in any case of inguinal lymphadenopathy. If the node is fluctuant and aspirated or is suppurative and ruptures spontaneously, the pus should be examined by culture for aerobic and anaerobic bacteria. Lymph node involvement may reflect superficial lesions anywhere in the draining area, and a careful search for skin lesions on the legs, around the toes and nails, etc., should be performed. Recovery of bacteria from the pus does not rule out a diagnosis of LGV, for many of these nodes may be secondarily infected.

Occasionally a patient with lymphoma may present with a picture similar to that of LGV. In this case differential diagnosis can be established by biopsy and histopathologic examination of the specimen.

CHEMOTHERAPY

It should be noted that a specific, highly effective method of treating LGV is not available. One of the problems involved in assessing the effects of chemotherapy is the extremely variable natural history of the disease. Spontaneous remission does occur, as shown by one of our patients who developed acute lymphadenopathy without evidence of LGV infection early in his clinical course. His CF and Frei tests were initially negative; his lymph node enlargement resolved spontaneously in approximately 6 to 8 weeks. Because of the initial negative laboratory results, a lymphoma was suspected. After the lesion had resolved without treatment, the laboratory tests were repeated and found to be positive.

MacCallum and Findlay noted that the LGV agent was susceptible to sulfonamides (1938), and this was the treatment of choice until the broad-spectrum antibiotics became available. Most therapeutic trials for LGV have involved treatment with a single drug of choice, or a comparison of a standard treatment with a new drug. Almost all trials have a certain number of total treatment failures, as well as some patients who respond only after repeated courses, of either the same drug or other drugs. No extensive, controlled double-blind treatment trials have been done. The only major therapeutic trial attempted was carried out by Greaves et al. (1957), who evaluated three antibiotics (chloramphenicol, oxytetracycline, chlortetracycline), sulfadiazine, and symptomatic therapy with aspirin in a group of patients with LGV. Recognizing the highly variable course of the disease and their inability to predict complications, they decided to measure only progression or remission of the buboes and to follow CF tests on the patients' sera. The duration of the buboes of the 25 patients who finished the course of antimicrobial treatment was significantly less than that of the control group (31 days versus 69 days). The investigators felt that all the drugs were somewhat beneficial, with an indication that perhaps sulfadiazine or oxytetracycline might be somewhat better than the other two antimicrobials, but the number tested was too small to provide conclusive results. In addition, there appeared to be a somewhat greater rate of complications in the symptomatically treated patients as compared to those receiving antimicrobial drugs (but again the number tested was too small to be conclusive). Antibody titers spontaneously decreased in 7 of 17 patients, while all those receiving antimicrobial therapy appeared to show some decline in antibody level one year after treatment.

In general, the feeling has been that treatment early in the disease has a better chance of success than treatment initiated at a later, chronic stage. Many authors claim that essentially all their patients get better with whatever drug they happen to be using, but careful reading of the literature indicates that in virtually all series, a few cases have required two, three, or more courses of therapy.

All of Abrams's (1968) patients responded well, but all of these cases appeared to be relatively acute. Our experience agrees with his, although some of our patients have required two courses of therapy. In general, results indicate that the sulfonamides and tetracyclines are equally effective in treating LGV. At least some of the earlier treatment failures probably reflect inadequate dosage. Our standard course of therapy has been 250 mg of tetracycline q.i.d. for 21 days. Alternatively, sulfisoxazole may be used with a loading dose of 4 gm followed by 1 gm q.i.d. for 21 days. We tend to use tetracycline because there are some indications that sulfonamides may not be effective in all cases; one chlamydia (*C. psittaci*), which we isolated from a patient with clinical LGV (Schachter, 1967a), was completely resistant to sulfa drugs. It is recognized (Shaffer et al., 1944; Hurst, Peters, and Melvin, 1950; Jones, Rake, and Stearns, 1945) that different LGV strains may show differing sensitivities to sulfa drugs. In addition, resistance to sulfonamides may develop following exposure in laboratory systems (Jones, Rake, and Stearns, 1945; Schachter and Meyer, 1969a). Chloramphenicol should not be considered as an alternate treatment, as it is relatively ineffective and may produce dangerous side effects.

In the chronic or tertiary stage of LGV it is very difficult to assess response to chemotherapy. Perhaps a series with biopsies performed before and after treatment would help to resolve this problem. Some studies have shown that at least two courses of therapy (with a tetracycline) resulted in absolute failure to improve at least 25% of patients. Improvement in the other patients was extremely difficult to assess (Greenblatt, 1952). It is probable that patients with inflammatory strictures may show some improvement if much of the inflammatory reaction is not due to secondary bacterial infections, while those patients who have fibrotic lesions are beyond the stage where chemotherapy is of use. It is obvious that surgical repair of these lesions must be considered.

Some workers have used a changing or decreasing CF titer as a measure of response to chemotherapy. This is probably not a valid criterion, since there is a tendency for spontaneous remission in some patients, and some studies have shown absolutely no effect of therapy on CF titers, although there was good clinical response. In some patients, CF titers decrease spontaneously.

LGV AND CANCER

A number of clinicians have observed coincident cases of carcinoma in patients with lymphogranuloma venereum. It was probably Liccione (1936) who first suggested that LGV might be a precancerous infection. He followed two cases with rectal strictures; both developed rectal adenocarcinoma at the site of the stricture. Cardwell and Pund (1940) extended this observation to include LGV infection of the penis and the vulva as lesions which had been seen preceding the development of carcinomas at the involved site. The possibility that LGV could be a precipitating factor in the development of carcinoma is obviously an intriguing one, and Pund and Lacy (1951) presented such an analysis of 135 cases of carcinoma of the penis, vulva, and ano-rectum. Their analysis suffered from a bias in that white patients tended not to be tested for LGV while all the black patients were tested. Among the latter group, 18 (72%) of the 25 penile carcinomas, 8 (42%) of the 19 vulvar carcinomas, and all 5 of the anal-rectal carcinomas were Frei-test positive. Some of these patients had long histories of LGV, and biopsies were often suggestive of active lymphogranulomatous lesions. Pund and Lacy felt that the coexistence of LGV and the carcinomas in these patients was not fortuitous, and pointed out that this association was much higher than observed in other venereal diseases such as chancroid or granuloma inguinale.

Rainey (1954) described 95 cases of coincidental carcinoma and LGV, and, in following 220 cases of uncomplicated LGV, he found that 11 (4.5%) developed carcinoma. Unfortunately, this latter study is the nearest thing to a prospective study presently available, and the true relationship of LGV and the carcinoma is not clear. But many workers (Levin et al., 1964) have felt that the late lesions of LGV are associated with an increased incidence of carcinoma.

Many studies have suggested that ulcerative venereal disease may lead to carcinoma. Since LGV is a chronic granulomatous disease that results in hyperplastic cell responses, it does not seem unreasonable to consider that some of the changes associated with LGV are also changes associated with early malignant lesions. Fortunately today we do not see very much late untreated LGV, and it is likely that the true role, if any, of LGV in human cancer will never be clearly elucidated. At this stage, the only thing which clearly emerges is that the clinician should be aware of the possible high association of malignancy with chronic active LGV, carefully examine the patients for possible malignancies, and, of course, biopsy any lesion which seems persistent.

DIAGNOSTIC METHODS

The Frei Test

In 1925 Frei made a significant contribution to the establishment of a specific diagnosis of LGV when he showed that pus, aspirated from a bubo of a patient with LGV and then heated in the laboratory, could elicit a delayed skin reaction when it was inoculated intradermally into another patient suffering from LGV. Heating these human antigens for one hour at 56° to 60° C on three successive days presumably inactivated the LGV agent as well as any other pathogens that might have been present. In view of our current knowledge of the transmission of hepatitis virus and other pathogens, it is obvious that such precautions cannot be considered adequate.

After the LGV organism was cultivated in the laboratory, potent Frei-test antigens were prepared, first from infected monkey brain and then from infected mouse brain. These preparations had an activity similar to that described by Frei for the human material. In 1940 a significant advance was made in standardizing and preparing the antigen with the use of yolk sac-grown LGV agent (Grace, Rake, and Shaffer, 1940; Rake, McKee, and Shaffer, 1940). This antigen,

Lygranum®, was simply a partially purified, killed elementary body suspension. Today one can only speculate, but it appears that the original human pus material, although not standardized, was probably a more potent antigen than the material currently available.

The antigens responsible for the group-specific tests — CF or skin test — appear to be lipopolysaccharide complexes. They are heat stable and sensitive to the action of periodate. When Barwell (1952) treated LGV suspensions with dilute acid, he felt he had developed a highly purified and specific skin test antigen. Although his observation has been confirmed, the antigen has not found large-scale clinical applicability.

Currently the Frei test is performed by parallel intradermal inoculation of 0.1 ml of the test preparation and 0.1 ml of a control preparation. The test is read in approximately 48 to 72 hours and erythematous zones are ignored. Only the papule or area of induration is measured. A 6-mm zone of induration is considered a positive reaction with no positive reaction in the control. If the control reacts, the test zone must have a reaction zone at least 6 mm greater than that seen in the control. Occasionally, in an extremely sensitized individual, the site of the skin test may become necrotic. There have been cases of axillary lymph node involvement or inflammation following skin tests in the antecubital area. Some workers have pointed out that skin testing in the highly reactive individual may precipitate systemic complications such as cutaneous manifestations and arthritic involvement.

The Frei test will produce a positive reaction within a few weeks of the initial infection. (The CF test usually becomes positive a few days before the Frei test does.) The Frei test is not specific for LGV, and is occasionally also positive in patients with trachoma, oculogenital chlamydial infections, or psittacosis. In fact, potent Frei-type antigens can be prepared with psittacosis strains, and have been shown by Pollard and Witka (1947) to react at least as well as the LGV antigens. The skin test reaction may be temporarily abolished by steroid administration (Grace, Frank, and Wyse, 1952) and may be permanently abolished if early, intensive, and effective chemotherapy is initiated. Once positive, the skin test appears to be positive for many years, possibly for the life of the individual. Thus, in a group of patients followed for up to 40 years in Finland, two-thirds of the patients were still positive at the long-term follow-up (Sonck, 1972).

The skin test can be repeated without interfering with either serologic testing or further skin testing. All evidence indicates that exposure to the antigen does not sensitize the patient to subsequent testing or result in CF titer increases. Occasionally, repeated testing will indicate conversion from negative to positive; however, this is usually not the case, and when it does occur, the initial test had usually been administered relatively early in the course of the disease. In Abrams's (1968) study, 5 of 20 patients became skin test positive while under observation.

Today, most patients with LGV are seen in VD clinics or in public health hospitals serving merchant seamen. They usually present a considerable length of time after initial infection. Thus, if the patient has a one-week incubation period for the primary lesion, followed by a one- to two-week incubation period for the development of lymph nodes or buboes, he will have been infected for at least two to three weeks before coming to the clinic. By this time most patients who will eventually develop a positive Frei test will be reactive.

Some workers have cast doubts on the reliability of the Frei test. Alergant (in Liverpool) summarized his experience of many years by pointing out that approximately one-third (16/51) of his patients with LGV did not have positive Frei tests (1957). Only one-third of our patients with a presumed diagnosis of LGV have had positive Frei tests, although two-thirds had positive CF tests. Although some of these patients may not have had LGV, LGV agents were recovered from some patients who had negative skin tests (Schachter et al., 1969). Perhaps if these patients had been repeatedly skin tested for many months, their skin tests might have become positive, but such unrealistic testing procedures certainly do not indicate a useful diagnostic test.

Because of the lack of specificity of the reaction, the possible delay in development, and the presentation of many patients who are never positive, one must conclude either that the Frei test is not as useful as once thought or that the currently available antigens are just not potent enough. At any rate, a positive Frei test supports a clinical diagnosis of LGV but does not prove it, and a negative Frei test does not exclude a diagnosis of LGV.

Serologic Diagnosis, Complement Fixation Test

The complement fixation (CF) test for LGV using infected mouse brain preparations as antigen was described in the 1930s and later replaced by yolk sac-grown antigen (Meyer, Eddie, and Schachter, 1969). The CF test is group specific, and may be performed with either psittacosis or LGV antigens. The preparation of the antigens usually destroys type-specific antigens. Since it is group reactive, it will measure antibodies to any chlamydial infection; thus, cross-reactions with psittacosis, trachoma, and the oculogenital infections are to be expected.

In LGV, the CF test probably becomes positive within the first week or two following infection, slightly before the Frei test (Alergant, 1957; Erskine, 1958), and may be positive for variable periods (Greaves and Taggart, 1953). In the untreated patient, it may remain positive for life; in the treated patient, the CF titer may fall dramatically following treatment. Some workers consider the persistence of CF titer to reflect the persistence of agent. On these speculative grounds, some workers have considered a falling CF titer indicative of therapeutic success, with a high titer meaning failure. However, the fact is that patients who have responded to therapy may very well retain their titers for years, possibly for life. It is impossible to disprove the contention that the maintenance of titer means maintenance of either adequate antigenic stimulus or viable agent, but such a situation is unlikely (Goldberg and Banov, 1956).

Early intensive therapy may abolish a CF response in man or animal (Wall, 1947). An ideal serologic conversion would have a four-fold or greater increase in the titer of paired serum acute and convalescent samples. Practically, this situation does not often occur, although in Abrams's study seven patients converted during the period of observation. His experience with a military population probably allowed earlier examination and closer follow-up than is usually feasible. In general, the patient with LGV is available for one, occasionally two, samples separated by a week or more. Usually the patient has a high titer by the time he is tested; significant rises during the test periods are rare and may indicate progressive disease in the chronic stage. While there is usually agreement between the CF titer and the Frei test, it is the feeling of some workers that the CF test is a more specific and sensitive index of LGV infection. Thus, Alergant found high CF titers in most of his patients (53/54), although a significant number had a negative Frei test; Sigel (1962) found that 97% of his LGV patients had high CF titers. Our experience supports this position; we have never recovered an organism from a bubo or other site in a patient with a negative CF test (Schachter et al., 1969).

There may be a significant quantitative difference in CF titers in patients with LGV compared to patients with the trachoma or TRIC agent oculogenital infections. For example, in a simple uncomplicated TRIC agent infection (either of the eye or of the eye and genital tract) we have never seen patients with CF titers above 1:64, whereas at least half of the patients with LGV have CF titers in excess of 1:64, usually 1:256 or higher. Positive CF titers of patients with TRIC agent infections are usually 1:8 and 1:16, and at least 50% of the patients do not have CF titers this high. In fact, in male patients with proven TRIC agent infections of the urethra, approximately 70% have negative CF tests. The high CF titers usually found in LGV may also be found following psittacosis infection or may be observed in some patients who have both Reiter's syndrome and TRIC agent infections. The reason for this latter finding is not clear, but may reflect a heightened reactivity of these patients to antigenic stimuli. However, only 10% of the patients with Reiter's syndrome will show CF titers this high.

Thus, it appears that a highly positive complement fixation test is the best commonly available laboratory aid to the diagnosis of LGV. It must be emphasized that such a reaction merely supports the clinical diagnosis and does not prove it. A high CF titer may occur in the absence of LGV and LGV may occur in the absence of a high CF titer. The only laboratory proof available is agent isolation (Figs. 3, 4). But this procedure (Chapter 11) is not yet routine.

Serologic Diagnosis, The Microimmunofluorescence Test

In 1970 Wang and Grayston described a microimmunofluorescent test for the detection of antichlamydial antibodies. The test was first utilized in typing chlamydial isolates, although it has also been applied to human serology, in genital tract infections, by at least four laboratories. The test is extremely sensitive and it may allow for a highly specific identification of infecting serotype. However, the LGV agents are very broadly immunoreactive. All patients with proven lymphogranuloma venereum have high titers when tested by this indirect fluorescent antibody test which uses yolk sac-grown elementary body suspensions as antigens. For example, our patients with isolate-positive LGV have had micro-IF titers usually on the order of 1:2 to 1:4,000, broadly reactive with all TRIC agent antigens. Wang and Grayston (1974) and Philip et al. (1974) have shown similar results. The former group used sera from our patients for their LGV test, the latter used sera from patients, in Washington, D.C., with LGV. Based on the idea that IgM antibody (presumably reflecting very recent or current infection) in patients with LGV would be highly supportive of the diagnosis of LGV, Philip looked for this antibody in his patients. However, IgM antibody was demonstrated in only two of the seven patients available for study. We have occasionally observed a short-lived (approximately one month) IgM antibody response in some of our patients with LGV. Often this means that the patient is being examined at the time when the IgM antibody levels begin to decline.

The micro-IF and the CF tests measure different antibodies, and it has been found that one test may be positive while the other is negative. The tests may have different developmental time courses. We find that the two are not totally unrelated, however, in that statistical analysis of the correlation between results from the two tests in patients with genital tract infections gives a correlation coefficient ranging from 0.5 to 0.7, depending on the patients studied. When one is elevated, the other is also exalted; and where there is disparity, it is usually the more sensitive micro-IF test which is positive.

The micro-IF test has been used to serotype LGV agents, and three different serotypes (L-1, L-2, and L-3) have been identified (Wang and Grayston, 1971a; Treharne et al., 1972). Insufficient numbers of isolates have been typed to yield information concerning geographic distribution, although one would assume no localization because so many cases are imported. Type L-2 appears to be the most common. There is no information concerning biological differences among types.

Agent Isolation

Although any involved site may be tested, the most rewarding specimen for isolation attempts in LGV is pus aspirated from a fluctuant lymph node. Chlamydiae are rarely recovered from sexual contacts.

It is possible to isolate the chlamydiae in mice, embryonated hens' eggs, or tissue culture systems. Wall (1946) showed that yolk sac inoculation of fertile eggs was more sensitive than intracerebral inoculation of mice. We have confirmed this observation (Schachter et al., 1969). Tissue culture systems are probably the methods of choice as we have found the LGV agent can be readily recovered (Fig. 4, Plate 1). The methods are presented in detail in Chapter 11. Isolation of the chlamydiae is the definitive laboratory test in proving the diagnosis of LGV.

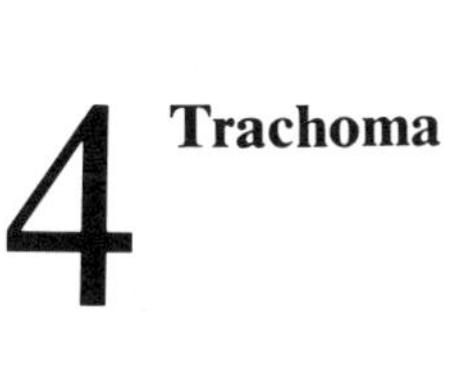

Trachoma, a chronic inflammation of the mucous membranes lining the eyelids and eyeball, is still the leading cause of preventable blindness in the world today. Blinding trachoma is a major public health problem in North Africa and sub-Saharan Africa, in the Middle East, in the drier regions of the Indian subcontinent, and in Southeast Asia. In addition, pockets of blinding trachoma exist in Australasia, the Pacific Islands, and Latin America. The disease has always been worse in poorer populations and, with economic development, becomes milder or may disappear entirely.

HISTORICAL ASPECTS

Trachoma has been known since antiquity. The treatment for trichiasis was described in China in the twenty-seventh century B.C. Medical treatment and surgical therapy were described in the Ebers Papyrus in the nineteenth century B.C. in Egypt (Thygeson, 1962a; Duke-Elder, 1965). The disease was common in the Mediterranean basin in classical times. The name trachoma (Greek: rough swelling) was first known in the first century B.C. It was well described in the medieval manuals in Greek and Arabic. In the Middle Ages, trachoma was disseminated by the crusaders returning from Palestine. The disease burst on the European scene following the Napoleonic campaigns in Egypt in 1798 and 1799. The Egyptian ophthalmia, as it was called, was rampant in the English and French troops in Egypt at that time and became endemic in both the civilian and military populations during the Napoleonic era. It was identified as a major cause of blindness in the English military population.

During the nineteenth century, trachoma was widespread in Europe, and most ophthalmic textbooks of the time devoted considerable space to the description and treatment of the disease. The course of the malady was well characterized; the focal "granulation" was recognized as lymphoid follicles similar to those of the intestine, and the conjunctival scarring and superficial corneal vascularization were considered sequelae of the chronic disease process. The chlamydial inclusions were identified by Halberstaedter and von Prowazek (1907a,b) in conjunctival scrapings from orangutans that had been infected with human trachomatous scrapings. The trachoma inclusions were finally established as the etiologic agent despite claims for a bacterial origin (e.g., *Bacterium granulosis* by Noguchi, 1928) for the following reasons:

1. The agent could be demonstrated in cases of endemic trachoma in many areas of the world.
2. Material from trachomatous eyes, when inoculated into subhuman primates, produced a follicular conjunctivitis and many new inclusion bodies in the inoculated conjunctival epithelium (Thygeson and Richards, 1938).
3. Bacteria-free filtrates of conjunctival scrapings from trachoma cases, when inoculated into human volunteers, produced all the signs of the clinical disease: lymphoid follicles and scarring of the conjunctiva, neovascularization in the cornea, and the formation of new inclusion bodies in the conjunctival epithelial cells (Thygeson and Proctor, 1935).

Despite the widespread cultivation of psittacosis and lymphogranuloma agents in eggs during the 1930s, the first accepted isolation of trachoma was not reported by T'ang and his associates in Peking until 1957. It is probable that Macchiavello, working in Peru, successfully isolated the trachoma agent and inoculated a volunteer with the cultivated agent in 1944, but his work was not accepted or was ignored by other workers in the field (Thygeson, 1962a).

Prior to the introduction of sulfonamides, the most widely used therapy for trachoma was the application of copper sulfate solutions or abrasion of the conjunctiva with copper sulfate crystals. Soon after its introduction, sulfanilamide was found effective when administered either by mouth or by the topical application of powder to the conjunctival cul-de-sac. The systematic application of sulfonamides among American Indians before 1942 led to the complete eradication of the disease in some tribes and to its marked suppression in others, especially in tribes of the Southwest (Forster and McGibony, 1944). In the early 1950s, the tetracyclines, notably chlortetracycline and erythromycin derivatives, were shown also to be effective when applied topically (Mitsui and Tanaka, 1951; Mitsui et al., 1954). In a number of clinical trials under the auspices of the World Health Organization, it was found that the prevalence of the disease could be reduced by topical chemotherapy given continually for 60 days or by the so-called intermittent method — chemotherapy administered 5 consecutive days each month for 6 months (Reinhards, Weber, and Maxwell-Lyons, 1959). However, in many areas, notably Yugoslavia and among the southwestern American Indians, it was found that orally administered sulfonamides or tetracyclines were more effective (Blagojevic, Savic, and Litricin, 1973; Dawson and Hanna, 1971). Advances in the microbiologic study of the agent have had little direct impact on public health control measures up to the present time; on the contrary, effective trachoma treatment methods have come about entirely due to independent developments in the use of chemotherapeutic agents.

CLINICAL DESCRIPTION

In the early stages, trachoma appears as a chronic follicular conjunctivitis, with particular involvement of the upper tarsal conjunctiva, and a varying degree of papillary hypertrophy and inflammatory infiltration of the conjunctiva. Conjunctival follicles appear as elevated avascular lesions that may be yellowish to grey-white, or occasionally translucent (Fig. 1, Plate 2). They vary in size from 0.2 to 2 mm in diameter. Histologically, they consist of lymphoid germinal centers. Conjunctival follicles may appear in response to a number of infectious agents or other foreign substances. As trachoma progresses, the scarring of the conjunctiva appears as fine linear scars in mild cases and as broader confluent scars in more severe cases (Figs. 2–7, Plates 2, 3). While the presence of scarring is sometimes thought to be necessary for healing, some cases with marked conjunctival scarring continue to have severe, persistent, active disease with follicular hypertrophy and conjunctival infiltration. Tear deficiency syndrome and stenosis of the lacrimal (outflow) duct can occur as late complications in patients with severe scarring. The major, potentially blinding sequelae, however, are distortion of the lids, particularly the upper lid, and trichiasis or entropion, the misdirection of the lashes so that they grow at an angle directed toward the eyeball itself (Fig. 8, Plate 3). The constant abrasion of the cornea by the wirelike lashes and occasional foreign body injuries in a relatively dry eye frequently result in corneal ulceration, followed by scarring and visual loss (Fig. 9, Plate 3).

The involvement of the cornea in trachoma includes punctate erosions of the epithelium (epithelial, keratitis), small cellular infiltrates of the peripheral central corneal epithelium and anterior stroma, superficial vascularization (vascular pannus), shallow peripheral ulcers, swelling of the limbus (corneal-scleral border), and the formation of lymphoid follicles at the limbus with the resultant scar called Herbert's pits (Figs. 10, 11, Plate 3). Rarely, patients will have a double row of these Herbert's pits where follicles have formed in the pannus itself. Typically, the epithelial keratitis of trachoma occurs more commonly in the upper half of the cornea, although it is not limited to this area. Inflammatory infiltrates of the cornea range in size from lesions so small that they can be seen only by a slit lamp, to large trachoma pustules (actually small corneal ulcers) at the site of an infiltrate. The trachoma pannus consists of a fibrovascular membrane and associated cellular infiltration and scarring. This vascular pannus is superficial and is usually more marked at the superior limbus, although it is present in all the corneal meridians.

In addition to the specific trachomatous involvement of the cornea, there is a high incidence of other corneal disease in trachomatous populations. Superficial foreign body scars are very common in association with the corneal vascularization. Avascular pearl-like excrescences, called Salzmann's nodular dystrophy, may form on the corneal surface. Bacterial ulcers of the cornea caused by trichiasis and entropion or by foreign body injuries are not infrequent. Individuals with allergic conjunctivitis (particularly vernal catarrh) in conjunction with trachoma present a particularly severe problem in management, since the corneal involvement is difficult to control by either antibiotic or steroid therapy alone.

The diagnosis of trachoma, according to the Third Expert Committee of the World Health Organization (1962), can be made if two of the following signs are present:

1. Lymphoid follicles on the upper tarsal conjunctiva
2. Typical conjunctival scarring
3. Vascular pannus
4. Limbal follicles or their sequelae, Herbert's pits

The presence of at least two of these should be regarded as the minimal criteria for the clinical diagnosis of disease. To establish that trachoma is endemic in a population, these minimal signs should be demonstrated in a significant proportion of suspected cases examined in a community. There are a number of other conditions (see below) that closely resemble trachoma but, with two minor exceptions — Axenfeld's chronic follicular conjunctivitis and chronic follicular keratoconjunctivitis of Thygeson — they are never endemic in a community. It is felt at the present time that limbal follicles or Herbert's pits are the only clinical signs unique to trachoma, although these signs do not occur in every case.

Trachoma cases are usually classified in "stages" according to the *MacCallan classification* (MacCallan, 1936). Although corneal signs must be present to make a diagnosis of trachoma, the MacCallan classification is based on findings in the conjunctiva alone (WHO III, 1962).

Stage 0	No signs of trachoma
Stage I	Immature follicles present on the upper tarsal plate, including the central area, but without conjunctival scarring (Fig. 1, Plate 2)
Stage IIa	Mature follicles present on the upper tarsus with moderate papillary hypertrophy
Stage IIb	Marked papillary hypertrophy of the upper tarsus obscuring the tarsal vessels (Fig. 12, Plate 3)
Stage III	Follicles present on the tarsus and definite scarring in the conjunctiva (Figs. 2–5, Plate 2)
Stage IV	No follicles present on the tarsal plate but definite scarring in the conjunctiva (Figs. 6, 7, Plates 2, 3)

"Mature" follicles are defined as "soft" or "necrotic," liable to rupture under light pressure, and leave a conjunctival scar. At various times in the past the MacCallan classification has been extended to include "trachoma dubium," a term which was used to indicate cases lacking enough follicular hypertrophy and keratitis to make a definite diagnosis of trachoma (WHO III,. 1962). The term "prototrachoma" has consistently been used to indicate cases with no definite signs of trachoma but with laboratory evidence of infection with a chlamydial agent.

The MacCallan classification has been of little use in evaluating the impact of trachoma on a community, since it fails to differentiate among varying degrees of inflammation and yields no data on visually disabling lesions. For this reason it has been necessary to evaluate trachoma endemic in a community in terms of individual clinical signs, particularly follicular reaction, conjunctival scarring, trichiasis/ entropion, and corneal scarring. In a series of recent studies, classification of intensity of active inflammatory disease in individual cases was based on the scoring of lymphoid follicles (F) and papillary hypertrophy (P) in the conjunctiva of the upper tarsus (Dawson, Jones, and Darougar, 1976). This intensity scale consists of four categories: Severe, moderate, mild, and insignificant or inactive (Table 1).

Table 1
Intensity Scale

Intensity	Follicle Score (F)	Papillary Hypertrophy Score (P)
Severe	F 1, 2, or 3	P 3
Moderate	F 3	P 2
Mild	F 2 (or F 3 if the follicles are less than 0.5 mm in diameter)	P 1 or 2
Inactive or insignificant	F 0 or 1	P 1 or 2

For the scoring of upper tarsal follicles, the upper tarsal conjunctival surface is divided into approximately equal thirds referred to as zones. These zones are divided by two imaginary lines, approximately parallel with the upper tarsal border, the curve upward toward their lateral extremities, as viewed on the everted tarsal surface. Zone 1 includes the entire upper tarsal border and adjacent tarsal surface. Zone 3 includes the tarsal conjunctiva adjacent to the central half of the lid margin and, at its center, covers just less than half the vertical extent of the tarsal surface. Zone 2 occupies the intervening area and extends to the lateral quarters of the lid margin.

The scores for *upper tarsal follicles* (F) are designated as follows:

F 0   No follicles present
F 1   Follicles present but no more than 5 follicles in zones 2 and 3 together (Figs. 6, 7, Plates 2, 3)
F 2   More follicles than F 1 but fewer than 5 follicles in zone 3 (Figs. 1, 2, Plate 2)
F 3   Five or more follicles in each of the 3 zones (Figs. 3, 4, 5, 12, Plates 2, 3)

The scores for upper tarsal papillary hypertrophy and diffuse infiltration (P) are as follows:

P 1   Minimal: normal deep subconjunctival vessels on the tarsus not obscured (Figs. 1, 2, 6, Plate 2)

P 2   Moderate: normal vessels appear hazy, even when seen by the naked eye (Figs. 3, 4, 7, Plates 2, 3)

P 3   Pronounced: conjunctiva thickened and opaque, normal vessels on the tarsus are hidden (Figs. 5, 12, Plates 2, 3)

The scores for follicles and papillary hypertrophy should be recorded and the grading of intensity made by the observer at the time of examination.

The *potentially disabling, irreversible lesions* are (1) distortion of the eyelids due to conjunctival scarring, and (2) trichiasis and/or entropion. Previously trichiasis and/or entropion have been recorded as conjunctival scarring, grade 4 (C 4). To emphasize disabling lesions and to provide a more direct indication of the risk, it is useful to record trichiasis/entropion separately from conjunctival scarring.

The *disabling lesion* is severe central corneal scarring (CC 3). The scores for these irreversible lesions have been modified as follows:

Conjunctival scarring (C):

C 0   No scarring on the conjunctiva (Figs. 1, 12, Plates 2, 3)

C 1   Mild: fine, scattered scars on the upper tarsal conjunctiva (Fig. 6, Plate 2)

C 2   Moderate: More severe scarring, but without shortening or distortion of the upper tarsus (Figs. 3, 4, Plate 2)

C 3   Severe: Scarring with distortion of the upper tarsus (Figs. 2, 5, 7, Plates 2, 3)

Trichiasis and/or entropion (T/E):

T/E 0   No trichiasis or entropion

T/E 1   Lashes deviated toward the eye but not touching the globe

T/E 2   Lashes touching the globe but not rubbing on the cornea

T/E 3   Lashes constantly rubbing on the cornea (Figs. 8, 9, Plate 3)

Corneal scarring (CC):

CC 0   Absent

CC 1   Minimal or not involving the visual axis, with no visual loss

CC 2   Moderate scarring involving the visual axis

CC 3   Severe central scarring with gross visual loss (Fig. 9, Plate 3)

The potentially disabling lesions are severe conjunctival scarring with distortion of the upper tarsus (C 3), and any trichiasis and/or entropion (T/E 1, 2, or 3). The disabling lesion is severe central corneal scarring (CC 3).

In areas where it is endemic, *blinding trachoma* can be recognized in a population by the presence of persons with severe visual loss due to corneal opacity and a substantial prevalence of potentially disabling trachomatous lesions, particularly trichiasis/entropion. These irreversible changes probably result from long, continued inflammatory disease of moderate or severe intensity. Nonblinding trachoma may result in a low prevalence of potentially blinding lesions, but it does not lead to a substantial prevalence of visual loss in a community.

In communities with blinding trachoma, chlamydial infection is always present even though other ocular bacterial pathogens appear to contribute significantly to the intensity of trachoma and to the lesions that impair vision. Indeed, relatively mild cases are referred to in the French literature as "trachome pur" (Nataf, Lepine, and Bonamour, 1960). From the public health point of view, trachoma is important as a cause of preventable blindness; the failure to distinguish blinding and nonblinding trachoma leads to confusion in determining priorities and selecting areas for public health programs. This has been particularly true in recent years, when the emphasis was on minimal clinical diagnosis and diagnosis through microbiologic methods, neither of which relates to the prevalence of blinding disease in the communities studied.

EPIDEMIOLOGY

Trachoma has a worldwide distribution. At present, blinding trachoma is a major public health problem in adults in a geographic area extending from North and sub-Saharan Africa to the Middle East, and to the drier regions of the Indian subcontinent and Southeast Asia (WHO Statistics, 1971). Pockets of blinding trachoma exist in Australasia, the Pacific Islands, and Latin America. Nonblinding trachoma is present in these same areas as well as in a much broader region that includes most of the drier, subtropical, and tropical countries. In North America, trachoma is limited to certain ethnic and cultural groups among whom trachoma was once endemic and who continue to have relatively low living standards. In the United States the disease occurs among Mexican Americans and Chinese and Japanese immigrants, as well as among American Indians, Samoans, and Filipinos (Thygeson, 1963). In addition, individuals of Scots-Irish extraction who grew up in the American trachoma belt of the Middle South, Oklahoma, and Texas may have recurrences of the disease, and their children may rarely have active disease (Siniscal, 1957). In Europe at the beginning of this century, trachoma was prevalent in the Mediterranean region, eastern Europe, and Russia, as well as in western Ireland (Bietti and Werner, 1967). Due to a rising standard of living and to active control programs carried out since World War II, the disease has disappeared for practical purposes in those European countries formerly affected (Blagojevic, Savic, and Litricin, 1973). Individuals or families migrating from trachoma-endemic areas to the developed countries of Europe and North America have not acted as reservoirs to reintroduce the disease to these countries. It would appear that under the living conditions of the industrialized countries trachoma is rarely transmitted, even to younger family members, and, if the disease is acquired, it is mild (Detels, Alexander, and Dhir, 1966). In persons with healed trachoma, however, there may be recurrence of active disease due to a number of causes, among which are extreme old age, allergic conjunctivitis, or administration of topical corticosteroids; but these disease patterns do not present a significant public health risk.

In communities where trachoma is endemic, the highest rate of active infection is found among children under 10 years of age. In one community with severe endemic trachoma, it was found that all children were infected by the age of 2 years, and, starting at age 5, the prevalence of disease declined steadily until the age of 15; about 5% of adults, however, had signs of active disease (Dawson et al., 1976). Because children constitute such a large proportion of the population in hyperendemic trachoma areas, this active childhood disease represented the reservoir in this community. Older children and adults appeared to have active disease because of their exposure to these younger children.

The intensity of trachoma in any particular child appears to be relatively stable — that is, children with severe disease continue to have severe disease on follow-up examinations despite the administration of one or more courses of chemotherapy, and mild or inactive disease rarely progresses to become severe. It can be assumed that the intensity of disease in any one individual is a result of environmental factors (Dawson et al., 1976).

It has also been observed that children with severe or moderate disease are more likely to develop conjunctival scarring of a degree sufficient to distort the eyelids and cause trichiasis or entropion. The scarring that occurs in early childhood produces increasingly more distortion of the eyelids, even though the infectious process no longer produces inflammation, probably because the scars shrink and contract. It should be noted that corneal vascularization associated with active trachoma rarely if ever extends to the pupil and obscures vision.

Those individuals with central vascularization and corneal scarring appear to have suffered from another disease process, probably corneal ulceration that could be due to a variety of causes.

Visual loss attributable to trachoma may be found in young adults in affected communities, but there are usually more blind persons in older age groups. With the natural decrease in the tear function with age, those adults with potentially blinding lesions are more subject to the consequences of dry eye syndrome, with subsequent breakdown of the corneal epithelium and ulceration of the cornea.

In less severely affected communities, two patterns may occur. In one instance relatively few families may be involved with the severe blinding disease; although the total reservoir of infectious agent is reduced for the community, those affected families continue to produce individuals who develop blindness. The second pattern, noted in Taiwan by Assaad and his associates, is that the onset of manifest disease occurs later and the disease itself is progressively milder so that it rarely, if ever, leads to visual loss, even though a substantial portion of the population may be affected (Assaad, Sundaresan, and Maxwell-Lyons, 1971; Assaad et al., 1971).

The intensity of trachoma is influenced by the size of the community. Nomads, for example, are known to have less severe disease in those countries where trachoma is endemic, probably because their mobility necessitates small, widely separated family units. Similarly, the disease is less severe in very small communities (i.e., those with a total population under 300), where the number of children is apparently not high enough to sustain the level of endemic disease.

In communities with trachoma, the disease is always associated with chlamydial infection, almost invariably of serotypes A, B, Ba, or C (Grayston and Wang, 1975). Not infrequently more than one serotype is found in the same community (Nichols, von Fritzinger and McComb, 1971). Serotype Ba is found most frequently among American Indians and has been found in Ethiopia (Wang and Grayston, 1971a). Serotypes A and C are common in North Africa and the Middle East. In such communities, however, bacterial infections also play an important role in the pathogenesis of the disease (Maxwell-Lyons, 1953; Huet, 1958). The common ocular pathogens that can be identified in such communities are *Haemophilus influenzae* and *H. aegyptius* (Koch-Weeks bacillus), pneumococci, *Moraxella* species, *Neisseria meningitis,* and *N. gonorrhoeae,* and *Staphylococcus aureus* (Vastine et al., 1974). Each of these organisms can cause disease acting alone. *H. influenzae* causes a mild, mucopurulent conjunctivitis; *H. aegyptius* causes a more severe purulent conjunctivitis. The two *Neisseria* species cause a hyperacute conjunctivitis with marked discharge and may progress to peripheral corneal ulceration. Epidemic gonorrheal ophthalmia has been reported most frequently in Egypt and is found in the oases of Arabia (Maxwell-Lyons, 1947; Meyerhoff, 1911). Pneumococci cause a purulent conjunctivitis and are found more frequently during the cold winter months. *S. aureus* is found more commonly on the lid margins; it causes a chronic blepharitis and chronic conjunctivitis in some individuals. It may be associated in varying degrees with corneal involvement but only rarely does it cause corneal ulceration.

In many areas with endemic trachoma, seasonal epidemics of purulent bacterial conjunctivitis begin in the spring, reach a peak in the fall months, and decrease precipitously with the onset of cooler weather. These epidemics are most frequently associated with *H. aegyptius*. To complicate matters, however, in such communities there is often a high carriage rate of ocular bacterial pathogens in children who do not have overt conjunctivitis, as well as the presence of large numbers of bacteria not known to be pathogenic for the eye, particularly *Streptococcus viridans* and diphtheroids (Vastine et al., 1974). It has been assumed that these ocular bacterial pathogens contribute to the disease process, but the exact mechanism is not known. In a recent series of studies in Tunisia, the highest rates of chlamydial infection were found in children with severe intensity trachoma and a lower prevalence in those with trachoma of moderate intensity. The same pattern (Table 2) existed in those cases that were *Chlamydia* negative, a higher prevalence of Koch-Weeks bacilli being found in severe and moderate cases. This was also true for the association of *Chlamydia* and Koch-Weeks bacillus with corneal inflammation (Table 3). It is probable that bacterial infection contributes to the intensity of the conjunctival reaction, thus enhancing the tendency towards scar formation. The bacterial infection would also enhance

Table 2
Chlamydial Agents and Koch-Weeks Bacillus As Factors
in Trachoma Intensity, Tunisia, October 1972

Inclusions*	K-W†	No.	Trachoma Intensity		
			Severe	Moderate	Mild
+‡	+	11	82%§	9%	9%
+	−	19	84%	11%	5%
−	+	28	68%	25%	7%
−	−	80	28%	60%	12%
Total		138	48%	42%	10%

*Trachoma inclusions in Giemsa- and immunofluorescent-stained smears.
†Koch-Weeks bacillus in Giemsa-stained smears.
‡+ organism found; − organism not found.
§Percent of patients with both inclusions and Koch-Weeks bacillus.

74

Table 3
Keratitis in Endemic Trachoma (1) — Relation of Inclusions and Koch-Weeks to Corneal Infiltrates, Tunisia, October 1972

Inclusions*	K-W*	No.	Infiltrates (%)
+	+	10	90%
+	−	18	83%
−	+	28	75%
−	−	77	47%

*Detected in Giemsa-stained conjunctival smears.

corneal inflammation, leading to a greater amount of corneal neo-vascularization. There was no evidence in this study that bacterial infections enhance the growth of the chlamydial agent.

The flies which cluster on children's eyes and feed on ocular discharges are another factor in the epidemiology of trachoma. In the southeastern and southwestern United States, these are usually *Hippelates* species (eye gnats); in North Africa and the Middle East they are usually the larger *Musca* species. Jones found that fluorescein-stained ocular discharges are transferred to the eyes of other children in the same family within 15 to 30 minutes (Jones, 1975). Flies taken from the faces of Egyptian children were found to harbor the ocular bacterial pathogens as well as coliform bacilli (McGuire and Durant, 1957). It is highly probable, then, that these flies can act as a passive vector, carrying chlamydial and ocular bacterial pathogens from one child to another in an affected community.

It has long been known that trachoma is associated with poverty and that economic development appears to eliminate or reduce the severity of the disease. It is difficult to identify with certainty those environmental features of greatest importance, but among them, the presence of young children in the household, crowding, and the unavailability of water for household use must be considered. With the presence of flies, these conditions lead to a condition described by Jones as "ocular promiscuity . . . the indiscriminate mixing of ocular discharges" (Jones, 1975).

DIFFERENTIAL DIAGNOSIS

The early active phase of trachoma is a form of follicular conjunctivitis in which lymphoid follicles contribute prominently to the disease process. The later stages of trachoma may be considered as one of the forms of cicatricial conjunctivitis and superficial corneal vascularization. Any follicular conjunctivitis that persists for more than 15 days may be regarded as a *chronic follicular conjunctivitis*. Such syndromes may have an acute onset with persistent disease or may develop insidiously. The conjunctivitis may persist for months or years. The syndromes to be considered for patients with chronic follicular conjunctivitis include:

1. Folliculosis
2. Trachoma
3. Inclusion conjunctivitis and other ocular chlamydial infections
4. "Toxic" follicular conjunctivitis
    a. Molluscum contagiosum
    b. Drug-induced
    c. Eye cosmetics
5. Bacterial: *Moraxella* and others
6. Axenfeld's chronic follicular conjunctivitis
7. Chronic follicular keratoconjunctivitis of Thygeson
8. Parinaud's oculoglandular syndrome
9. Vernal catarrh

Folliculosis is a condition most frequently found in young children. Follicles are found in the conjunctiva in the absence of any other inflammation, hyperemia, or discharge. Marked folliculosis is most common in children between the ages of four or five years and adolescence, but the presence of a few follicles in the conjunctivas of adults is not unusual.

Trachoma may be regarded as a prototype of other forms of follicular conjunctivitis in which the chronic lymphoid follicle formation and inflammation of the conjunctiva are accompanied by superficial erosions of the corneal epithelium, inflammatory infiltrates of the superficial cornea, and superficial corneal vascularization. In addition, many of these syndromes progress to conjunctival scarring.

Inclusion conjunctivitis and other ocular chlamydial infections are discussed in Chapters 5 and 9.

Toxic follicular conjunctivitis is a syndrome that occurs following chronic exposure of the conjunctiva to some foreign substance for prolonged periods. This syndrome occurs when molluscum contagiosum nodules in the lid margin spill their contents into the conjunctiva, thus exposing it to virus protein, even though the molluscum virus itself does not grow in the conjunctiva. Most commonly the molluscum nodules are on the lid margin itself (Fig. 13, Plate 4), although in the occasional case the nodule may be elsewhere on the lid or brow. In cases that have been allowed to progress untreated, a fleshy, superficial vascular pannus of the cornea may occur that occasionally extends into the pupillary area. Conjunctival scarring may occur in particularly prolonged cases. These cases are best treated by eliminating the molluscum nodule either by direct surgery, excision, or cryotherapy, or by creating a stab wound in the nodule, allowing blood to gain access to it. This last method is preferred in lesions of the lid margin.

Toxic follicular conjunctivitis may also be the result of prolonged use of a number of eye medications, particularly atropine, eserine, pilocarpine, idoxuridine (IDU), and difluorphosphate. Characteristically these drugs are used to treat chronic eye conditions, so the drug is administered over long periods. After a certain length of exposure (varying from 39 to 102 days in the case of IDU), the conjunctiva develops a follicular conjunctivitis that involves the entire conjunctival surface, including the upper tarsus. There may be marked swelling of the limbus and corneal vascularization with accompanying keratitis. Some cases may even progress to conjunctival scarring. Treatment for this condition consists of discontinuing the offending medication.

In women who apply cosmetics to the lids and to the eyelashes, some of the cosmetic is often seen in the conjunctiva, and a follicular response with mild inflammation may occur. The dark granules of the cosmetic appear to become incorporated in the follicles. Like folliculosis, this condition is rarely symptomatic and should not require treatment unless there is secondary infection.

Bacterial follicular conjunctivitis may occur occasionally with *Moraxella lacunata*. This *Moraxella* usually produces an angular blepharitis, and was once relatively common in American Indian children and in children in institutions (Fig. 14, Plate 4). The follicular conjunctivitis is occasionally seen in adolescent girls, who apparently acquire it through the exchange of ocular cosmetics. Although the *Moraxella* will respond to ¼% zinc sulfate, the usual topically applied chemotherapeutic agents such as sulfonamides, tetracyclines, or erythromycin are even more effective. If this diagnosis is suspected, scrapings of the lateral canthus should be examined for the typical large square diplobacillus. The infection is often mixed with *Staphylococcus aureus*.

Axenfeld's chronic follicular conjunctivitis (Fig. 15, Plate 4) has been reported primarily in institutionalized children, thus the name "orphan's conjunctivitis" (Nataf, Lepine, and Bonamour, 1960). It has an insidious onset and is accompanied by a scanty discharge in which mononuclear cells (lymphocytes) predominate. The follicles involve the entire conjunctiva, including the upper tarsal plate, but are firm and do not break up when pressure is applied. The cornea is not involved and probably for this reason the disease is asymptomatic. In one experimental transmission, the French ophthalmologist Victor Morax inoculated himself, and the ensuing disease had an incubation period of 10 days. It was relatively severe at onset but subsided spontaneously in two years without scarring. At its height, the disease was diagnosed by several eminent ophthalmologists of the day as trachoma (Nataf, Lepine, and Bonamour, 1960).

Because Axenfeld's chronic follicular conjunctivitis is not associated with florid corneal involvement and does not produce conjunctival scarring, it has been classified as a disease entity separate from trachoma. The descriptions of it, however, are compatible with the mild, chronic trachoma found in American Indian schoolchildren. The few observations of Axenfeld's follicular conjunctivitis made with the slit lamp revealed small degrees of keratitis. Moreover, in the mild trachoma of American Indians, inclusions are rarely demonstrated in smears, and the disease produces little, if any, scarring. It is possible, then, that Axenfeld's conjunctivitis is a particularly mild form of trachoma that runs a self-limited course under the relatively hygienic conditions of a children's institution. In such cases, a regular course of trachoma therapy (i.e., oral tetracycline) should be administered (Thygeson and Okumoto, 1967).

Chronic follicular keratoconjunctivitis of Thygeson is an entity characterized by:

1. A follicular hypertrophy most marked in the fornices but occasionally involving the tarsal plate
2. A punctate superior epithelial keratitis
3. Moderate exudate in the conjunctiva
4. Foreign body sensation and photophobia
5. Subacute or insidious onset
6. Duration of four to five months
7. No secondary bacterial infection
8. Occasional micropannus formation
9. Spontaneous remission with conjunctival or corneal scars

An epidemic of this disease occurred in a California high school in which some trachoma cases were found in Mexican-American students. Moreover, most of the cases were girls who had been trading eye make-up (Thygeson and Okumoto, 1967). There was a possibility, then, that this may also be a particularly mild form of trachoma.

Parinaud's oculoglandular syndrome (Fig. 16A and B, Plate 4) is characterized by four cardinal features:

1. A localized lesion of the conjunctiva with follicles and deeply seated yellowish lesions
2. An enormously enlarged preauricular lymph node on the side of the involved eye, often with large nodes in the ear region as well
3. Possible fever and malaise

4. A frequent history of specific exposure to an animal, usually a cat

Biopsy of the conjunctiva usually reveals that the deep yellow lesions are a granulomatous reaction. The disease is usually of sudden onset, with redness, lid swelling, and discharge in the infected side accompanied by an enormous engorgement of the regional lymph node (1 cm or more in diameter). In most cases the patients report that a cat sleeps with them at night or on their pillow during the day. The etiology of this syndrome has not been determined, but special histologic stains have revealed actinomycetes in biopsy specimens (Verhoeff, 1940), a finding that has not been repeated in other pathology laboratories. It would appear that the syndrome associated with cats is a variant of cat scratch fever.

If there is a known exposure to wild rabbits, which may have transmitted tularemia to the patient, the patient should be treated with streptomycin. Other causes of Parinaud's oculoglandular syndrome include syphilis, tuberculosis, sarcoid, glanders, Pasteurellosis, lymphogranuloma venereum, soft chancre, and other granulomatous diseases.

Vernal catarrh and atopic keratoconjunctivitis (Fig. 17, Plate 4) are manifestations of classic atopic allergy and may persist for many years. Vernal catarrh commonly occurs in young children. Adult patients with atopic dermatitis will frequently present with a conjunctivitis similar to that of vernal catarrh. The milky hyperemia of the tarsal conjunctiva in those chronic allergic diseases is quite characteristic.

Papillae form as inflammatory response where the conjunctiva is bound down to the upper tarsus and, to a lesser extent, to the inferior tarsus (Fig. 17, Plate 4). Initially these appear as vascular tufts with surrounding infiltration. In the severe papillary hypertrophy of vernal catarrh, the conjunctival infiltration becomes very marked with hypertrophy of the conjunctiva and the formation of giant or cobblestone papillae.

LABORATORY DIAGNOSIS

Since the specific laboratory procedures and fundamental aspects of the biology are described elsewhere (Chapters 10 and 11), these subjects will only be referred to here as they pertain to infection in man. Laboratory studies of trachoma in humans are used for a number of reasons: to support the clinical diagnosis of the disease in individual cases; to measure the prevalence of agent in a community where trachoma is endemic (i.e., to estimate the force of infection); to monitor individuals or communities for the effect of therapy; to estimate the total exposure of a population to chlamydial infection; to monitor for shifts in serotypes in a given population that might indicate the influx of agent from outside the community or from a genital reservoir.

Bacterial studies must be considered an integral part of the laboratory evaluation of individuals or communities with trachoma. The major ocular bacterial pathogens include *Haemophilus* species, pneumococcus, *Neisseria* species, *Moraxella* species, and *Staphylococcus aureus;* in studies on trachomatous populations (Vastine et al., 1974; Haddad and Ballas, 1968; Huet, 1958) other pathogens such as gram-negative rods and beta streptococci are rarely found. The primary methods used in the past to detect bacterial pathogens in trachomatous populations were Gram-stained or Giemsa-stained conjunctival smears. Until recently, the other method available, bacterial culture, showed little correlation with findings from the smears. A simple technique for bacterial cultures suggested by Vastine and associates has been successful in isolating most ocular pathogens, although it is relatively insensitive for *Neisseria* species. It involves the use of a broth or saline-moistened cotton swab which is first rubbed gently over the conjunctiva and then streaked directly onto a sheep's blood agar plate. The streak is inoculated at three sites with *Staphylococcus epidermidis* and the plates incubated 48 to 72 hours (Vastine et al., 1974). If *Neisseria* are suspected, a second plate of Isovitalex-enriched chocolate agar may be inoculated and incubated in CO_2 (Vastine et al., 1974). This Isovitalex mixture has proven particularly successful for passing strains of isolated *Haemophilus*.

As would be expected, the bacterial culture techniques are much more sensitive than examination of direct smears. In trachoma-endemic regions with seasonal epidemics of conjunctivitis, there is a high carrier rate of *Haemophilus* in the eyes of children (Maxwell-Lyons and Amies, 1949). The intensity of trachoma or the presence of conjunctivitis does correlate clearly with the presence of *Haemophilus* in conjunctival smears (Vastine et al., 1974).

The laboratory procedure selected for use depends on the purpose of the test, the techniques available, and, finally, relative costs. Individual tests useful in diagnosis of chlamydial infections have been reviewed elsewhere (Chapter 11). It should be pointed out, however, that the cytologic examination of conjunctival scrapings represents a direct sampling of the affected tissue; Giemsa or immunofluorescent staining of conjunctival smears will yield semiquantitative data on the amount of chlamydial agent actually present in the conjunctival scraping. One clear-cut advantage of Giemsa stain is that the original specimen (i.e., the stained smear) can be stored indefinitely and examined repeatedly without damage to the specimen. Smears stained by this method can be sent to specialized laboratories for confirmation of suspected inclusions, whereas fluorescent antibody (FA)-stained smears must be examined within 24 to 48 hours after staining. Moreover, Giemsa-stained smears can yield valuable information on the presence of bacterial pathogens and associated conditions such as atopic conjunctivitis.

The relative specificity and sensitivity of the two tests varies considerably from one population to another. In American Indians, for example, studies carried out over the last 10 years have revealed that inclusions are found only very rarely in Giemsa-stained smears, but are relatively common in FA-stained smears (Hanna, 1968; Schachter et al., 1971). Indeed, these stains showed that the prevalence rates of trachoma agent in FA-stained smears were only slightly higher in active trachoma cases than in those with inactive trachoma in the endemic population, indicating that there was a high carrier rate (Jawetz et al., 1967). This marked difference between the two tests may have been a reflection of previous chemotherapy. On the other hand, studies carried out in North Africa and Egypt (Tarizzo, Nabli, and Labonne, 1968; Dawson, et al., 1974a,b) have shown that the Giemsa-stained smears show a high degree of correlation with clinical intensity of active disease. Surprisingly, in these latter studies the FA technique was only slightly more sensitive than Giemsa (Yoneda et al., 1975).

The relative cost of performing the FA test is considerably higher, since trachoma agent must first be cultivated, rabbits immunized with the cultivated agent, the agent grown in yolk sac or tissue culture, and tests carried out to measure the antibody titer of the immune serum. This serum must then be conjugated with fluorescein, or a commercial fluorescein-conjugated antiglobulin must be obtained. Although the cost of the fluorescent miscroscope is little more now than that of a good research microscope, the examination of the FA-stained smear requires considerable skill and represents a substantial investment in the training of technicians. This process can be shortened somewhat by using serum from patients who have a high titer against lymphogranuloma venereum (Nichols et al., 1963, 1967). The advantages of the FA test are most marked in mild trachoma and in infections with relatively little agent demonstrated.

Using the Giemsa stain, however, is relatively simple, since the stain may be purchased commercially and good quality preparations are easily obtained. Some training is required for technicians carrying out the examination of Giemsa-stained smears, but this is easily communicated since a number of publications are available showing the cytologic features to be observed (Yoneda et al., 1975; see Chapter 11). Once the cytologist is aware of the forms of "pseudo-inclusions," the Giemsa stain is less likely to have false positives, and the test is probably more specific than the FA test. Moreover, if only smears with a suggestive cytology are selected for extensive examination, it may be that the Giemsa technique is less time consuming than the FA technique.

The two isolation techniques — inoculation of the yolk sac of embryonated hens' eggs and specially treated cell cultures — yield strains of agent which can be studied further in the laboratory. The egg technique gives no idea of the initial amount of agent in the inoculum, although the positivity or negativity of the specimen may be correlated with the intensity of disease (Tarizzo, Nabli, and Labonne, 1968). In cell culture it is possible to count the number of inclusions found in the initial inoculation. This may be misleading because of other factors, such as variations in the size of the initial inoculum (i.e., number of epithelial cells obtained), and the ability of a particular strain to grow in cell culture (Jones, 1974). It would appear, for example, that isolates from the eye in either trachoma or adult inclusion conjunctivitis grow less readily than those obtained from the genital tract (Kuo, Wang, and Grayston, 1975).

The egg isolation technique was the first available and is a relatively straightforward laboratory procedure requiring a level of skill available in most hospital bacteriology laboratories. A source of fertile hens' eggs from a flock known not to have been fed with antibiotic-containing feeds, an egg incubator, appropriate stains, and a good microscope are all that are required. The cell culture technique is rather more sophisticated, requiring a maintenance of cells in tissue culture in the absence of many of the usual antibiotics used for this purpose, and often some special treatment (irradiation, idoxuridine) before the cells are planted in small tubes or coverslips. A modern, preferably refrigerated, centrifuge must be available to spin the inoculum onto the cell sheet. The iodine staining and microscopic examination of the inoculated cell covers are relatively simple matters.

Because of the necessity of having large numbers of fertile eggs and holding each specimen through the equivalent of six weeks' incubation time, the egg technique is more expensive, although less technically demanding. If tissue culture facilities are not readily available, however, and media is difficult to obtain, the cost of the tissue culture technique in terms of material and staff time may rise astronomically, particularly in many developing countries (Grayston and Wang, 1975).

The two serologic methods — complement fixation and micro indirect immunofluorescence — primarily give evidence of past infection with a chlamydial agent. The relatively low prevalence of CF titers in a population with widely disseminated severe trachoma indicated that this test is relatively insensitive in endemic disease

(Schachter et al., 1973). Micro-IF, however, is much more sensitive and there is a good correlation with intensity of active inflammatory disease. The micro-IF also yields information on the serotypes of the infecting agent, particularly in longitudinal studies on individual families or communities (Grayston and Wang, 1975; Hanna et al., 1973). Micro-IF can be performed with either blood or tears, although tears are a much less sensitive indicator in many cases than blood. At the present time, venous blood specimens are required (a distinct disadvantage when working with children), but the micro methods developed for analyzing tears should be equally applicable to blood specimens obtained by finger-prick. The micro-IF is a relatively demanding test — the laboratory must be able to maintain a number of serotypes of chlamydial agent, be thoroughly versed in fluorescent antibody staining techniques, and have the necessary experience to carry out the microscopic interpretation of the stained antigens. It is certainly the most sophisticated procedure in the armamentarium of chlamydial laboratory tests. Such skills are necessary in only a few laboratories, however, since the tear or serum specimens can be frozen (e.g., in liquid nitrogen), so specimens may be stored and shipped for considerable distances.

Serologic studies have been used to draw epidemiological inferences on the distribution of infection with various strains of *Chlamydia* (Briones et al., 1974). In individual cases that have a broad serologic response, specific absorption may be performed to identify the infected serotype.

The use of these tests in several specific situations will be considered. For individual cases, fluorescent antibody staining may be slightly more sensitive than Giemsa staining. If facilities are available, isolation attempts should certainly be carried out so that serotype of the infecting agent may be eventually identified. The presence of one of the "genital" serotypes would suggest that the disease might have been acquired through sexual activity, and that the patient's sexual contacts and family members should also be examined. The micro-IF serology would also be useful for the same purpose.

For public health purposes the simplest and least expensive test to support field activities is the examination of Giemsa-stained smears of the conjunctiva. With such smears both the trachoma agent and pathogenic bacteria can be identified, and their presence correlates well with trachoma intensity. If facilities are available, efforts should be made to isolate the trachoma agent for serotyping and possibly determination of antibiotic sensitivity. Micro-IF serology can be done to determine the prevalence of antibody in a population and the relative frequency of infecting serotypes in the population under consideration.

IMMUNIZATION

Since naturally occurring active trachoma subsides in older children, it was supposed that some degree of immunity occurred. After the isolation of the chlamydiae associated with trachoma, vigorous efforts were made to produce a vaccine. Although these attempts did not lead to a useful vaccine, the clinical trials and animal experiments have made a significant contribution to understanding the immunology of trachoma. Most of the work on vaccines was carried out by four groups: (1) The Medical Research Council (MRC) Trachoma Unit headed by Leslie Collier, at the Lister Institute in London and at a field station in The Gambia; (2) Grayston and his colleagues at the University of Washington in Seattle and the Naval Medical Research Unit 2 (NAMRU 2) in Taiwan; (3) the group at the Harvard School of Public Health working with Aramco in Saudi Arabia; and (4) the Italian group with Bietti and Ghione. In the course of vaccine development, all these groups carried out both clinical studies and animal research on the immune mechanisms.

At the outset, these workers faced a common set of problems: How to produce a vaccine — what chlamydial strains should be used; how should they be purified; should they be used live or killed; how should they be standardized? How to measure potency — by antibody response in humans, primates, and other species and/or by resistance of primates to challenge infection? Finally, how to test vaccines in the field — should use be prophylactic or therapeutic; what age groups should be tested; how would the effect be measured? Since producing vaccine, testing for safety and efficacy, and field testing are slow procedures, the technology underlying a particular vaccine often lagged behind available knowledge when the vaccine was finally field-tested.

It is necessary then to review each group's efforts separately. In their initial studies of immunized baboons, the MRC Trachoma Unit found that: (1) immunization produced resistance to challenge eye infection with the same strain of agent; (2) immunity was short-lived; (3) crossprotection to challenge with heterologous strains was minimal; (4) there was no relation between antibody (CF) response and resistance to challenge; and (5) adjuvant vaccines failed to increase the serum antibody response and may have led to enhanced eye disease on challenge, possibly as a manifestation of hypersensitivity (Collier and Blyth, 1966a,b, 1967). An initial clinical trial by this group in The Gambia suggested that immunization led to a short-term (8- to 17-week) improvement in the clinical disease. A second trial with a live vaccine prepared from a Gambian trachoma strain and administered with adjuvant failed to produce a clinical or microbiological effect compared to a placebo (Sowa et al., 1969). A third trial in The Gambia used a live vaccine prepared from two "fast killing" strains (subsequently shown to be similar to LGV rather than to other TRIC strains [Wang and Grayston, 1971b]). These fast strains were later found to multiply in the skin and spleen when injected into guinea pigs and primates. In this trial the vaccine had neither "protective" nor therapeutic effect and may have adversely affected the disease (although this effect may be an artifact of the clinical scoring system used). Finally, another trial carried out in Iran using both killed and live vaccine showed a significant degree of protection in children with no trachoma at the time of vaccination. Protection lasted for up to one year after vaccination, although it was no longer found at two years (Jones, 1975). Thus these workers showed a short-lived protective and therapeutic effect of some vaccines, but possible deleterious effects due to hypersensitivity with other preparations.

The most thorough experiments on trachoma vaccines have been carried out by Grayston and his colleagues working with the NAMRU 2 laboratory in Taiwan and at the University of Washington in Seattle. This group tested a number of vaccine preparations in the *Macaca cyclops,* the only monkey native to Taiwan where many of the experiments were perform d (Wang, Grayston, and Alexander, 1967; Grayston et al., 1971). These animal experiments revealed: (1) adjuvant but not alum vaccine provided protection to challenge with the same strain but only partial protection to challenge with a heterologous serotype; (2) formalin treatment of vaccine preparations did not affect their potency; (3) hypersensitivity (more severe disease) resulted in animals immunized with low-dose vaccine and some high-dose vaccine; (4) purified vaccines induced pannus formation on homologous and heterologous challenge in some animals; (5) when vaccines with high titer were used, protection decreased by nine months and disappeared by two years; (6) a purified vaccine preparation was associated with a hypersensitivity and more severe disease on challenge with the homologous strain.

From their animal experiments, this group concluded that the sensitizing effect of vaccines could be induced with low doses, and that it persisted longer than the protective effects. Moreover, protection appeared to be strain-specific, although the hypersensitivity was not (Grayston et al., 1971). In some of these immunized Taiwan monkeys, the complete trachoma syndrome was reproduced — follicular conjunctivitis, corneal vascularization, conjunctival scarring, trichiasis, and entropion (Gale, Wang, and Grayston, 1971).

Field trials of these same vaccines were carried out in Taiwan and India. The first clinical trial in Taiwan utilized an alum-absorbed elementary body ("PEB") vaccine; this vaccine was given to the younger siblings of first-grade school children with active trachoma (Woolridge et al., 1967). On serial follow-up examinations, conversion to trachoma was accepted by two consecutive clinical diagnoses of active disease or by laboratory proof of infection. This vaccine had a protective effect, but it began to disappear within a year of the final booster vaccine dose; no effect was noted in the subsequent 3½ years. A second study on Taiwan utilizing mineral oil adjuvant vaccines showed a modest protective effect with vaccine which included two serotypes, while a monovalent vaccine was associated with a higher trachoma rate than the placebo group (Woolridge et al., 1967). The design of these studies was excellent, since the selected subjects (non-diseased preschool siblings of infected first-graders) were known to be at risk. It should be pointed out, however, that the prevalence and intensity of trachoma was declining during the period of these studies (1959–1966), due to the rapid economic growth on Taiwan. Thus there may have been a steadily declining exposure to infection over the period of study.

The University of Washington-NAMRU 2 group conducted another clinical trial in India to test two high-titer, purified vaccine preparations (Dhir et al., 1967). This study was carried out in a group of villages in northern India with holoendemic trachoma (88% of children five years and under had active trachoma). Only children under five without active trachoma were included in the study. By eight months after the final booster dose, 15% of the vaccinated subjects and 37% of controls had converted to active trachoma (a statistically significant effect). The degree of severity of those trachoma cases that did occur in the vaccine group was no higher than that in the placebo group. In this trial the selection of trachoma-free children in a holoendemic area was logical, even though these children would be at least risk of developing disease since they had escaped previous infection.

Grayston concluded that "unfortunately in no case has a trachoma vaccine been developed that is effective and practical for routine field use. . . . We doubt whether further concentration of elementary bodies will provide a practical, effective vaccine. . . . Hope for the control of trachoma would seem to lie in the explosive advances being made in immunology" (Grayston, 1971).

The group at the Harvard School of Public Health first conducted clinical trials in Saudi Arabia and subsequently carried out animal studies in New World monkeys. Their major clinical trial was performed in an area of Saudi Arabia where trachoma was holoendemic (Nichols et al., 1966, 1969). Only children under age three were included; on the basis of clinical examination before vaccination, they were diagnosed as having active trachoma, non-trachomatous conjunctivitis, or no conjunctivitis. A bivalent vaccine containing serotypes B and C was administered to 1,259 subjects; a placebo vaccine, to 1,193 subjects. The placebo injection was either typhoid vaccine or tetanus toxoid mixed with purified yolk sac constituents (Nichols et al., 1966).

Three vaccine groups were included: one received 0.2 or 0.4 "arbitrary vaccine units" (AVU) of an aqueous preparation; a second group received 2 to 4 AVU of aqueous vaccine; and a third group received 0.25 AVU of adjuvant vaccine. Some subjects in all three groups received booster doses of aqueous vaccine at 6-month intervals. The adjuvant vaccine did not prevent the appearance of trachoma in previously uninfected children (Nichols et al., 1966), nor did it reduce the prevalence of inclusion-positive smears, although there were fewer inclusions in those vaccinees with positive smears than in controls (Nichols et al., 1969). Both aqueous vaccines, however, had a statistically significant effect in preventing the onset of clinical disease at 6 months; this beneficial effect was noted at 12 but not at 18 months with the higher dose vaccine. Only the higher dose vaccine reduced inclusions to a marginal degree (Nichols et al., 1969). Moreover, among those children who were clinically normal at the beginning of the trial and received the higher dose aqueous vaccine, three times as many (29%) developed disease as did those receiving control vaccine (11%). Thus the protection against infection afforded by this more potent vaccine was also linked to a higher attack rate of clinical disease.

These bivalent vaccines did have some modest effect in preventing the onset of disease and in reducing the amount of agent recovered. The protective effect could not be maintained, even though booster immunizations were given at six-month intervals. The most effective vaccine (high dose aqueous) reduced the onset of active disease and microbial infection.

The Harvard group subsequently carried out a series of experiments in owl monkeys (*Aotus trivirgatus*) which were highly susceptible to the trachoma serotypes (B and C) of *Chlamydia*. They found that previously unexposed animals developed acute infection with numerous inclusions and acute disease (Murray et al., 1971). Following initial infection, the monkeys become resistant, for at least two months, to challenge infection with homologous or heterologous serotypes. Since this resistance was associated with tear antibody, attempts to induce local resistance were made by applying chlamydial antigen directly to the conjunctival surface in gel foam sponge to increase exposure time (McComb et al., 1971). The experiment was further complicated by the presence of pre-existing tear and serum antibody in some animals. Nevertheless, it was concluded that "serum and eye secretion antibody titers were associated with a diminution in inclusion rates after challenge" (McComb et al., 1971). A later experiment by this group confirmed this finding and extended the period of resistance to challenge infection up to 18 months (Fraser et al., 1975).

The vaccine field trials carried out by the Italian group were the earliest to be done and among the most extensive ever described. Since most of the early reports appeared in the Italian language or in journals not easily accessible to other European and American workers, these studies have been somewhat neglected. The studies are well described in English in the book by Bietti and Werner (1967), and in the article by Guerra et al. (1967). The vaccines consisted of a formalin-treated suspension of purified egg-grown elementary bodies of a single trachoma strain. When they were evaluated in monkeys (*Cercopithecus* sp.), a water-in-oil vaccine provided partial protection, but there was no effect with aqueous or alum-absorbed vaccines.

Similar experiments were then carried out in human volunteers. In the first experiment, aqueous vaccine appeared to protect against challenge infection, but water-in-oil and alum-absorbed vaccines did not. In a second experiment, immunized and control subjects were challenged with 0.25, 2.5, or 25 egg LD_{50} of the same strain used to prepare the vaccine. All but one control subject developed conjunctivitis. Both the water-in-oil and alum-absorbed vaccines protected completely against infections with 0.25 and 2.5 egg LD_{50} and partially against 25 egg LD_{50} of agent. Eye disease was not more severe in vaccinated subjects who developed disease.

These vaccines were then evaluated in a series of field trials around Asmara and Addis Ababa, Ethiopia, in 1960, 1961, and 1962. Vaccinations were administered to children two to four years old regardless of whether they were free of trachoma or had active disease; they were administered to children under the age of two only if they were disease-free. Thus the trial evaluated both the therapeutic and the prophylactic effect of the vaccines. The immunization consisted of an initial injection of adjuvant vaccine with 5×10^8 elementary bodies (EB) followed by booster injections with aqueous vaccine (2.5×10^8 EB) after 40 days and six months.

This schedule of immunization had a significant preventive effect, with 37% of vaccinees and 70% of controls developing active disease. There was also a therapeutic effect, with 65% of vaccinees and 31% of controls improving.

In 1964–1965 two larger trials were carried out in Eritrea and Ethiopia involving 10,000 subjects (Bietti and Werner, 1967; Guerra et al., 1967). Newly acquired disease developed in 17% of vaccinees and 23% of controls; this difference was significant with these large numbers of subjects. Similarly, in active disease, 59% of vaccinees and 43% of controls improved, a significant therapeutic effect. In a final trial utilizing the clinical scoring system suggested by WHO (Fourth Scientific Group, 1966), 330 subjects received either vaccine, placebo, or no treatment (controls). The vaccine had both a therapeutic and a preventive effect on clinical disease. Moreover, trachoma inclusions in smears and isolations in yolk sac were significantly reduced only in the vaccine group. Some of these studies were also complicated by changes in the standard of living in the test area.

These studies were, however, encouraging enough so that a vaccine was produced by Farmitalia Pharmaceutical Company (Milan) on a commercial scale. Bietti concluded that vaccine would be useful in trachoma-endemic areas for several purposes: (1) to prevent infection in newly exposed persons (e.g., medical personnel, teachers); (2) to be used in association with chemotherapy; (3) to prevent reinfection; (4) to prevent initial infection of young children.

Thus several groups have shown the vaccines have a short-lived and modest effect in preventing the onset of trachoma and in reducing intensity of established disease. The occurrence of longer lasting hypersensitization induced by some trachoma vaccines would appear to overshadow the beneficial effects, particularly since sensitization is longer lasting than protection (Gale, Wang, and Grayston, 1971).

At the present time, then, there is no effective vaccine that could be recommended for use in human populations.

If a safe, effective vaccine were available, it would have a use in the control of blinding trachoma if it were given to children up to age 10 in holoendemic areas and combined with antibiotic treatment programs. The most critical property of any new preparation must be that it does not induce hypersensitivity and thus aggravate the disease.

Meanwhile the immunologic response of man and other primates to chlamydial infections must be studied in greater depth, and vaccines consisting of purified fractions should be evaluated. Another possibility is "immunomodulation" mentioned by Jones (1975), in this case the administration of levamisole or other agents which enhance cellular immunity.

TREATMENT AND CONTROL

Since blinding trachoma is a disease endemic in economically underdeveloped communities where health services are limited, considerations of treatment must extend far beyond a discussion of the effect of chemotherapy or surgical intervention on the inflammatory disease. The primary goal of control programs is the prevention of blindness in communities where there is the possibility of visual impairment due to trachoma. Eradication of the disease in a particular population must be a secondary goal. Thus trachoma therapy must be approached as a public health problem.

Trachoma control programs are based on the following assumptions:

1. Trachoma causes blindness. The inflammatory disease of childhood leads to scarring of the conjunctiva. This scarring produces distortion of the lids, causing the in-turned lashes to constantly abrade the cornea. The accompanying deficient tear production, the persistent abrasion of the lashes, other minor ocular trauma, and the ever-present bacterial pathogens lead to corneal ulceration with opacity and visual loss.
2. The inflammatory phase of trachoma must be over a certain degree ("threshold") of severity and duration to produce visual disability.
3. The inflammatory disease results from infection with both chlamydial and bacterial pathogens.
4. The surgical correction of trichiasis reduces the risk of blindness. The tear deficiency state cannot be easily corrected, however, and patients so affected still have a high risk of developing visual loss.
5. Economic development is usually followed by a reduction in the overall trachoma intensity in a community, causing the severity of the disease to fall below the minimum threshold needed to produce potentially blinding scarring. The blinding consequences of previously severe disease may continue to cause visual loss for another 20 to 50 years after active disease has been controlled in a community.

Sulfonamides applied topically as (sulfanilimide) powder or systemically were the first effective chemotherapy (Gradle, 1938; Richards, Forster, and Thygeson, 1939; Freyche, 1949–1950). The success of sulfonamide treatment in American Indians (Forster and McGibony, 1944) and elsewhere led to its widespread application in the 1940s and 1950s (Bietti, Pannarale, and Milano, 1967; Freyche, 1949–1950). The long-acting oral sulfonamides were enthusiastically accepted because the less frequent dosage schedule (as seldom as once a week with some compounds) allowed greater efficiency in control programs (Bietti, Pannarale, and Milano, 1967; Shukla et al., 1966). When the tetracyclines became available in the early 1950s, chlortetracycline was found to achieve 80% cure rates when applied topically two to three times daily for 50 days and was also effective when administered intermittently over a six-month period (Reinhards, Weber, and Maxwell-Lyons, 1959; Reinhards et al., 1968). Erythromycin and other macrolide antibiotics have also been shown to be effective by the topical route (Nataf, Daghfous, and Tarizzo, 1965; Agarwal, Saxena, and Gupta, 1955; Dawson et al., 1974a). Topical rifampicin may have a distinct theoretical advantage but is no more efficacious clinically than other antibiotics (Dawson et al., 1974b, 1975; Becker et al., 1969). Moreover, resistance to rifampicin developed rapidly in laboratory strains of *Chlamydia* exposed to the drug (Keshishyan, Hanna, and Jawetz, 1973).

The most extensive studies on chemotherapy have been reported by Reinhards and associates in Morocco, and by Bietti and his colleagues in Morocco and Libya, areas where blinding trachoma is endemic (Reinhards, Weber, and Maxwell-Lyons, 1959; Reinhards et al., 1968; Bietti, 1963). The first studies reported by Reinhards, Weber, and Maxfield-Lyons (1959) compared various schedules of treatment with topical chlortetracycline applied only to schoolchildren. In the first test, treatment three times daily for 60 working days led to a striking decrease in active trachoma, but there were more treatment failures in the younger children (20%) than in the older (4%). In a second trial, treatment two or three times daily for 60 days was compared to an intermittent dosage given twice daily, 3 consecutive days every 4 weeks for 20 weeks; all three treatments had an equivalent effect. The third trial compared twice-daily dosage for 60 days with the intermittent administration; again the two treatments were both effective with a failure rate of about 11%. These studies established the value of a type of intermittent treatment by which three to five times as many children could be treated with the same personnel and amount of ointment as the continuous therapy.

The same workers described the effects of public health programs for trachoma control carried out in more remote rural areas suffering from particularly severe disease (Reinhards et al., 1968). This study emphasized the pattern of seasonal epidemics of bacterial conjunctivitis, and its containment by fly control and self-treatment over a 10-year period. In the initial trial, it was found that a single four-day course of oral sulfonamides was as effective as a six-month course of intermittent (three-day cycle) chlortetracycline in reducing purulent conjunctivitis, but that intermittent therapy was better for reducing the intensity of trachoma; the greatest effect was achieved by using the two drugs together. This effort was changed to one of self-treatment by families, and a community survey was made 8 years later; there had been a reduction in the prevalence of active trachoma, the average age of onset, and severe cicatricial sequelae. Nevertheless, in older age groups, there was an apparent increase in the prevalence of trichiasis and demand for trichiasis surgery. In two related field studies, self-treatment was seen to be less effective among 1- to 8-year-olds compared to treatment by a mobile team.

In summary, these studies established the value of an intermittent treatment schedule of tetracyclines applied topically (Reinhards et al., 1968). They also set the pattern which has been followed in other endemic areas: treatment of schoolchildren by auxiliary health workers, but self-treatment for families. The need for ongoing programs of trichiasis surgery is particularly critical since ". . . a mass campaign against trachoma does not immediately lead to reductions in complications due to excessive cicatrization" (Reinhards et al., 1968). It also appears that distribution of ointment directly to families, with instructions on its use, is good strategy in mass chemotherapy programs.

The role of oral sulfonamides or antibiotics was evaluated extensively by Bietti and his associates (Bietti, 1963). A long-acting tetracycline derivative (demethylchlortetracycline) given every 2 to 4 days for three months produced a significant reduction in disease, but longer intervals (7 days) or shorter treatment periods (one month) were substantially less effective. A preliminary trial in Sardinia of a long-acting oral sulfonamide, sulfamethoxypyridazine (Kynex®), given every 7 to 10 days for three months showed a favorable result, particularly when combined with topical tetracycline. In Libya an extensive comparison of dosage schedules and drugs revealed that good results were achieved with higher doses of Kynex®, but that a rapidly excreted sulfa, sulfisoxazole (Gantrisin®), and topically applied tetracycline alone were much less effective. The best results were achieved from combined treatment with oral sulfonamide and topical tetracycline. An even larger trial confirmed the efficacy of once weekly doses of Kynex® given for three months alone or in combination with tetracycline ointment, and the very limited effect of intermittent topical tetracycline alone (Bietti, 1963).

Combined oral sulfonamides and topical chlortetracycline were also effective in children who had not responded to a previous course of topical antibiotic (Reinhards et al., 1968). A recent study in Iran showed that a single dose monthly for six months of doxycycline, a long-acting tetracycline, led to a marked reduction in the presence of *Chlamydia* in village schoolchildren and families (Jones, 1975). Thus it appears that systemically administered chemotherapeutic agents are very efficient in controlling trachoma in hyperendemic areas.

92

Serious doubts of the efficacy of chemotherapy were raised, however, when Foster, Powers, and Thygeson reported in 1966 that clinical cures occurred as frequently in American Indian children receiving no treatment as in those treated with topical tetracycline or systemic Kynex®. Similarly, in a controlled trial in Taiwan schoolchildren, topical antibiotics or oral sulfonamides were found to offer no advantage over a placebo (Woolridge et al., 1967).

Because of these disturbing observations, a series of controlled chemotherapy trials was carried out in American Indian schoolchildren with a low prevalence of mild trachoma and no blinding complications. During these trials, the children remained in a single environment (boarding schools), and serum antibiotic levels were monitored in both drug- and placebo-treated groups (Dawson and Hanna, 1970). In addition, three clinicians examined each child independently to minimize observer variation, and conjunctival smears for trachoma agent and bacterial cultures were taken (Dawson and Hanna, 1971). The results of these trials are summarized for the time when maximum effect of chemotherapy was observed (Table 4).

Table 4
Chemotherapy Trials in Treatment of Trachoma

Treatment	(No. Tested)/ Percent Cured	P Value (chi square)
Topical tetracycline (Dawson, Hanna, and Jawetz, 1967)	Drug (41)/59% Placebo (40)/35%	<0.05
Oral sulfisoxazole (Gantrisin®) (Dawson, Hanna, and Jawetz, 1967)	Drug (30)/67% Placebo (31)/48%	N.S.
Oral triple sulfas (Dawson et al., 1969)	Drug (18)/67% Placebo (18)/17%	<0.05
Oral tetracycline (Dawson et al., 1971)	Drug (31)/68% Placebo (29)/28%	<0.05
Oral tetracycline vs. oral doxycycline (Ostler et al., 1971)	Tetracycline (42)/88% Doxycycline (43)/82%	N.S.

To achieve a significant therapeutic effect in this mild disease, it was necessary to administer drugs orally in full doses for at least three weeks. Topical tetracycline given twice daily for six weeks was also effective (Dawson, Hanna, and Jawetz, 1967). Sulfisoxazole, a rapidly excreted sulfa, was no better than placebo, but the sulfa blood level (2.6 mg/%) was lower than the minimum (5 mg/%) needed for most infections even when given for three weeks. With oral triple sulfonamides and adequate blood levels (7.6 mg/%), there was a significant suppression of active trachoma (Dawson et al., 1969).

With the well-organized programs for trachoma treatment in American Indians, untoward reactions to the sulfonamide occurred in a substantial portion of patients (Hoshiwara, 1971). Oral tetracycline given for three weeks suppressed trachoma activity as well as sulfonamides did and had very few side effects in these otherwise healthy children (Dawson et al., 1971). Doxycycline was as effective as tetracycline, but offered the significant advantage of only one daily administration; this resulted in a significant saving in personnel costs which compensated for the higher costs of doxycycline (Ostler et al., 1971; Hoshiwara et al., 1973).

In these trials there was usually a large degree of improvement in the placebo-treated groups. This may have been due in part to the improved hygienic standards of the boarding schools where the trials were carried out. Moreover, this relatively mild trachoma is characterized by remissions and exacerbations; since only children with active inflammatory disease were selected, the only fluctuation possible was toward milder disease. In none of the trials was antibiotic *better* than placebo in suppressing the rate of infection with *Chlamydia* (Dawson and Hanna, 1971).

In recent years, a series of small, carefully controlled trials of topical chemotherapy has been carried out in Tunisia by the Institut d'Ophtalmologie of Tunis and the Francis I. Proctor Foundation in San Francisco. While trachoma has disappeared from most of Tunisia, it continues to be a problem in the southern desert areas despite school-based control programs of the last 20 years (Dawson et al., 1976). In these therapeutic trials, the clinical effect of treating schoolchildren has been evaluated with the slit lamp by three independent observers, and laboratory studies have been done to follow changes in the prevalence of chlamydial agent and bacterial pathogens (Vastine et al., 1974; Dawson et al., 1974b). Following an initial examination, groups of first-grade schoolchildren with active trachoma were treated with an antibiotic ointment or boric acid ointment. All children were retreated with a standard course of topical tetracycline following the end of the trial. The control (boric acid-treated) group was necessary because of changes in disease activity with the seasons and with increasing age.

In the first trial, topical chlortetracycline, erythromycin, and boric acid were administered twice daily for 60 days (Dawson et al., 1974a). Both antibiotics were considerably more effective than boric acid in suppressing disease for 4 weeks and 17 weeks after treatment.

While both antibiotics reduced the prevalence of trachoma agent at 4 weeks, a significant decrease was found at 17 weeks only with erythromycin. A subsequent trial compared 60 days of treatment with topical tetracycline or rifampicin to boric acid ointment (Dawson et al., 1975). The greatest effect of the two antibiotics was noted 5 weeks after the end of treatment, but by 19 weeks only the tetracycline groups had significantly less inflammatory disease than the controls. There was marked suppression of chlamydiae by both antibiotics. Thus rifampicin offered no advantage over tetracycline. In both studies, recurrent disease, probably due to reinfection in the home environment, limited the effect of this school-based treatment.

In a third trial, the intermittent treatment with tetracycline or erythromycin was compared to boric acid (Whitcher et al., 1974). There was a barely detectable effect on clinical disease by the end of the sixth month of treatment, and after another six months without treatment there were no differences between the antibiotic and control groups, again due probably to reinfection. Yet another trial compared three-week treatment regimens by topical tetracycline with the same drug administered by an ocular delivery device ("Ocusert") or by ointment. The devices were as effective as conventional therapy.

In all these trials, the suppression of chlamydial agent following treatment has persisted even after there has been a recurrence of clinically detectable inflammatory disease (Dawson et al., 1976) so that transmission of the agent may be interrupted to a greater extent than is apparent in terms of disease suppression. These trials emphasize once again the necessity to treat the entire community, particularly preschool children, in order to substantially reduce the total load of ocular microbial pathogens and the disease they generate.

The optimal choice of chemotherapeutic agent and of route of administration is not entirely clear. Sulfonamides carry unacceptably high risks when administered orally (Hoshiwara, Powers, and Krutz, 1970) and are ineffective locally. The tetracyclines, particularly the long-acting preparations, are effective when given systemically, but their use must be severely limited in children under seven years (a prime target group for treatment) and in pregnant or nursing mothers. Moreover, the almost certain selection of tetracycline-resistant intestinal pathogens (an important cause of childhood mortality in trachomatous populations) would militate against such use. Topically administered tetracyclines will continue to be the mainstay of trachoma chemotherapy programs, but there is an urgent need for studies on better methods of drug delivery (e.g., higher concentrations, more persistent ointment bases, ocular delivery devices, etc.). Erythromycin ointment is a suitable substitute for tetracycline. Short-term use of orally administered erythromycin or doxycycline to the entire population under treatment might be considered once yearly at the beginning of the conjunctivitis season.

Trachoma control programs are still needed in areas where trachoma continues to be a blinding disease. Such programs should incorporate the following elements:

1. Preliminary assessment should determine priority in different geographic regions of a country, and ongoing assessment should evaluate the efficacy of the program. The limited resources available should be concentrated in the areas of greatest need.

2. Chemotherapy programs should concentrate on children under 10 years of age, especially preschool children. In addition to school programs, village health aides should distribute drugs to families and instruct the mothers of young children in drug use.

3. The surgical correction of lid deformities has a more immediate impact than antibiotic treatment on preventing blindness; identifying cases for surgery and follow-up of surgical results should be another part of the assessment program. Surgical programs might have to be extended to regions in which active trachoma is no longer a problem, but where the accumulated scarring acquired by adults when they were children still causes eyelid deformity and visual loss.

4. The immediate treatment of bacterial corneal ulcers is an important measure, since corneal ulcers are the most common antecedent of visual loss and are relatively frequent — an estimated 18 per 10,000 population per year in Morocco (Reinhards et al., 1968). Village health aides should be instructed in the diagnosis of and urgent need for treatment of corneal ulcers so that patients can be sent to central hospitals for definitive treatment.

Most of these programs can be carried out by public health nurses and health aides who need relatively little special training. Specific surgical skills are needed for the correction of deformed lids, but simple lid procedures are presently being performed by surgically trained nurses in northern Nigeria and East Africa. Such programs will attain their effect by thorough organization, concentration of resources, and planning, rather than by novel approaches or technological breakthroughs. These programs must be kept within the limits dictated by the available financial resources. Outside technical assistance is most important in organization of the efforts, although specific items such as mobile eye units for surgical teams may be obtained through technical assistance programs. In the final analysis, trachoma control programs should be aimed initially at preventing blindness, but they can be the beginning of a sustained effort to deliver continuing eye health care to rural populations.

5   Adult Inclusion Conjunctivitis

Since the chlamydial agent that causes inclusion conjunctivitis (IC) is genitally transmitted, the disease is limited to those who would come in contact with genital tract secretions — newborns and sexually active young adults. Because inclusions of the agents of trachoma and IC look morphologically identical, there has been long and acrimonious debate concerning the identity of the two agents and the nature and epidemiology of the clinical syndromes associated with them (Thygeson, 1971; Jones, 1964, 1975; Grayston and Wang, 1975). Lindner (1911) first proposed that IC be referred to as "genital trachoma," an idea supported to some extent by Jones in London (1975) and lately by Grayston and Wang, who propose calling all ocular chlamydial infections "trachoma" (Grayston and Wang, 1975). This view has been most emphatically opposed by Thygeson, who has pointed out that IC in newborns and adults does not lead to the blinding complications associated with true trachoma, that IC is dependent upon genital transmission with occasional eye infection, and that in subhuman primates the genitally transmitted agents cause much more severe disease than do strains from classic trachoma cases

(Thygeson, 1971). Throughout these debates there has been a tendency to classify the microbial agent (i.e., the chlamydiae) on the basis of clinical syndrome or, conversely, to classify the clinical disease by the microbiological properties of the agent.

When dealing with a patient presenting with eye infection, the physician's main problem is one of etiologic diagnosis, since a number of other clinical syndromes resemble chlamydial infection of the eye. Chlamydial infections respond to antibiotic treatment, so it is important to make this etiologic diagnosis. Since these infections can only be definitively diagnosed on the basis of laboratory tests, which are rarely available to ophthalmologists, chlamydial infections still cause an amount of morbidity out of proportion with their frequency.

HISTORICAL ASPECTS

While an abacterial form of neonatal ophthalmia was recognized as early as 1884, and in 1903 was described by Morax as "conjonctivite amicrobienne," the adult syndrome was not as readily recognized. A mild type of "trachoma" was described by Schultz in 1899 as an epidemic among the clients of a swimming pool in Berlin (Kroner, 1884; Schultz, 1899, 1900; Morax, 1903). It was correctly deduced by Fehr that this syndrome was quite distinct from trachoma, and he described it as "endemische Bad Konjunktivitis" (Fehr, 1900).

The chlamydial agent was first identified from an adult with eye disease by Huntemüller and Padderstein, who successfully infected the eye of a monkey with it (1913). The particular issue of swimming pool conjunctivitis continued to be confusing, however, since a shorter-lived form of follicular conjunctivitis (now known to be caused by adenoviruses) was also associated with swimming pools. At the turn of the century it was thought that infection of the eye probably occurred through genital discharges coming in contact with the eye, a view confirmed by Morax in 1933, in his monograph "La Conjonctivite Folliculaire."

It is of interest that much of the work on extra-ocular infection was done by ophthalmologists such as Thygeson and Mengert, who reported the apparently self-limited nature of the genital infection (1936), and Braley, who showed that the transitional epithelium of the cervical os supported the growth of the chlamydial agent in experimentally inoculated baboons (1939). Identification of the agent in the genital tract of a 10-year-old girl with chronic vaginitis was reported both by Thygeson and Stone (1942) and Hardy (1941), an observation repeated only in recent years by Mordhorst, who found a similar infection in prepubescent girls in Copenhagen (1967). The occasional infection of a gynecologist from patient's genital material or eye-to-eye transmission in a glaucoma clinic were reported by Thygeson and Mengert (1936).

In the late 1940s and early 1950s, the earlier reports of conjunctival scarring and inclusion conjunctivitis in newborns and keratitis in adults were forgotten or overlooked, and it was supposed that adult IC was not associated with a serious involvement of the cornea or subsequent corneal scarring (Lindner, 1911; Aust, 1929–1930). Isolation of the chlamydial agent led to the observation by Jones and his group that some genitally transmitted chlamydial infections met the criteria established by the World Health Organization for the diagnosis of trachoma, namely, presence of lymphoid follicles on the upper tarsal plate, significant pannus formation (superficial corneal vascularization), and presence of an inclusion agent in conjunctival scrapings (WHO Trachoma Expert Committee Third Report). This led to a proposal to revive Lindner's (1911) term "paratrachoma" for any sexually transmitted chlamydial infection of the eye or genital tract (WHO Trachoma Expert Committee Fourth Report).

The diagnosis of "acute trachoma" was applied to the cases of acute follicular conjunctivitis with pannus that occurred in urban environments (Thygeson, 1949). While some of these patients were from endemic trachoma areas, many of them were young adults living in urban areas who may well have acquired their infection from a genitally transmitted agent. In the early 1960s it was pointed out by Jones and his associates that the disease caused by the genitally transmitted chlamydia could manifest as adult IC without corneal involvement, as classic trachoma with conjunctival scarring and pannus, or as an intermediate syndrome, TRIC agent punctate keratoconjunctivitis (TPK) (Jones, 1964). Similarly, Mordhorst and later Grayston and Wang reported a small series of cases of classic trachoma with pannus, conjunctival scarring, and follicles in girls who had apparently acquired the infection during the neonatal period but had continued to have chlamydial infection and manifest disease of the genital tract and eye into adolescence (Mordhorst, 1967; Grayston and Wang, 1975).

During this same period the rapid evolution of methods of serotyping chlamydial isolates led to the observation that isolates from patients with trachoma in endemic trachoma areas had been limited to serotypes A, B, Ba, and C, whereas isolates from the genital tract have, for the most part, been serotypes D through K with a few types C, B, and Ba, all of which have considerable immunologic overlap with other genital strains. Primate inoculations first performed with material from human cases (Thygeson and Crocker, 1956), and later with isolated chlamydial strains, showed that the genital chlamydial strains appeared to be more pathogenic for the eyes of monkeys and other subhuman primates than did classic trachoma strains (Dawson, Mordhorst, and Thygeson, 1962; Grayston and Wang, 1975).

Thus the controversy seems to have arrived at an unsatisfactory conclusion: the eye diseases associated with genitally transmitted chlamydiae may at times resemble classic trachoma; on the other hand the serotypes of chlamydial agents obtained from cases of endemic trachoma appear to be limited in number and may differ from the genitally transmitted agents in other microbial characteristics (e.g., primate pathogenicity). Since the epidemiologic settings in which the two diseases occur vary so greatly, it does not seem justified to make any judgments on the microbiological character of the organisms on the basis of the clinical syndromes.

EPIDEMIOLOGY

It has been pointed out elsewhere in this volume that the chlamydial agents are transmitted as a venereal infection involving the epithelium of the cervical os and rectum in women and the urethral epithelium in men. Recent studies have emphasized that inclusion conjunctivitis in sexually mature individuals is almost always the result of sexual activities, and is usually accompanied by infection of the genital tract of the patient or of the patient's sexual consort (Jones, 1964; Dawson and Schachter, 1967; Schachter, Rose, and Meyer, 1967; Schachter et al., 1967, 1970; Dawson et al., 1970b; Mordhorst, 1967). The eye rarely acts as a source of transmission of the infection to others, although a few cases of eye-to-eye transmission have been documented (Jones, 1964; Mordhorst, personal communication).

Most patients with genitally acquired chlamydial infection of the eye are between the ages of 15 and 30 (Jones, 1964; Dawson and Schachter, 1967; Thygeson and Stone, 1942). These patients have often had multiple sexual consorts and a history of other venereal disease, particularly gonorrhea or pubic lice. Moreover, many of the men in our series in San Francisco had participated in oral-genital sexual acts, thus exposing their eyes directly to infectious discharges. It has been our experience that eye infections are frequently acquired by one or both members of a consort pair within the first two to four months of their sexual relationship.

At present it is difficult to ascertain if the swimming pool conjunctivitis described by Schultz (1899, 1900), Fehr (1900), and Morax (1933) was indeed due to exposure to infected genital discharges in the swimming pool or was acquired during sexual encounters. The cases described by Morax were relatively young for this latter possibility (ages 13 and 15 years), although overt sexual activity cannot be ruled out.

Despite the high rate of venereal disease in male homosexuals, we have not seen, nor are there any reports in the literature of, chlamydial eye infection in this group. There was one case of ocular chlamydial infection in our series, in a female homosexual, but this woman had also had heterosexual intercourse.

A small number of cases have been reported in older adults who were exposed to newborn infants with inclusion blennorrhea (Jones, 1964). Thygeson reported several gynecologists who acquired chlamydial eye infection after being struck in the eye by genital material while performing surgery, e.g., dilatation and curettage (Thygeson and Mengert, 1936; Thygeson and Stone, 1942). He also reported a small epidemic of chlamydial infection among older patients in a glaucoma clinic, apparently transmitted through an infected tonometer.

There have been a few case reports of neonatal eye infection in which the disease persisted up to the sixteenth year of life (Jones, 1964). The cases reported by Mordhorst in young girls had a combination of vaginal infection and eye disease, apparently acquired at birth (Mordhorst, 1967). Other cases of vaginal infection in prepubertal girls have been reported by Thygeson and Stone (1942), Hardy (1941), and Dunlop et al. (1966a,b). Moreover, Mordhorst has observed the apparent eye-to-eye spread of infection among children and staff in a nursery school (Mordhorst, personal communication). Most likely the index case was a child with an undetected eye infection acquired at birth. Thus it is possible that genitally transmitted chlamydiae may rarely cause outbreaks of eye disease in prepubertal children as well.

The role of chlamydial genital infection in classic endemic trachoma areas has not yet been determined. The most suggestive finding was that of the Lister Institute group working in The Gambia who identified a case of neonatal inclusion conjunctivitis in a village with endemic trachoma (Sowa, Sowa, and Collier, 1968). Later studies, however, showed that the isolate from this infant was a typical genital strain, type F, but that the trachoma prevalent in the community was associated with serotypes A and B, typical trachoma strains (Collier, 1973).

Since trachoma in endemic areas has a high prevalence in children from infancy up to five years of age and disappears in adolescence, it is unlikely that genital exposure or reinfection is a major epidemiologic pathway. It is possible, however, that chlamydial infection of the genital tracts of adults would serve as a reservoir for limited reinfection of children. The almost universal absence in classic trachoma of those serotypes that cause the great majority of genital infections would again suggest that there is not a genital reservoir of chlamydiae in endemic trachoma.

CLINICAL DISEASE

In the adult, genitally acquired chlamydial infection of the eye usually presents as an acute follicular conjunctivitis. With renewed interest in the microbiology of the chlamydial agents in the 1960s, detailed studies of naturally acquired infections and of a large number of experimental inoculations in humans were carried out.

In volunteers inoculated with genital chlamydia (types D and F), conjunctivitis developed within 2 to 19 days after inoculation depending on the concentration of the inoculum, the incubation period being shorter with higher concentrations (Dawson et al., 1966). At onset there is a slight foreign body sensation ("gritty sensation"), with hyperemia, mucoid discharge, papillary hypertrophy, and epithelial keratitis (Jones and Collier, 1962; Dawson et al., 1967). The conjunctivitis becomes progressively more intense, typically reaching a peak 13 to 17 days after inoculation (Dawson et al., 1967, Figs. 1 and 2, Plate 5). Soon after the onset of conjunctivitis, ptosis develops and small lymphoid follicles become evident in the inferior fornix along the border of the upper tarsus as does a slight to moderate mucopurulent discharge. Preauricular lymphadenopathy accompanies symptoms in the eye. The lymphoid follicles become particularly prominent in the lower conjunctiva, but are often present in the upper tarsal conjunctiva also. The conjunctivitis may subside slightly, to recur in increasing intensity. In many inoculated volunteers the disease appeared to subside gradually, and in some instances it healed without chemotherapy.

In volunteer inoculations and in naturally occurring cases, corneal involvement is a regular feature of ocular infection with genitally transmitted chlamydial agents. Diffuse punctate epithelial keratitis and swelling of the limbus are present in almost all cases. Discrete subepithelial infiltrates occur at the corneal limbus and central cornea without preceding epithelial keratitis (Fig. 3, Plate 5). These are not unlike the corneal infiltrates found in association with bacterial conjunctivitis.

Particularly with dense and persistent marginal infiltrates near the corneal-scleral junction (limbus), there may be corneal neovascularization (Fig. 4, Plate 5). This neovascularization is occasionally so extensive that it resembles a trachoma-like pannus. In a few volunteers (12%), large persistent subepithelial infiltrates were noted that first appeared 20 to 34 days after initial inoculation and in some instances occurred as long as 7 to 11 days after oral sulfonamide therapy had been initiated (Dawson et al., 1967). These opacities resembled those found in epidemic keratoconjunctivitis, and they are found immediately beneath the epithelium in the anterior stroma. They persist for up to 21 months and do not have overlying lesions in the corneal epithelium, except in the initial phase (Dawson et al., 1967). Interestingly enough, the recurrence of corneal infiltrates seems to precede the peaks of recurrent conjunctivitis by a few days.

Reports by Jones and his group have emphasized the occurrence of conjunctival scarring both in adult oculogenital chamydial infections that are naturally acquired and in experimental cases (Jones, 1964, 1975; Freedman et al., 1966). Our group in San Francisco has seen three adults presumed to have inclusion conjunctivitis with conjunctival scarring. All these cases had had a prolonged course, probably due in part to topical corticosteroid therapy. They had received antibiotic therapy by the time we examined them, however, so the agent was not isolated. In general, most cases in adults subside with or without treatment and do not ordinarily leave conjunctival scarring or its complications, trichiasis and entropion. Jones reports that among 92 adults with genitally transmitted chlamydial infection of the eye, 14% had inclusion conjunctivitis (i.e., no keratitis), 32% had TPK, and 54% had typical trachoma (Jones, 1975).

In volunteers whose initial infection had been limited to one eye, the degree of conjunctivitis following bilateral reinoculation was less severe in both eyes than in the primary infection (Dawson et al., 1966). Thus the partial resistance to reinfection appeared to be mediated by systemic rather than local immune mechanisms. In contrast, the corneal disease appeared three to six days earlier in reinfected volunteers than it had in the primary infection. When both eyes were reinoculated in volunteers with a unilateral primary infection, the keratitis in the previously uninfected eye appeared no earlier than in the primary infection. Thus keratitis appears to be mediated by local factors and might be considered as a manifestation of hypersensitivity (Dawson et al., 1967).

In adult IC, the clinical appearance of the conjunctiva and cornea depends on the duration of the disease: in the first two weeks, the hyperemia, infiltration, and discharge of the conjunctiva dominate the clinical picture; after two weeks, the conjunctival lymphoid follicles and superficial keratitis become more prominent features; in cases that have persisted for several months, the follicles may be less prominent, but corneal neovascularization and conjunctival scarring may occur.

Iritis (anterior uveitis) is an uncommon complication of adult IC that has been observed both in naturally acquired disease and in volunteer inoculations (Dawson et al., 1967; Dawson et al., 1970b).

In this latter group, iritis occurred late in primary infection or a few days after reinfection. The uveitis was characterized by moderate flare, numerous cells in the anterior chamber, and fine to medium white keratic precipitates, but posterior synechiae have not been observed. Topical corticosteroids and cycloplegics have produced a prompt disappearance of the uveal disease. This iritis is similar to but less severe than that seen in patients with Reiter's syndrome (Dawson et al., 1970b), and may represent a form of hypersensitivity in individuals with a particular genetic susceptibility associated with the HLA-B27 marker (Brewerton et al., 1973, 1974).

Middle ear inflammation is a relatively common complication of ocular inclusion conjunctivitis, and occurred in 14% of infected volunteers (Dawson et al., 1967). There is usually a complaint that the ear on the infected side is "stopped" or "plugged." Occasionally there is a definite earache (Dawson et al., 1967). These more severe cases have been diagnosed as serous or secretory otitis media, and are usually accompanied by enlarged, slightly tender lymph nodes at the angle of the jaw or in the posterior cervical chain. In one case of naturally occurring inclusion conjunctivitis seen by an otolaryngologist and diagnosed as "serous otitis media and diffuse lymphoid hyperplasia in the nasopharynx with eustachian tube blockage," the fluid drained from the outer ear by ear myringotomy yielded chlamydiae by isolation (Dawson and Schachter, 1967).

In another case the conjunctivitis was followed one week after onset by a dramatic bilateral hearing loss (Gow, Ostler, and Schachter, 1974). The demonstration of agent in middle ear fluid and in the throat scrapings from some of these patients suggests that the chlamydial agent can infect tissues other than those of the conjunctiva and genital tract.

DIFFERENTIAL DIAGNOSIS

Since adult inclusion conjunctivitis usually presents as an acute follicular conjunctivitis, the differential diagnosis of IC should include the following entities:

1. Adenovirus acute follicular conjunctivitis
   a. Pharyngoconjunctival fever
   b. Epidemic keratoconjunctivitis
2. Herpes simplex follicular conjunctivitis
3. Newcastle disease virus conjunctivitis
4. Acute hemorrhagic conjunctivitis (enterovirus type 70)
5. Other chlamydial infections

Adenovirus follicular conjunctivitis was originally described as Béal's follicular conjunctivitis (Morax, 1933). There are two major forms of the syndrome, pharyngoconjunctival fever (PCF) and epidemic keratoconjunctivitis (EKC). As the name implies, PCF is a syndrome that combines an upper respiratory infection, fever, and conjunctivitis (Thygeson and Dawson, 1971). Typically, the conjunctivitis is of unilateral onset and is often associated with a small, nontender preauricular node on the side of the infected eye. The second eye may not be involved or may develop disease some days after the first eye; both eyes heal at the same time. The eye disease is usually associated with a watery discharge. Follicles may be very small at first and are rarely as florid as in inclusion conjunctivitis (Figs. 5 and 6, Plate 5). There may be minor degrees of epithelial keratitis and occasionally some corneal epithelial infiltrates. The eye disease rarely lasts more than two weeks. The upper respiratory infection and fever are most prominent during the first week of the illness. This disease is now the most common form of swimming pool conjunctivitis (Caldwell et al., 1974; Cockburn, 1953).

In adults and older children, EKC is usually not accompanied by fever or respiratory symptoms (Dawson et al., 1963). The disease is often unilateral at onset, with milder symptoms developing in the second eye. The distinguishing feature of EKC is the local keratitis that develops the second week of the illness and progresses to form small (0.5 mm) subepithelial opacities that persist long after the conjunctivitis has subsided at the end of 15 days (Dawson et al., 1970a). EKC is frequently associated with a membranous conjunctiva followed by conjunctival scarring (Figs. 7, 8, Plate 6) (Dawson, Hanna, and Togin, 1972). This syndrome is usually caused by adenovirus types 8 or 19. In the past EKC has been spread by ophthalmologists or others treating eye disease, who transfer the causative agent from infected patients to the eyes of other patients on their fingers, on instruments, or in eye drops (Dawson and Darrell, 1963). Recent epidemics of adenovirus 19, however, appear to be spread in the community without the help of medical personnel (Taylor et al., 1975). In young children, adenovirus type 8 may produce a severe upper respiratory infection and otitis media (Dawson and Darrell, 1963). Like PCF, the conjunctivitis of EKC usually subsides in 15 days, although the corneal opacities persist for months after the acute episode. Thus, both PCF and EKC differ markedly from IC in their self-limited course.

The laboratory tests useful in the diagnosis of adenovirus infections include Giemsa-stained conjunctival smears, virus isolation procedures, and antibody titers. Giemsa-stained conjunctival smears from adenovirus conjunctivitis cases usually show numerous lymphocytes and few polymorphonuclear cells, although EKC cases with conjunctival membranes have many polymorphonuclear cells. This contrasts with the cytology in IC, where an equal number of PMNs and lymphocytes are found. Isolation of the virus or a rising antibody titer are, of course, definitive means of demonstrating adenovirus infection.

Herpes simplex virus (HSV) keratoconjunctivitis is much less frequent than adenovirus eye infections and IC. The conjunctivitis caused by herpesvirus resembles that with adenovirus in that the disease is usually unilateral, with watery discharge, the follicles are less prominent than IC, and the course is self-limited (Fig. 9, Plate 6). Usually there are herpetic vesicles on the lids or lid margins, although these may be so small as to be overlooked. Corneal involvement does not always occur, but may start several days after the conjunctivitis and appear as irregular punctate corneal epithelial erosions ("coarse epithelial keratopathy") or typical linear branching ulcers of the corneal epithelium ("dendritic ulcers"). Like all herpes simplex virus infections, the conjunctivitis may be recurrent. Since corticosteroids enhance HSV corneal infections, often with disastrous results, these compounds should never be used in treating episodes of acute follicular conjunctivitis.

The laboratory diagnosis of HSV follicular conjunctivitis depends on isolation of the virus from the conjunctiva. The cytology is much like t' of adenovirus conjunctivitis, with a predominance of lymphocy'

Newcas lisease virus (NDV) causes an infection of chickens which is of great importance in commercial poultry farming. Human eye infection occurs in persons exposed to infected birds in poultry processing plants, and in veterinarians and others exposed to the live virus used in vaccinating young birds. NDV conjunctivitis is an acute conjunctivitis characterized by watery discharge, preauricular lymphadenopathy, and epithelial keratitis (Hales and Ostler, 1973). The eye disease lasts 7 to 10 days and no sequelae have been reported.

Acute hemorrhagic conjunctivitis (AHC) was first described in 1969 in epidemics in Africa and Asia. The eye disease presents as an acute conjunctivitis with watery discharge, and numerous hemorrhages that are punctate at first but quickly become confluent, particularly on the bulbar conjunctiva (Fig. 10, Plate 6). The conjunctival inflammation is accompanied by the formation of small follicles and subsides in 4 to 5 days, but the hemorrhages do not resolve for 7 to 10 days (Whitcher et al., 1976). There is frequently a fine epithelial keratitis. In all but one epidemic, enterovirus 70 (a member of the picornavirus group) has been identified as the etiologic agent (Kono et al., 1974).

AHC has occurred in large scale epidemics in the developing countries of Africa and Asia and in a few clinic outbreaks in Europe. The disease has not yet (1976) been reported in the Western Hemisphere. AHC due to enterovirus 70 is apparently a new disease; the clinical syndrome has not been reported previously. In epidemics, both young and old and both rural and urban populations are affected. The virus has not previously been identified. In the laboratory, the virus grows best at 33° C, the approximate temperature of the conjunctiva.

In outbreaks in eye clinics, the incubation period has been as short as 18 to 24 hours, and patients are most infectious the first day of the disease (Whitcher et al., 1976). These nosocomial infections are apparently spread by direct transfer of the virus on fingers, instruments, and medications that come in contact with the eye. Since most of the community-based epidemics have been in developing countries, the transfer of infection probably only occurs under conditions of close personal contact and crowding.

The only reported complication of AHC is a lumbar radiculomyelitis which was reported in Taiwan and in the Bombay epidemic, where 20 cases of this nervous system involvement were noted in an estimated 500,000 AHC cases (Kono et al., 1974). This complication leads to partial paralysis of the involved limb. In primate experiments, enterovirus inoculated directly into the spinal cord has about the same pathogenicity as vaccine strains of poliovirus, producing a localized inflammation of the spinal cord (myelitis) (Kono et al., 1974).

Conjunctival infections with *Chlamydia psittaci* (psittacosis and feline pneumonitis agents) have occurred, causing follicular conjunctivitis in humans. In one accidental laboratory infection, a technician developed a follicular conjunctivitis with a slight keratitis and preauricular lymphadenopathy (Fig. 11, Plate 6) (Schachter et al., 1968). The disease responded to systemic tetracycline, although the chlamydial agent continued to be isolated from the eye for two weeks after systemic tetracycline therapy had been started. We have seen two cases of follicular conjunctivitis caused by the feline pneumonitis agent (Schachter, Ostler, and Meyer, 1969; Ostler, Schachter, and Dawson, 1969). In one case, an adult male was exposed to a young cat who regularly slept on his bed. The cat had had discharge from the eyes and was found to have feline pneumonitis agent in the conjunctiva. The patient did not have corneal involvement, but did develop a phlyctenular nodule (a manifestation of delayed hypersensitivity) at the limbus. The second case was in a 7-year-old girl who had taken a stray kitten with eye discharge as a pet (Fig. 12, Plate 6). In both cases there was no corneal involvement, and the disease responded to systemic tetracyclines.

LABORATORY TESTS

The laboratory diagnosis of adult IC can be made definitively by demonstrating the agent in conjunctival specimens or presumptively by demonstrating the presence of chlamydial antibody in serum or tears. In proven eye infections, specimens taken before treatment showed that, in conjunctival smears, the agent was detected more often by fluorescent antibody (FA) staining (80%) than by Giemsa staining (60%), and that iodine staining was much less effective (32% positive) (Dawson and Schachter, 1967; Schachter et al., 1967; Schachter et al., 1970). In Giemsa-stained smears, there are often no more than one to five inclusions even in very florid cases, so a prolonged search for the agent is necessary. Moreover, minimal treatment (e.g., two or three applications of topical sulfonamides) either eliminates the agent or produces bizarre forms impossible to diagnose as inclusions. In this same series, the agent was demonstrated by egg isolation in about 60% of cases. While there is no direct comparison of egg isolation and cell culture isolation in eye specimens, cell culture appears to be more sensitive and is certainly less expensive and quicker (Jones, 1974; WHO, 1975). Isolation in cell culture has the added advantage that it does not require personnel with the special training necessary to examine conjunctival smears for inclusions.

Serological evidence of chlamydial infection is, of course, indirect proof of etiology of the eye disease. The CF test is positive more frequently in adults with both eye and genital tract infection (50% of men and 85% of women with titers of more than 1:16) than in those with disease limited to the genital tract (28% in men and 50% in women) (Dawson and Schachter, 1967). In adult IC, the CF titers rarely exceed 1:32 to 1:64. Since the antibody levels detected by the microimmunofluorescence test (Wang and Grayston, 1970) are elevated in most patients with genital tract infection, failure to detect antibodies by the micro-IF would tend to exclude the diagnosis of IC. All of the laboratory-confirmed cases we have tested have been antibody positive. Since genital tract infection probably occurs some time before eye infection, most patients have developed serum antibodies by the time they seek care for an eye infection, so rising antibody titers are hardly ever detected.

TREATMENT

Adult IC responds promptly to treatment with systemic tetracyclines. Within 48 hours, the discharge decreases, and symptoms from keratitis and hyperemia diminish (Dawson et al., 1967, 1970b). Doses of 1 gm tetracycline a day (250 mg four times daily) for persons under 150 pounds and of 1.5 gm daily (500 mg three times daily) for those more than 150 pounds given for three weeks have been effective in curing the disease and eliminating infection. Courses of treatment shorter than one week have been associated with recurrences.

Since IC in adults is acquired through sexual activities, the patient's sexual consorts should be treated with the same dose of tetracycline at the same time to prevent reinfection. Most treatment failures of IC occur when the sexual consort has not been treated. The other tetracyclines, such as doxycycline, are equally efficacious but must be given in full doses for the full three-week period. While effective treatment reduces the keratitis, conjunctival infiltration (papillary hypertrophy), and discharge, the follicles may persist for several months before gradually disappearing.

In patients who have sensitivities or undesirable side effects to tetracyclines (e.g., *Candida* vaginitis) or in whom these drugs are contraindicated (e.g., pregnant women, nursing mothers, or children under seven years), erythromycin may be used. Since the erythromycins may cause nausea and the estolate sometimes causes cholestatic hepatitis, they are not the first drug of choice. Like tetracyclines, erythromycin derivatives must be used in full recommended doses for three weeks.

Oral sulfonamides have also been effective in the treatment of IC. Studies with volunteers showed clearing of disease and infection with very low doses of sulfisoxazole (Gantrisin) given for two weeks (Dawson et al., 1966). Since IC strains vary in their sensitivity to antimicrobial drugs and only two strains were employed in those studies, such low dosages cannot be recommended. At one time IC was treated with full doses of triple sulfonamides (3 gm per day), but the occurrence of manifest side effects (skin rash, headache) was so high that the use of sulfonamides should now be considered only under unusual circumstances (Dawson et al., 1970b).

Topical antimicrobials, usually tetracycline, appear to have a limited effect in adult IC, with partial but not complete clearing of symptoms. Topical antimicrobials have an effect on the chlamydial agent in conjunctival smears. A few applications produce inclusions with bizarre forms, and longer topical therapy leads to suppression of the agent detectable by Giemsa or FA staining or by isolation. Despite this effect on the agent, the disease resolves only partially with topical therapy. Keratitis and follicular conjunctivitis are only partially suppressed and may persist even after six weeks of topical therapy. Moreover, topical therapy would have no effect on the genital infection which usually accompanies adult IC. Since systemic treatment brings such prompt clearing of disease, we have not found that topical antibiotic offers any additional benefit.

The occasional episode of iritis has responded promptly to the application of topical corticosteroids four times daily without residual lesions (e.g., posterior synechiae). The iritis has not been recurrent (Dawson et al., 1970b). Otitis media with adult IC subsides after a few days of treatment with systemic tetracycline.

6 Inclusion Conjunctivitis of the Newborn and Chlamydial Pneumonia in Infants

The appalling results of conjunctivitis of newborns in the mid-nineteenth century are almost beyond our comprehension today. Before Credé prophylaxis was introduced, 10% of all newborn infants developed eye disease, chiefly caused by gonococcal infections (Howe, 1896). Too often, the accompanying corneal ulceration led to loss of the eye or severe corneal scarring. The immediate post-partum cleansing of the lids and conjunctiva with silver nitrate solutions advocated by Credé (1884, 1963) was one of the early triumphs of scientific medicine. Before the antibiotic era, however, neonatal ophthalmia was so frequent that many hospitals set aside a ward to treat these cases by frequent washing of the conjunctival sac and instillation of silver nitrate solutions. With the availability of effective chemotherapeutic drugs to treat overt venereal disease in the parents, blinding eye infections of the newborn have become medical rarities, and, when present, the disease in newborns now receives prompt attention. There is a real danger, however, that the current popularity for deliveries in the home may lead to a resurgence of serious eye infections

112

in newborns, particularly when coupled with the cavalier attitude and ignorance of many physicians today regarding this disease.

HISTORICAL ASPECTS

By 1884, it was recognized that there was a form of ophthalmia neonatorum without apparent bacterial infection (Kroner, 1884), and Morax labeled this "conjonctivite amicrobienne" (1903). By 1909, the typical cytoplasmic inclusion was found in conjunctival scrapings from newborns (Lindner, 1909; Stargardt, 1909), from the genital tract of their mothers, and from the urethras of their fathers (Halberstaedter and von Prowazek, 1909; Fritsch, Hofstätter and Lindner 1910; Lindner, 1911). Material from infants with inclusion conjunctivitis inoculated into primates produced follicular conjunctivitis (Fritsch et al., 1910) identical to that obtained with material from adults with follicular conjunctivitis (Huntemüller and Padderstein, 1913). Thus the etiology and epidemiology of the disease was well established soon after the disease in infants was defined.

EPIDEMIOLOGY

The infant acquires the infection from the mother's genital tract shortly before or during birth. The genital infection in adults is, of course, spread as a venereal infection. Rarely, other family members (siblings, grandparents) will acquire infection from the infant. Of babies born to mothers with documented chlamydial infection of the cervix, about one-third develop the eye disease. Inapparent infection of the infant's eye has not been reported.

In female infants, infection of the genital tract may develop as a vulvovaginitis (Dunlop et al., 1966a,b). Others have reported chlamydial infection in girls 4, 5, 10, and 15 years of age, all of whom had no sexual contact and the last with an intact hymen (Dunlop et al., 1966a,b; Thygeson and Stone, 1942; Hardy, 1941; Mordhorst, 1967). In most of the cases, the genital infection was discovered because of accompanying eye disease.

The rate of neonatal chlamydial infection of the eye has been reported as ranging from 1.4 to 4.4 cases per 1,000 live births (Watson and Gairdner, 1968; Allen, 1944; Hansman, 1969; Thygeson and Stone, 1942).

Chandler and Alexander and their respective colleagues have performed a prospective trial on development of chlamydial infection in neonates (Alexander et al., 1977; Chandler et al., 1977). They studied 142 unselected pregnant women and found 18 (12.7%) to have chlamydial infection of the cervix. Of the 18 infants born to these women, 9 (50%) developed conjunctivitis and 12 (67%)

developed serum antibodies against chlamydiae. In San Francisco, the results of a study performed by us differed slightly — only 5% of the pregnant women studied yielded chlamydiae from the cervix — but the attack rate was similar: 10 of the 25 infants at risk developed laboratory-proven inclusion conjunctivitis (ICN). The results of these two pilot studies suggest that approximately 40% to 50% of the infants exposed develop conjunctivitis. If the range of chlamydial carriage in the cervix is between 5% and 13%, then 2% to 6% of all newborns in the U.S., a very significant proportion, will acquire this chlamydial infection at birth. The prospective studies suggest that the incidence of ICN is much higher than previous estimates.

CLINICAL DISEASE

The incubation period of inclusion conjunctivitis of the newborn is said to be 5 to 12 days after birth, but early infection can result if the placental membranes rupture before delivery (Thygeson and Stone, 1942). In a carefully followed series, Freedman et al. (1966) found that 14 of 38 neonates had ocular discharge the first day of life and 6 more developed discharge the second to fourth day. In this same series, 8 infants had an onset of the disease from 10 to 13 days of life and 1 infant exhibited infection during the third week. Thus the incubation period is not a sure indicator of chlamydial conjunctivitis in the newborn, although it is assumed to be 5 to 12 days. Moreover, prophylaxis with antibiotics might delay the onset of disease beyond the "normal" range.

Infected infants first show a slight watery discharge which becomes progressively more purulent. The eyelids are swollen and bulging. The conjunctiva becomes reddened throughout and the portion lining the lid is thickened with diffuse infiltration manifest as papillary hypertrophy on the upper tarsus (Fig. 1, Plate 7). In some cases, "pseudomembranes" develop as an inflammatory exudate closely adherent to the conjunctival surface. The conjunctiva has no lymphoid layer at birth, but follicular conjunctivitis develops after several weeks; Freedman et al. (1966) noted lymphoid follicles as early as three weeks and in 7 of 23 infants by six weeks. If untreated, the disease persists for 3 to 12 months, although occasional cases persist longer; in one case of Freedman et al. (1966) a membranous conjunctivitis persisted for 16 months, and a chlamydial agent was isolated when the child was two years old.

The reports noting conjunctival scarring published prior to 1930 (Lindner, 1911; Aust, 1929–1930) were overlooked, and it was generally accepted that the neonatal disease had no cicatricial sequelae (Thygeson, 1962b). The conjunctival scarring and superficial corneal vascularization which occurred in 10 patients in the series reported by Freedman and colleagues in 1966 again brought attention to such scarring. These observations were confirmed by several other workers (Watson and Gairdner, 1967; Forster, Dawson, and Schachter, 1970; Mordhorst and Dawson, 1971; Goscienski and Sexton, 1972). The conjunctival scarring was usually seen as broad ("sheet") scars or long linear scars (Fig. 2, Plate 7). In no instance were lid deformities reported. The corneal vascularization has usually been less than a 2-mm extension of vessels from the limbus. Mordhorst and Dawson (1971) noted that these signs occurred only in children who were treated with tetracycline after the twelfth day of life or who had received only silver nitrate or chloramphenicol. One patient in the series of Freedman et al. (1966) had persistent disease and was noted to have scarring, tarsal follicles, and pannus in one eye typical of stage III trachoma.

A mucopurulent rhinitis occurs in some infants with inclusion conjunctivitis. A chlamydial agent was isolated from nasal material in four of nine attempts and from the throat in one of six attempts in one series (Freedman et al., 1966).* Dunlop and his associates (1966a,b) observed vulvovaginitis in 6 of 14 newborn girls with chlamydial eye infections. One patient with trachoma III also had a membranous vulvovaginitis from which *Chlamydia* was isolated. These authors isolated a chlamydial agent from the vulva of a 6-year-old girl whose parents both had genital infection. The infection was "possibly transmitted by hands, towels, face-flannels or similar means" (Dunlop et al., 1966b).

Mordhorst (1967) reported chlamydial infection in two girls whose eye disease was first recognized at four years of age. One girl had typical trachoma III (tarsal follicles, conjunctival scarring, and corneal vascularization); Giemsa-stained conjunctival scrapings showed typical inclusions and the chlamydial isolate from her vagina was serotype G (Grayston and Wang, 1975). The second patient had trachoma III (tarsal follicles, corneal vascularization), and a chlamydial isolate from her eye was also type G (Grayston and Wang, 1975). Both of these children were the only children in their family, neither had been outside Denmark, and both of their fathers were in the Danish merchant marine. It might be postulated that their chlamydial infection was acquired at birth and that genital tract infection served as a source of agent to infect the eye.

Obviously some of these children with genital tract infections could have been victims of sexual abuse. However, it is far more likely that the chlamydial infections were contracted at birth. The persistence of infection and severity of the eye disease are of par-

---

* Despite a later retraction, these results are probably valid.

ticular interest. Of significance is the possibility that such infections may result in child-to-child transmission, causing outbreaks of conjunctivitis.

One infant with neonatal inclusion conjunctivitis who subsequently developed pneumonia was found to have chlamydial agent in his sputum (Schachter et al., 1975d). His eye disease had cleared after topical therapy. Thus, in this infant, pneumonia may have been caused by a chlamydial agent whose portal of entry was the eye.

DIFFERENTIAL DIAGNOSIS

The following organisms and drugs may produce inflammation of newborn infants' eyes during the first three weeks of life: *Neisseria gonorrhoeae; Staphylococcus aureus;* pneumococci; *Haemophilus* sp.; *Pseudomonas; Klebsiella* and other gram-negative rods; *N. meningitidis;* alpha and beta hemolytic streptococci; *Herpesvirus hominis* and other viral eye infections; silver nitrate toxicity. For the management of ophthalmia neonatorum, gonococcal infection must be established or ruled out. Commonly, gonococcal conjunctivitis starts two to five days after birth with a copious, yellow, purulent discharge and marked swelling of the lids. Chemical conjunctivitis due to silver nitrate prophylaxis occurs during the first 24 hours of life but has much less discharge and lid swelling.

Conjunctivitis with staphylococci and pneumococci often begins after the second day. Since the other forms of nongonococcal neonatal ophthalmia, including chlamydial infections, have a similar clinical pattern of reddened, swollen conjunctiva, lid swelling, and purulent discharge, laboratory studies are necessary to select appropriate therapy. Most *Staphylococcus* infection is acquired by the infant during the hospital stay and conjunctivitis in newborns is one of the common manifestations of hospital-acquired staphylococcal infection. Gram-negative organisms, particularly *Pseudomonas* and *Klebsiella,* are the other common nosocomial infections. In contrast, contact with family members probably accounts for neonatal conjunctivitis with streptococci, pneumococci, *N. meningitidis, Haemophilus,* and other nasopharyngeal bacteria.

Like gonococcal and chlamydial infections, neonatal herpes simplex blepharoconjunctivitis is acquired from the genital tract of the mother during birth. The prominent herpetic skin vesicles distinguish this infection from the bacterial infection of the newborn eye. Herpetic eye infection of the newborn has a much higher risk of causing visual damage than the more common bacterial infections. In neonatal herpetic eye infections, topical antivirals should be given to prevent corneal involvement.

116

There is one report of adenovirus type 8 infection of the new-born eye which presented as a moderately severe neonatal ophthalmia (Dawson et al., 1960). Like adult adenovirus infections, this neonatal infection was self-limited. There was no residual scarring, but the patient did have minimal corneal vascularization when examined at age seven.

LABORATORY TESTS

In infants with chlamydial conjunctivitis, the single most useful method to detect the agent is the microscopic examination of Giemsa-stained conjunctival smears.The major source of diagnostic error has been the failure to obtain adequate smears; specimens without enough epithelial cells are inadequate, and new specimens must be collected. To detect chlamydial agent in other sites (nose, throat, vagina) isolation is probably more sensitive.

In all cases of ophthalmia neonatorum it is *absolutely mandatory* to search for gonococci. Swabs moistened with sterile broth or saline should be used to collect material from the infant's conjunctiva. Swabs should be streaked immediately onto appropriate media but may be sent to the laboratory on transport media if necessary. The swabs should be streaked onto blood agar plates and enriched (Isovitalex) chocolate agar plates which should then be incubated with CO_2. For immediate diagnosis, conjunctival scrapings stained with Gram's and Giemsa stains should be examined for gonococci. Treatment with systemic penicillin should be given if there is any suggestion of *Neisseria* infection, and treatment should not be delayed until the organism is identified as gonococcus or meningococcus. Since so many cases of neonatal inclusion conjunctivitis are accompanied by bacterial infections, cultures are also vital to determine appropriate antibiotic therapy.

TREATMENT

Neonatal inclusion conjunctivitis responds to topically applied sulfonamides, tetracyclines, or erythromycin given four times daily for two to three weeks (Freedman et al., 1966). Unfortunately, oint-ments are relatively difficult for parents to apply to their children's eyes, and tetracycline and erythromycin for ocular use are available only in this form. It would be reasonable to supplement treatment by ointment with sulfonamide drops administered before each dose of the ointment. In patients whose eye disease does not respond to topical treatment or who have chlamydial infection at other sites, a two- to three-week course of oral tetracycline or erythromycin has been recommended (Freedman et al., 1966). Most treatment failures are thought to be a result of inadequate application of the drug by the parent. In current studies we are finding a failure rate of close to 50% for topical therapy.

PNEUMONIA IN INFANTS

Chlamydial infection in the newborn is of greater concern in the light of recent observations by Beem and Saxon that *C. trachomatis* can be recovered from nasopharyngeal and tracheobronchial aspirates collected from infants with a distinctive pneumonia syndrome (Beem and Saxon, 1977a). This pneumonia is characterized by an afebrile course, chronic diffuse lung involvement, tachypnea, and elevated serum IgG and IgM levels. A distinctive cough was observed in many of the infants and some had a slight eosinophilia. Of 20 infants with this syndrome, 18 (90%) yielded chlamydiae from the tracheal-respiratory tract. Histories and examinations revealed that 11 of these 20 had conjunctivitis. Respiratory tract colonization was not restricted to infants with respiratory disease: chlamydiae were also recovered from the nasopharynx of 10 of 12 infants with ICN who had no respiratory manifestations. The infants with both respiratory disease and chlamydial infection differed from those with ICN alone in having significantly higher antichlamydial antibody levels.

Because of the high recovery rate of and very high antibody levels to *C. trachomatis* in infants with this pneumonia syndrome, Beem and Saxon have suggested that these chlamydiae are etiologically associated with the syndrome and might be a significant cause of respiratory disease in infants. Support for chlamydial etiology of the respiratory disease has come from isolation of the organism from an open-lung biopsy of a child in Denver with similar disease (Frommell, Bruhn, and Schwartzman, 1977) and from another one tested at the Hooper Foundation in San Francisco. The pneumonia syndrome seems to be relatively common in Chicago, where Beem has been able to expand his study group to approximately 50 infants, and results confirm his initial findings. From his observations of the expanded group, Beem feels that chlamydiae might be involved in the etiology of the excessive secretory otitis media and obstructive nasopharyngeal problems he has seen (personal communication, 1977).

The Beem and Saxon report is typical of many new findings that promise to be of great significance in that it raises intriguing questions that we cannot presently answer (Schachter, 1977). For instance, the infants with pneumonia are under three months of age, but the incubation period for respiratory disease, although somewhat uncertain because of the chronic nature of the condition, appears to be considerably longer than the incubation period for ICN. Why? Does it reflect two incubation periods, or does it reflect an insidious onset? Preselecting conditions have not been identified, but it is tempting to postulate that in at least some cases a more severe pneumonia may result from a double infection with cytomegalovirus and chlamydiae (both acquired from the infected mother).

The study by Beem and Saxon was performed with a highly selected population. Prospective studies must be done to define the incidence and spectrum of the disease. Approximately one half of Beem and Saxon's patients had ICN. The percentage of infants with ICN who develop respiratory tract infections, the percentage with respiratory tract infection who had antecedent ICN, and whether respiratory tract disease can occur in the absence of antecedent conjunctival infection are all questions of significance.

The most immediate question to be answered, however, is: How should the disease be managed? It appears that in many of these infants the disease resolves itself without intervention. However, some of the infants appear to be quite seriously ill, and lung X-rays seem to show a severe pneumonitis, indicating that the disease process may be more severe than the clinical condition of the patient suggests. In fact, in some of these infants, slight breathing difficulties are the only symptoms. Systemic chemotherapy may well be indicated, but it will be difficult — because of the variable nature of the disease, and ethical considerations — to perform double-blind treatment trials, particularly with a placebo. Tetracycline is generally considered the drug of choice for treatment of chlamydial infections, but it is contraindicated in this pediatric population. Erythromycin and sulfonamides are currently the most acceptable alternate drugs (Beem and Saxon, 1977b).

The infants with ICN in the Beem and Saxon series received topical tetracycline, but when seen for respiratory tract infection, most (11 of 12) still had chlamydial infection of the conjunctiva. It is obviously important to determine whether these figures reflect failure of topical tetracycline treatment or inadequate administration of the drug, or whether persistent chlamydial infection of the respiratory tract allows reseeding of the conjunctiva. Other studies have also pointed out that treatment failures with topical therapy are common (Rowe et al., 1977). Thus, one should consider whether or not infants with ICN should receive systemic rather than topical treatment.

The prospective studies on ICN mentioned above do not provide any information on the incidence of respiratory disease in infants with conjunctivitis. They were not designed to study respiratory disease, and while it is possible that some cases were missed, only one case was found (Schachter et al., 1975d). The number of infants at risk (previously estimated at 5% to 13% exposed to an infected cervix, or 2% to 6% if pneumonia is a sequela of conjunctivitis) represents a substantial population: a small risk could provide a very large number of cases and a major public health problem. If the risk of developing pneumonia is sufficiently high and the spectrum of neonatal disease broad enough to include severe respiratory disease, and possibly otitis or nasopharyngeal obstruction, another series of questions arises: Should efforts be made to routinely screen pregnant women for chlamydial infection of the cervix? Should these women be treated, and if so, what would the optimum treatment regimen be? Should efforts be made to develop Credé-like prophylaxis for chlamydial infection if the eye is found to be the seeding site for systemic infections?

One must also consider the possibility that the Beem and Saxon report describes only the beginning of an expanded clinical spectrum of neonatal chlamydial infections. Initially they found that eye infection or neonatal exposure may result in infection of the respiratory tract. Now there are suggestions that secretory otitis or nasopharyngeal obstruction may result from chlamydial infection. If these sites are infected, is it not likely that infective material reaches the gastrointestinal tract and that chlamydiae may cause disease there?

It is clear from natural models of *C. psittaci* infection in animals that the gastrointestinal tract is a common site for chlamydial infection in mammals (Storz, 1971). Although *C. psittaci* is considered to be a more invasive agent, capable of systemic infections, all information to date suggests that *C. trachomatis* (the agent causing ICN) grows only in columnar epithelial cells. These cells, which are found in the conjunctiva, the cervix, and the urethra, are also found in the respiratory tract, the gastrointestinal tract, and the rectal mucosa. It would thus seem likely that in appropriate epidemiologic circumstances one could consider *C. trachomatis* infection in any anatomic site containing cells capable of supporting its growth. One could almost predict that chlamydial infection of the digestive tract will be found in some of the neonates at risk. It is likely that research during the next few years will provide considerable information on the public health significance of chlamydial infections in neonates, but the data at hand already suggest that there may indeed be highly significant pathogens in this population.

In an effort to answer some of the questions raised above, we and our colleagues have undertaken a number of studies on chlamydial pneumonia in neonates. At San Francisco General Hospital we have found approximately 4% of pregnant women to have chlamydial infection of the cervix. We have detected 2 cases of chlamydial pneumonia in a prospective study based on 500 pregnant women (Grossman, Holt, and Sweet, unpublished data, 1977).

Chlamydial pneumonia did develop in infants who never had detectable conjunctival infection. In addition, we found chlamydial infection of the vagina in female neonates and we found rectal infections and fecal shedding of chlamydiae to occur in infants with and without respiratory disease.

At Kaiser Hospital we have serologically diagnosed 4 cases of chlamydial pneumonia during a period when there were 1,350 births. During this time eight infants with pneumonia were admitted (Shinefield and Miller, unpublished data, 1977). Thus it would appear that *C. trachomatis* was responsible for approximately one half of the cases of pneumonia. Although the numbers are very small, a provisional estimate of incidence may be 3 to 4 cases of chlamydial pneumonia per 1,000 live births.

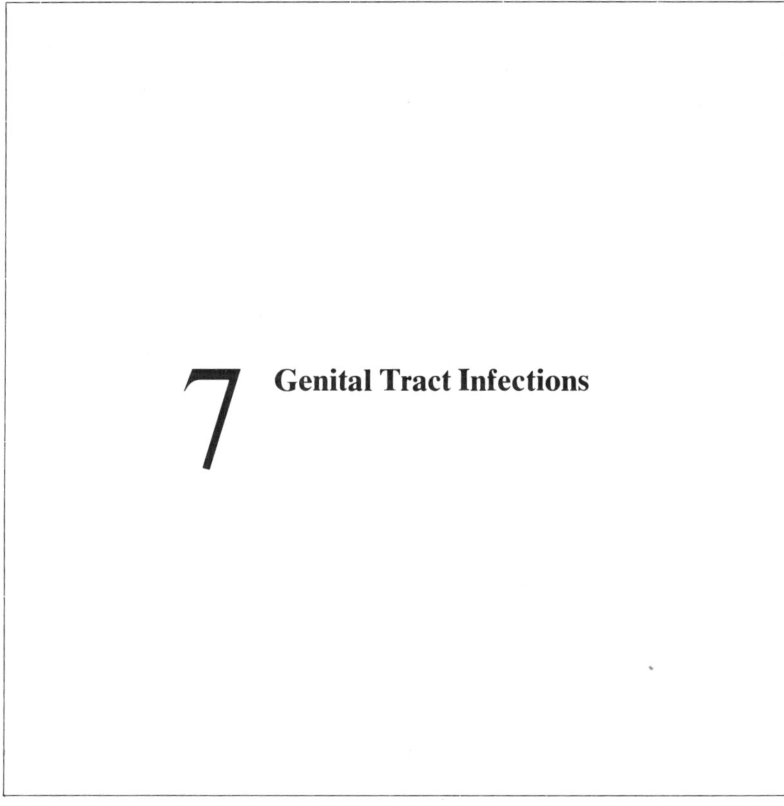

HISTORICAL ASPECTS

Although general interest in chlamydial infections of the genital tract is very recent, the association of these agents with genital tract disease has a long history. The chlamydial disease affecting the eye in the newborn led to the elucidation of the epidemiology of these infections in the first decade of this century. In the latter part of the nineteenth century, gonococci were thought to be the sole cause of neonatal conjunctivitis. But following the introduction of Credé prophylaxis, it became apparent that there were other causes of neonatal ophthalmia. Kroner (1884) reported on this nongonococcal form, and Morax described it as "conjonctivite amicrobienne" (1903). In 1907, Halberstaedter and von Prowazek (a,b) demonstrated typical intracytoplasmic inclusions in conjunctival scrapings from orangutans that had been infected with material collected from patients suffering from trachoma. Shortly thereafter, they found identical inclusions in conjunctival epithelial cells collected from infants suffering from ophthalmia neonatorum (Halberstaedter and von Prowazek, 1909). Many other workers soon confirmed their results (Stargardt, 1909;

121

Schmeichler, 1909; Heymann, 1909; Lindner, 1909). Heymann (1910) discovered inclusions in the cervix of the mother and in the urethra of the father of an infant with the disease now called inclusion blennorrhea.

There was speculation that these agents could be the potential causes of an amicrobial form of urethritis that had been described earlier (Guiard, 1897; Waelsch, 1904). Lindner performed tests on men with nongonococcal urethritis (NGU) and found typical inclusions in the urethral epithelial cells in 3 of 10 cases (1910), a proportion consistently found in studies being performed today. Thus, it was known that the agent of inclusion blennorrhea of the newborn and, soon thereafter, inclusion conjunctivitis of the adult (and possibly trachoma as well, since some of these authors had considerable problems with the differential diagnosis of these eye conditions) were sexually transmitted. The agent was known to infect the urethra of the male and the cervix of the female, and to cause eye disease when the infective genital tract discharges accidentally came in contact with the conjunctiva. The agents may be clinically inapparent in the genital tract, or they may cause cervicitis in the female or urethritis in the male. For all practical purposes, little has been added to the clinical and epidemiologic knowledge that existed in 1911. Nowadays, more cases may be studied and the diagnosis made by isolation rather than by tedious cytologic studies, but the end results are essentially much the same. Unfortunately, until very recently, the pioneering studies were ignored or overlooked by most workers.

Since the introduction of the yolk sac technique for isolation of trachoma and inclusion conjunctivitis agents, isolates have been obtained from the conjunctivae of adults and neonates and from the cervices and the urethras of epidemiologically related cases. The first recovery of chlamydiae from the genital tract was made in 1959 by Jones, Collier, and Smith, who isolated a TRIC agent from the cervix of the mother of a baby suffering from ophthalmia neonatorum. Chlamydiae were also recovered from the baby's eye. The first isolates from the male urethra were reported in 1964, when chlamydiae were recovered from the urethras of fathers of babies with inclusion blennorrhea, from men with adult inclusion conjunctivitis, and from the male sexual contacts of women with inclusion conjunctivitis (Jones, 1964; Dunlop, Jones, and Al-Hussaini, 1964; Rose and Schachter, 1964). The same workers also recovered chlamydiae from the cervices of women who had had sexual contact with male patients with eye disease.

In these initial isolation attempts, the index cases were patients with eye disease, and the studies expanded to include sexual contacts (Jones, 1964; Schachter, Rose, and Meyer, 1967). Dunlop et al. (1966b) then applied the same techniques to study men with nongonococcal urethritis (NGU), and 4 of the 10 patients were found to have chlamydial infection. Thus, by 1966 modern (and more expensive) techniques had merely confirmed the conclusions presented 56 years before!

Although it was clear that chlamydiae were obviously associated with genital tract disease, the cumbersome yolk sac technique made it very difficult to study large numbers of patients. Gordon and Quan (1965b) introduced a tissue culture method for the isolation of *Chlamydia*. A number of small-scale studies proved the feasibility of the method, and large surveys on chlamydial infection of the urethra and cervix were performed in a number of countries, particularly Great Britain (Tables 1 and 2).

Table 1
Recovery of Chlamydiae From the Male Urethra

			Percent of Patients Yielding Chlamydiae			
			NGU*	Gonorrhea	PGU†	Control
England	Dunlop	1972	44			
England	Richmond	1972	39	32	76	5
England	Oriel	1972	36			0
Canada	Ford	1971	5			
U.S.A.	Philip	1971	23	16		
U.S.A.	Schachter	1975	36	11		0‡
U.S.A.	Holmes	1975	42	19	60	7§
England	Oriel	1975		25	60	

* NGU = nongonococcal urethritis.
† PGU = postgonococcal urethritis.
‡ Patients with pyuria excluded.
§ Asymptomatic pyuria found in those tested.

Table 2
Recovery of Chlamydiae From the Cervix

			Percent of Patients Yielding Chlamydiae				
			Attending VD Clinic	Gonor- rhea	NGU Contacts	Cervicitis	Con- trol
England	Dunlop	1972			29		
England	Oriel	1972			67†		
England	Oriel	1974	18				
England	Hilton	1974	31	63	34		3
U.S.A.	Wentworth	1973	21				
U.S.A.	Kuo	1972	28			34	
England	Hobson	1974	20			63*	
U.S.A.	Schachter	1975				36(47*)	3
U.S.A.	Holmes	1975			68†		

* Cervical erosions.
† Contact of chlamydiae-positive NGU.

NONGONOCOCCAL URETHRITIS
IN MALES

Dunlop and his colleagues (1972b) isolated chlamydiae from 44 of 99 men with NGU (Figs. 1, 2, Plate 8). In a comparison of the methods used for collecting specimens from the male urethra, they found that either using endourethral swabs or scraping with a curette was essentially equivalent (37% versus 39% positive), but that collection from the meatus was considerably less efficient (26% positive).* Female sexual contacts were also studied, and 10 of 34 yielded chlamydial isolates (cervix, 10 of 33; rectum, 3 of 33; urethra, 2 of 11). Even though the women studied were often asymptomatic, only 5 had normal cervices; 21 showed some signs of mucosal change (Fig. 3, Plate 8), and 9 of these yielded isolates. The rectal isolates were obtained from women who showed signs of proctitis or inflammation of the anal-rectal mucosa, and the urethral isolates were obtained from women with either grossly inflamed urethras or pus in their urine. Five of the women had salpingitis (2 isolates).

These workers have noted that chlamydial infection of the genital tract may be associated with "follicle-like" lesions (Figs. 2, 3, Plate 8). These are grossly similar to the follicles seen in chlamydial conjunctivitis (Chapters 4 and 5).

In Richmond, Hilton, and Clarke's (1972) study of chlamydial infections in patients with NGU and gonococcal urethritis, 39% (40 of 103) of the NGU patients and 32% (32 of 99) of the patients with gonococcal urethritis yielded chlamydiae. One of the 40 of *Chlamydia*-positive NGU cases had conjunctivitis, as did one in the Dunlop group mentioned above. A "control" population of asymptomatic men had a chlamydial carriage rate of 5% (5 of 92). These men were also attending VD clinics and conceivably could have had low-grade urethritis. When the patients and controls were matched on the basis of types of recent sexual contact, the association of chlamydial recovery with urethritis was statistically significant. These workers also found an association between chlamydial carriage among patients with gonococcal urethritis and the development of postgonococcal urethritis (PGU); those who were initially *Chlamydia*-positive were more prone to develop PGU. It was suggested that *Chlamydia* may not be a primary cause of NGU, but that other types of urethral

---

* Our studies support these conclusions. In our early work we used curettes and separately scraped the four quadrants of the urethra. Chlamydiae were not recovered regularly from all four specimens — possibly suggesting focal infection. Urine and urine sediment have not proven to be useful specimens for chlamydial isolation.

inflammation activate a quiescent chlamydial infection. This interpretation certainly may be true in some cases, but on the basis of their own data, it is certainly subject to other, more likely interpretations. The 5% carriage rate in controls (which is higher than reported elsewhere) may not necessarily be indicative of the background of quiescent chlamydial infection, but could be due to poor selection of controls and failure to vigorously rule out urethritis. There is also the obvious possibility of simultaneous infection with two agents (gonococci and chlamydiae) that have different incubation periods.

This is not to suggest that latent or subclinical infections do not occur. They are probably relatively common. However, most of the clinically inapparent chlamydial infections of the male urethra have, in our experience, occurred in patients with white cells in their urine *and* a history of previous bouts with NGU; they had been given a treatment course which provided symptomatic relief, but one that we would consider inadequate for eradication of chlamydiae. More recent data on the prevalence of chlamydial antibodies in NGU patients and controls (Holmes et al., 1975) suggest that some of the previous failures to demonstrate differentially higher seroreactor rates among NGU patients than among patients with gonococcal and postgonococcal urethritis might reflect inadequate group specific tests and poor population selection. In addition, recent results suggest that chlamydiae are extremely common in patients attending VD clinics, so it is unlikely that these patients, who tend to be repeaters, would have antibodies to only the organism responsible for their current disease episode.

Oriel et al. (1972) studied 150 men with NGU. They recovered chlamydiae from 49 of 135 valid specimens but none from 34 men without urethritis. The use of either a urethral curette or swabs yielded essentially the same recovery rates (38% versus 35%). Sexual contacts of these men yielded chlamydial isolates from 13 of 38 cervical specimens and 8 of 38 urethral specimens. The agent was recovered from 12 of 18 contacts of *Chlamydia*-positive men but from only 1 of 23 contacts of *Chlamydia*-negative men. The authors concluded that this result provided further evidence for the sexual transmission of the chlamydiae. There was no apparent difference in the clinical disease in the *Chlamydia*-positive and *Chlamydia*-negative NGU cases although patients with chlamydiae may have had a slightly longer incubation period. Richmond and colleagues (1972) also found that the *Chlamydia*-positive men appeared to have longer durations of untreated discharge, both among patients with NGU and in patients with proven gonococcal infection.

In San Francisco, approximately 20% of 282 men seeking medical attention for genital tract symptoms were found to have chlamydial infections (Schachter et al., 1975b). Chlamydiae were only recovered from those with urethral symptoms or findings. The chlamydial recovery rate was particularly high (57%) in those who had NGU with frank, persistent discharge. The recovery rate was much lower in those with mild dysuria or asymptomatic pyuria (9%). These groups were all considered to have NGU, with the overall recovery rate at 36%. Chlamydiae were never recovered from the 57 men who had had normal urinalyses.

The lowest reported rate of recovery of TRIC agents in patients with NGU is 5% (8 of 151) by Ford and McCandlish (1971) in Canada. It is probable that this low rate was due to some technical deficiency in their method, since much higher rates have been reported in Seattle (Handsfield et al., 1972) and San Francisco (Schachter et al., 1975b) where the populations tested were probably similar to that of the Vancouver study.

In Taiwan, Gale et al. (1970) studied men attending a military VD clinic for urethritis cases and found only 10% to have chlamydial infections. In New Delhi, India, Mukhija et al. (1973) failed to isolate chlamydiae using the yolk sac technique on specimens from patients with nongonococcal urethritis. Although these studies are limited, they suggest that chlamydial genital tract infections may not be as common in areas of current or recent trachoma endemicity.

The single study presenting the most convincing data on the causative role of chlamydiae in NGU was performed by the group at the University of Washington (Holmes et al., 1975). Their chlamydial recovery rates were comparable to those obtained elsewhere: 42% (48 of 113) for NGU versus 19% (13 of 69) for GC and 7% (4 of 58) for men without overt urethritis. The higher infection rates were paralleled by higher serologic positivity rates. Microimmunofluorescent antibody rates were correlated with current and previous bouts of NGU. This latter also held true for a group of matched control men with no current urethritis. When paired sera were tested, it was found that the majority (9 of 17) of men without antibody titers who yielded chlamydiae did seroconvert. This result suggests that most of this symptomatic group had been infected shortly before attending the clinic.

In a later study by this group, chlamydiae were found in 26 of 69 men (38%) having a first episode of NGU, compared to only 1 of 39 men without urethritis (Bowie et al., 1977). Of 10 culture-positive men seen within the first ten days of symptoms, 9 demonstrated seroconversion to chlamydial antigens by the microimmunofluorescence (micro-IF) technique. Sixteen of 20 men (80%) with *Chlamydia*-positive NGU had IgM antibody to chlamydiae, compared to 3 of 39 (4%) with *Chlamydia*-negative NGU, and none of the 34 men without urethritis. In this study, all 13 patients with *Chlamydia*-positive urethritis who received a ten-day course of sulfisoxazole responded, while only 14 of 29 *Chlamydia*-negative, *Ureaplasma*-positive NGU cases responded (P < 0.002).

Bowie and co-workers (1976) further exploited the principle of differential therapy to elucidate the etiology of NGU by comparing clinical response and culture results. They treated men with NGU with either sulfisoxazole or an aminocyclitol. The sulfonamide is active against *C. trachomatis,* which was recovered from 40% of their NGU patients, but it is not active against ureaplasmas. The aminocyclitols have the opposite antibiotic activity. The responses to therapy in this group were essentially those to be expected if both ureaplasmas and chlamydiae were contributing to the etiology of NGU. Treatment with the aminocyclitols resulted in no clinical response for the 6 men who were *Chlamydia*-positive and *Ureaplasma*-negative, while 9 of 11 men who were *Chlamydia*-negative but *Ureaplasma*-positive responded. If the ureaplasmas persisted despite this therapy, the clinical response was poor. The sulfonamide resulted in the cure of all 7 men with *Chlamydia*-positive, *Ureaplasma*-negative NGU and produced clinical response in 5 of 19 *Chlamydia*-negative, *Ureaplasma*-positive NGU patients. Men with double infections responded poorly to single antimicrobial therapy.

These results further suggest not only that chlamydiae are a cause of NGU but also that (1) ureaplasmas contribute to this condition, (2) there is a spontaneous remission in at least some *Chlamydia*-negative NGU cases, and (3) some cases of NGU are caused by something other than these two organisms. In the first Bowie study, ureaplasmas were recovered more frequently (35/43; 81%) from *Chlamydia*-negative than from *Chlamydia*-positive NGU patients (11/26; 42%) (Bowie et al., 1977). They were also recovered frequently from men without urethritis (22/38; 59%). The ureaplasmas were also recovered at greater concentrations from *Chlamydia*-negative NGU patients. This was most marked at concentrations above 10^3 color-changing units per ml. Wong and co-workers (1977) also report a higher *Ureaplasma* recovery rate from men with *Chlamydia*-negative NGU than from those with either *Chlamydia*-positive NGU or no urethritis. Perhaps more meaningful, however, is their observation that while a statistically significant association of ureaplasmas and NGU was not found in an analysis of their entire population, such an association was found for *Chlamydia*-negative NGU.

Whether or not *Ureaplasma* infections cause some nonchlamydial NGU is of obvious practical import and has significant therapeutic implications. However, the studies of Bowie and colleagues have effectively dealt with the theory that chlamydiae may be "passengers" in the genital tract.

The fact that successful antichlamydial therapy is also generally effective in treatment of NGU supports the cultural and serologic evidence which implicates chlamydiae in the etiology of the condition.

DIAGNOSIS OF NONGONOCOCCAL URETHRITIS

Basically, NGU is a diagnosis which is reached by exclusion. The routine workup of male urethritis must always start with tests for gonococcal infection. In the absence of gonococcal infection, an effort (usually not rewarded) may be made to establish infection with *Herpesvirus, Trichomonas vaginalis,* or *Candida albicans.* Attempts to recover *Chlamydia* should be made in tissue cultures on urethral swabs inserted several centimeters into the urethra. Chlamydial isolation techniques, discussed in detail in Chapter 11, are not yet routinely available to most clinicians.

In general, the clinician will be attempting to establish a diagnosis in a patient who either has a discharge or complains of dysuria or frequency of urination. Discharge should be smeared, and the presence of white cells is adequate grounds to assume the existence of a urethritis. In the absence of discharge, other attempts must be made to determine the presence of urethral inflammation. The two techniques which can be used to establish urethritis (defined as the presence of leukocytes) would be microscopic examination of either a urethral scraping or a urine sample. Urinalysis should be performed on a first morning specimen or one collected several hours after previous urination. Some workers use direct leukocyte count on the first urine specimen, while others prefer a count of centrifuged urine sediment. In either instance a standardized procedure should be used, and, although the values applied in various studies are arbitrary (such as 20 white blood cells per high-powered field), they are necessary in order to supply an objective measurement of urethral inflammation and to allow for a laboratory test which can be used to determine response to therapy.

CERVICAL INFECTION WITH CHLAMYDIAE

Although it has been relatively easy to assign chlamydiae an etiologic role in NGU, it is more difficult to attribute a causative role to chlamydiae in cervicitis. Kuo et al. (1972) found a higher recovery rate in women with cervicitis than in women with normal cervices. Wentworth et al. (1973) confirmed the high chlamydial recovery rate (21.5%) in women attending the same venereal disease clinic. But the latter workers pointed out the complicated nature of the etiology of cervical disease. They found most of the women infected with more than one potential pathogen. The same might be said, of course, for gonococcal infections of the cervix — here, too, the bacteria can be recovered from both symptomatic and asymptomatic women in combination with other pathogens.

Oriel et al. (1974) studied chlamydial infections in 247 women attending a clinic for sexually transmitted diseases. Forty-five (18%) of these women yielded chlamydial isolates from cervical scrapings. Most of the positive tests came from women who either had gonorrhea or were contacts of men with NGU (36 of 45). A large proportion of these women (20 of 45, 44%) were free of symptoms. No association could be made between chlamydial recovery and the use of oral contraceptives. Only 1 of 49 women with negative history and negative routine tests for other sexually transmitted infections was *Chlamydia*-positive. Most of the *Chlamydia*-positive women had some abnormality of the cervix by clinical or cytologic criteria. Twenty-three of the 26 *Chlamydia*-positive women without gonorrhea or trichomoniasis had such findings. Of course, this was a high-risk population for such findings, and the numbers were inadequate to allow statistical analysis. Of the entire 318, 28% attended the clinic because their sexual contacts had had NGU.

Hilton et al. (1974) studied the prevalence of genital tract pathogens among 279 women attending a VD clinic and 63 attending a family planning clinic. Gonococci were recovered from 57 (20%), herpesvirus type 2 from 7 (3%), and chlamydiae from 86 (31%) of the VD patients. Only 2 (3%) of the control group were found to have chlamydiae. The chlamydiae were recovered at comparable rates from women attending the VD clinic for screening purposes and those attending because of symptoms. Herpesviruses were recovered more often from women coming for screening. Women with gonorrhea had a significantly higher isolation rate of chlamydiae (62%) than did other patients. Chlamydiae were more often recovered from women whose male contacts had nongonococcal urethritis (34%) than from women whose contacts were apparently asymptomatic (17%). Eighty-two percent of the women with uncomplicated chlamydial infections had abnormal cervical examinations, but in this VD clinic, 56% of the women with no demonstrable pathogen had abnormal cervices. A statistically significant higher rate of recovery (45%) was found for women taking oral contraceptives than for those not taking them (24%). Results of isolation attempts performed on pregnant women suggested that length of pregnancy might have a role in influencing the chlamydial isolation rate; all 5 pregnant women yielding chlamydiae were in the third trimester (17 tested), and none of the 16 in the first or second trimesters were positive.

Wentworth et al. (1973) studied 385 women attending a VD clinic in Seattle. In addition to chlamydiae and gonococci, they also tested for T strain mycoplasma, *Mycoplasma hominis,* cytomegalovirus, *Trichomonas vaginalis,* and *Candida albicans* in their study. They recovered chlamydiae from 21.5%, GC from 16.7%, and herpesvirus from 5.8%. A major point of this study was that at least 61% of the specimens yielded a multiplicity of agents that could be regarded as genital tract pathogens.

The recovery of chlamydiae from 20% of women attending another venereal disease clinic in England is quite similar to results elsewhere (Hobson et al., 1974). These workers found a higher recovery rate in women with hypertrophic cervical erosions, as 22 of 35 (63%) women with this diagnosis were *Chlamydia*-positive. After a three-week course of systemic tetracycline, all these patients were isolate-negative. Their findings for cervicitis are similar to our results in San Francisco, where we found a very specific association of chlamydial infection with cervicitis. Chlamydiae were recovered from 36% of the women with cervicitis, compared to only 4% recovery from women with vaginitis but no cervicitis (Schachter et al., 1975b). We, too, found an even higher chlamydial recovery rate from those women with cervical erosions. In this study, chlamydiae were the most common pathogens in a survey of 1,269 women. Chlamydiae were recovered from 3.5% of the 665 women undergoing routine examinations and from 15.6% of the 604 women who attended the clinics because of symptoms.

Perhaps the best evidence linking chlamydiae and cervicitis comes from Rees and colleagues (1977), who studied a selected population of 254 female contacts of men with NGU. Infection with *C. trachomatis* was associated with 87% of the hypertrophic cervical erosions and 84% of the mucopurulent endocervical contents observed in these women. After a three-week course of tetracycline, the erosions were no longer hypertrophic, but had become simple, and cervical secretion remained purulent in only one of the 45 women who had had this finding.

Sexual contacts of patients with nonspecific urethritis are usually found to have inflammatory changes demonstrable on cervical smears (Simmons and Vosmik, 1974). Obviously, most studies show that contacts of *Chlamydia*-positive nongonococcal urethritis are more likely to have chlamydial infections than other patients attending VD clinics; thus, it would appear this study also provides indirect evidence that the chlamydiae are causing some cervical inflammation.

The normal baseline of carriage in chlamydial genital tract infections is not known. Thygeson and Mengert (1936) estimated that 1% of normal pregnant women had cervical inclusions. Using yolk sac isolation procedures, Foy et al. (1967) found 2 of 149 pregnant women to be *Chlamydia*-positive, and Chiang et al. (1968) found 2 of 86 normal pregnant women in Taiwan to be carrying chlamydiae. More recent studies, using cell cultures, indicate that the baseline in women is less than 5%, with an even lower baseline in men. The Taiwan study is of particular interest because relatively small recovery rates were obtained in prostitutes (2 of 59), and no positive cultures or recoveries of chlamydiae were obtained in patients with nongonococcal urethritis. Similar low results were obtained with tissue culture methods for men studied in Taiwan (Gale et al., 1970). The possibility that there may be some differences between genital tract chlamydial carriage in trachoma-endemic areas and other areas or among different socioeconomic strata must be considered, although the possibility of self-treatment with antibiotics cannot be eliminated. However, Shaaban et al. (1971) found that 20% of the women (10 of 51) attending an outpatient clinic in Assiut, Egypt, where trachoma is endemic, had chlamydial infections of the cervix. Three of the isolate-positive women had had children who had developed inclusion blennorrhea. Unfortunately, no epidemiologic data on this population were presented.

It is not known how long the chlamydiae persist in the genital tract, but the observation that successive infants born to the same mother have developed inclusion blennorrhea suggests that infection may persist for as long as three or four years (Thygeson and Stone, 1942). We have documented carriage for at least a year in men and women.

POSTGONOCOCCAL URETHRITIS

Richmond et al. (1972), in their study on men attending a VD clinic, found that 32% of the men with gonorrhea also had chlamydial infections. In a prospective survey, they found that most (76%) of the PGU occurred in this doubly infected group. Oriel et al. (1975) confirmed this observation, feeling that in their population chlamydiae were responsible for most of the PGU. In the Seattle study, all 12 men with evidence of double infections with chlamydiae and gonococci developed PGU after treatment for gonorrhea (Holmes et al., 1975). Another 9 men, free of chlamydial infection, also developed PGU. The general consensus is that between one-fourth and one-third of all

132

men being treated with penicillin for gonorrhea develop PGU. It appears that chlamydiae may be responsible for close to two-thirds of this syndrome.

TREATMENT

Although the treatment regimen of choice is not known, it is clear that there can be a rapid clinical response to tetracyline and that prolonged therapy eradicates genital tract chlamydial infection. We treat the genital tract chlamydial infections with systemic tetracycline (250 mg q.i.d. for 21 days; see Chapter 5, Adult Inclusion Conjunctivitis). This has been the standard treatment used so successfully in most of the studies mentioned above. Courses of less than one week still allow chlamydial recovery in some patients and likely lead to relapse in a significant proportion.

Successful treatment implies microbiologic cure (eradication of chlamydiae) and reversal of the urethritis (failure to demonstrate leukocytes in urethral scrapings or urine). It is imperative that the partners of patients with chlamydial infection be treated in parallel with the patient. This is one of the reasons we recommend the full 21-day course of tetracycline. In some instances delay in treating the consort can lead to reinfection of the patient, who may be terminating a shorter course of therapy while the consort is just beginning a course and is still potentially infective.

Shorter courses may be successful if only men are to be treated because their consorts are not available. Handsfield and associates (1976) have evaluated the efficacy of tetracycline (500 mg four times daily for seven days) for the treatment of NGU. Both *Chlamydia*-positive and *Chlamydia*-negative NGU responded significantly better to tetracycline than to placebo: 10 *Chlamydia*-positive men who received placebo were isolate-positive at the end of the week's treatment, while none of the *Chlamydia*-positive men treated with tetracycline remained infected. The recurrence or persistence rate for pyuria was significantly higher in *Chlamydia*-negative cases (47%) than in *Chlamydia*-positive cases (17%). Some of the *Chlamydia*-positive NGU patients had recurrences at periods greater than six weeks after therapy and were again *Chlamydia*-positive. Since chlamydiae were recovered from 15 of 24 (62.5%) sex partners of men with *Chlamydia*-positive NGU, compared to only 1 of the 21 (5%) consorts of men with *Chlamydia*-negative NGU, it appears that these late recurrences represent reinfection rather than relapse — a strong indication that both sex partners should be treated at the same time.

The failure to treat nongonococcal urethritis as a venereal disease is probably a major reason that the disease has received a reputation for difficulty in treatment. In part this may stem from a previous, outmoded term for the condition: "nonspecific urethritis." By accepting the nonspecific nature of the condition there is an implicit denial of specific etiology. Currently, we recognize that chlamydiae are major causes of nongonococcal urethritis and that the infection is sexually transmitted. For men with chlamydial urethritis, we find 75% of their sexual contacts carrying chlamydiae in the cervix. Thus, epidemiologic treatment of sexual contacts is warranted for chlamydial urethritis just as it is for gonococcal urethritis.

We see no rationale for treating patients with chlamydial infections with very large doses (2 gm per day or greater) of tetracycline. It is likely that the most significant problem in treating the chlamydial infection is the maintenance of an adequate blood level for an adequate period of time. High blood levels do not seem to provide any improvement. Therefore, the major problem the clinician will have in treating the infection will be in patient compliance with a 21-day course of therapy. This is particularly true in patients with a very rapid clinical response to treatment. It is possible that the long-acting tetracyclines may have a role in treatment of NGU by requiring the patient to take only two doses a day, thus increasing the chances of patient compliance.

Oriel and associates (1975) have investigated the effect of minocycline (100 mg two times daily for 21 days) on NGU. Their test group included 133 men with objective signs of urethritis. Thirty-three (25%) had chlamydial infections. Approximately 90% of the patients were symptomatic. There was a rapid response to treatment: only 12% were symptomatic one week later, and after three weeks only 5% still had symptoms. However, inflammatory cells could be demonstrated in the urethras of approximately 24% of the men at the end of three weeks. There appeared to be no difference in the clinical responses of *Chlamydia*-positive and *Chlamydia*-negative patients. The minocycline treatment eradicated the infection in all 33 *Chlamydia*-positive men and in all 24 of their *Chlamydia*-positive female contacts. Side effects of treatment were noted in 3% of the men and 12% of the women. These vestibular effects were generally seen within the first week of therapy. Minocycline, which may offer some advantages in terms of patient compliance with its twice-a-day regimen, was found to be roughly equivalent to tetracycline in terms of therapeutic response.

Prentice, Taylor-Robinson, and Csonka (1976) also have studied the effect of minocycline on NGU. They found minocycline (1.3 g total in 6 days) highly effective in curing NGU when compared to a lactose placebo (89% symptom- and sign-free versus 28.5% symptom- and sign-free) in a one-week treatment regimen. The efficacy of minocycline was marked in treating chlamydial urethritis: 11 of

12 *Chlamydia*-positive patients responded to therapy, while only 2 of 13 *Chlamydia*-positive patients responded to placebo. These authors also found evidence suggesting that *Ureaplasma urealyticum* was a cause of some of the *Chlamydia*-negative NGU, although the treatment effect and supportive evidence were not as striking as was the evidence for chlamydiae in this syndrome, and some minocycline resistance was noted in ureaplasmas.

In patients who cannot take tetracycline because of side reactions or pregnancy, the treatments which can be substituted would be full doses of sulfonamides or erythromycin. It should be noted that therapeutic regimens successful in treating NGU are effective against both *C. trachomatis* and *Ureaplasma urealyticum* (the latter being the most likely etiologic agent in nonchlamydial NGU).

DISCUSSION

Their observation that chlamydiae probably had a major role in causing PGU led Richmond et al. (1972) to question the primary role of chlamydiae in NGU. They found a relatively high 5% of control men (who did not have urinalysis) harboring chlamydiae and reasoned that chlamydial infection may normally be quiescent until activated by a superinfecting pathogen. Thus, gonococcal infection would activate chlamydiae, resulting in PGU. They postulated that an unknown agent, the real cause of NGU, might be activating the chlamydiae, thus explaining the high rates of chlamydial recovery in NGU. They felt that the equivalent recovery rates of chlamydiae from men with gonorrhea or NGU were further evidence for this hypothesis. (It should be noted [Table 1] that American workers have found higher chlamydial recovery rates from patients with NGU than from patients with gonorrhea.) A further complication is the doubt of some workers that tetracyclines are effective in treating NGU. For example, it is estimated that 20% to 30% of NGU clears spontaneously during the time therapy would be in progress, and most NGU will resolve untreated in less than two months. The best estimates are that tetracycline actually benefits only one third to one half of NGU patients. (For a review, see Grimble and Amarasuriya, 1975.) And of course, venereologists are properly skeptical after disappointing experiences with previous candidates in the etiology of NGU, the most recent being the T strain mycoplasmas.

Similar arguments have been expressed concerning the role of chlamydiae in cervicitis. The clear association of chlamydial infection and cervicitis has been described above and appears to be generally accepted, but some workers do not accept a chlamydial etiology because of the complicated nature of the cervical flora as shown in the study by Wentworth and colleagues (1973). Other workers invoke "Agent X" — the unidentified but actual cause of cervicitis — which is often accompanied by a sexually transmitted, but relatively innocuous, chlamydial infection. (Some workers feel there is inadequate documentation of sexual transmission.)

The cervical lesion most often associated with chlamydial infection is an "erosion" or ectopy. Some feel that this lesion, which indicates extension of squamocolumnar cells, is caused by other factors (e.g., infection, trauma, hormones from birth control pills). An increase in columnar cells would suggest an increase in susceptibility to chlamydiae, because their parasitism is restricted to these cells. Thus the lesion would precede the infection. Support for this viewpoint may come from the recovery of chlamydiae from completely normal cervices.

Some of these arguments are reminiscent of discussions of past decades on the role of "the elementary body virus" in psittacosis or the inclusion in trachoma. Ironically, some early workers discounted the meaning of the inclusion in trachoma because similar "nonspecific corpuscles" could be found in genital tract infections. Rather than being concerned about the recovery of chlamydiae from normal cervices, we would be surprised if these agents were always associated with lesions. All known chlamydial infections (of man, lower mammals, or birds) have a subclinical component in the spectrum of host response to infection (see reviews by Meyer, 1965; Jawetz et al., 1967; Storz, 1971). Latency is characteristic of all chlamydial host-parasite relationships. It is not inconsistent for chlamydiae to act as either primary pathogens or as causes of inapparent infection in the same host species.

It seems to us that there are simpler explanations of the various results than invoking an unknown agent as the primary cause of NGU. It is probably erroneous to consider NGU as a single disease entity, and more reasonable to consider multiple causation. The recent studies by Bowie and associates (1976, 1977), discussed earlier, have provided compelling evidence that *C. trachomatis* is the most clearly identifiable cause of NGU. Thus, chlamydiae are probably responsible for 35% to 50% of NGU, most likely with a clinical spectrum ranging from asymptomatic pyuria to purulent discharge (although a serous discharge is probably typical). These infections do respond to tetracycline therapy, and doubt on this point represents unwarranted extrapolation from Jawetz's (1969) valid reflections on the efficacy of tetracyclines.

Other causes of NGU include *Herpesvirus hominis* in less than 5% of the cases and possibly *Trichomonas vaginalis* and *Candida*

136

albicans in a few cases. Thus, in approximately 40% of NGU there is no readily identifiable pathogen. The most likely candidates are still the mycoplasmas, particularly T strains. Virtually all studies have shown a high prevalence of these organisms in the genital tracts of sexually active men or women. However, most adequately controlled studies have failed to demonstrate a significant association with NGU. It is likely, however, that a reassessment of *Chlamydia*-negative NGU may lead to the identification of any mycoplasma-caused disease. There appears to be a general consensus that chlamydiae are responsible for approximately two of every three cases of PGU.

The effects of chlamydial infection on the cervix are less easily defined. Part of the problem is in the lack of precise clinical criteria for cervicitis. It is clear that clinically normal cervices may be infected with chlamydiae. In our series approximately half of the cervical infections detected during routine screening had no apparent cervicitis. Thus, in some clinics we find up to 50% of the infected women have clinically inapparent infections. Even women with abnormal cervical findings may not have symptoms, so patients are often unaware of the infection. This, of course, is similar to the situation with other microbial infections of the cervix.

In women, response to chemotherapy is also more difficult to assess. Inflammatory changes may resolve (as determined clinically, cytologically, and by biopsy), but ectopic changes persist for periods of at least 1 to 12 months after treatment. These changes may be permanent.

It is quite clear, however, that chlamydiae are a cause of cervicitis. In 1962 we began studies on genital tract chlamydial infections and had the opportunity of following some untreated cases. A few male patients had new sexual contacts after their infections had been identified, and we were able to follow these women through the development of cervical erosions and seroconversion as their chlamydial infections progressed (Fig. 4, Plate 8). Biopsies showed progressive nonspecific inflammatory lesions. We did not find inclusions in the sections, but Swanson et al. (1975) have been successful in demonstrating inclusions in cervical biopsies (Fig. 5). There is a spectrum of disease with chlamydial infection of the cervix, but it is not known what proportion of infections will be subclinical and what proportion will cause disease.

A point that must not be forgotten is that the genital tract chlamydial infections represent the reservoir of ocular disease that occasionally can be quite severe. With the majority of chlamydial studies now being carried out on patients in VD clinics (clearly the highest risk population), the eye disease may be ignored. Although most workers studying genital tract infections have stated that their

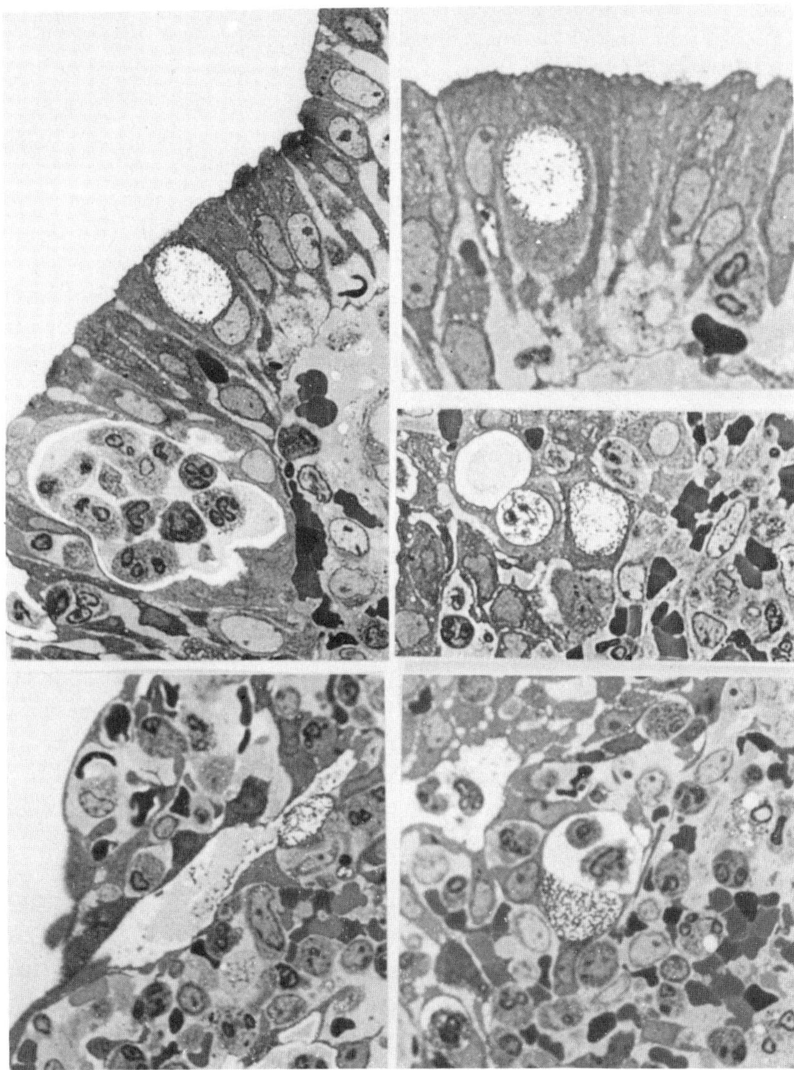

Fig. 5. Chlamydial inclusions in a cervical biopsy. Visualized by phase microscopy of toluidine blue-stained section. (From Swanson, et al., 1975)

patients did not have conjunctivitis, some have noted isolated cases. Our experience is somewhat different. In one study we isolated chlamydiae from the genital tracts of 173 individuals attending clinics at the University of California in San Francisco (Schachter et al., 1975b). None of these patients complained of ocular symptoms or was noted to have conjunctivitis during the examination given to patients upon entering the study. However, a review of these patients' charts revealed that four (approximately 2%) had been attending the

Eye Clinic for diagnosis and treatment of follicular conjunctivitis. In one ironic instance, a patient participating in a double-blind treatment trial informed us (correctly) that she knew she was receiving the tetracycline and not the placebo, not because her genital tract symptoms had improved, but "because my eyes don't stick together in the mornings anymore." Obviously some effort to rule out conjunctivitis should be made. More studies on the true prevalence of adult inclusion conjunctivitis are needed. With increasing genital tract infection we should expect to see more eye disease.

But of greater significance may be the neonatal infections (Chapter 6). In some of our clinics we are now finding the cervical carriage of chlamydiae in normal sexually active women to be as high as 11%. The risk of transmission to the newborn is not known (but from pilot prospective studies we estimate it to be in excess of 30%), and the potential for these agents to cause systemic disease in infants or adults is also uncertain. It is clear that prospective studies in these areas are needed before we can feel that we have defined the clinical spectrum and the public health significance of these chlamydial infections.

Another area needing further study is that of the potential role of chlamydiae in pelvic inflammatory disease (PID). The association was observed in the 1930s (Thygeson and Stone, 1942). Most studies have noted a few cases of PID in mothers of babies with inclusion conjunctivitis. Eschenbach et al. (1975) noted a rising titer of antichlamydial antibodies in some women with PID. We have had similar results and have recovered the organism from the cervix as the sole pathogen. Mårdh and colleagues (1977) have found that approximately 30% of women (6 of 20) with PID had chlamydial infection of the fallopian tubes (as sampled by laparoscopy) and 35.8% (19 of 53) had cervical infections. The study was performed in Sweden, where PID has been increasing and gonorrhea has been decreasing in incidence.

The clinical spectrum of venereally transmitted chlamydial infections is not known. In one study we found epididymitis associated with chlamydial infection of the urethra. However it does not appear fruitful to discuss complications of NGU until chlamydiae are recovered from the involved sites. We have found these agents associated with pharyngitis in adults with inclusion conjunctivitis (Dawson and Schachter, 1967) and in a patient without ocular involvement (Schachter and Atwood, 1975). The agents have also been recovered following myringotomy of a patient with otitis and conjunctivitis (Dawson et al., 1970b), and hearing loss has been documented (Gow, Ostler, and Schachter, 1974). A simplistic approach may be to assume that any anatomic site containing columnar epithelial cells may be susceptible to chlamydial infection and disease if a means of transmission exists.

It should be noted that the discussion in this chapter has been limited to the group of agents known as *Chlamydia trachomatis* (Group A). Some *Chlamydia psittaci* (Group B) strains have been recovered from the human genital tract, but the significance of these observations is not clear.

Nongonococcal urethritis is becoming an increasingly common diagnosis. Most cases of NGU are venereal in origin. Although the condition is being recognized with increasing frequency in the United States, it is very difficult to determine actual prevalence because it is not considered a reportable disease. Some clinics see approximately as much or more nongonococcal urethritis as gonococcal urethritis (Volk and Kraus, 1974). For example, in Seattle 62% of 585 consecutive cases of urethritis were nongonococcal (Holmes et al., 1975). It would appear that there are some socioeconomic differences in the incidence of NGU. It seems to be more prevalent among the more affluent and among college students (Jacobs and Kraus, 1975; McChesney et al., 1973). We have had similar results in studying chlamydial infections in patients attending clinics in the San Francisco Bay area. In VD clinics we find that approximately 60% of urethritis is gonococcal. However, in patients attending street or drop-in clinics, there is a higher rate of NGU, with approximately 60% of urethritis cases being nongonococcal. In patients coming to a hospital clinic, or in university students, gonococcal infections become more infrequent and between 80% to 90% of all urethritis is nongonococcal. In each of the clinics, chlamydiae are responsible for one-third to one-half of the NGU. In all but the VD clinic, chlamydiae are the most commonly recovered organism (Schachter et al., 1975a).

In England and Wales it has become apparent (because of their more accurate statistics) that NGU is now more common in men than gonococcal urethritis. For example, in 1970 there were 54,717 cases of gonorrhea reported for men, women, and children. In the same year 48,550 cases of NGU were reported, exclusively in men (Dunlop et al., 1972a). From these data, the public health significance of genital tract chlamydial infections becomes clear. Since a significant proportion of all GC infections are accompanied by chlamydial infections, and approximately 40% of NGU and 60% of PGU are caused by chlamydiae, it is time to seek specific measures for identification and control of chlamydial infections.

In addition, despite the advances of recent years, we have much to learn about chlamydial genital tract infections. Their natural history is still obscure. We need information on communicability, persistence of infections, and the potential clinical effects of long-term infection. We know nothing about immunity to these infections. It is probable that we know less about chlamydiae than about any other common, treatable pathogen.

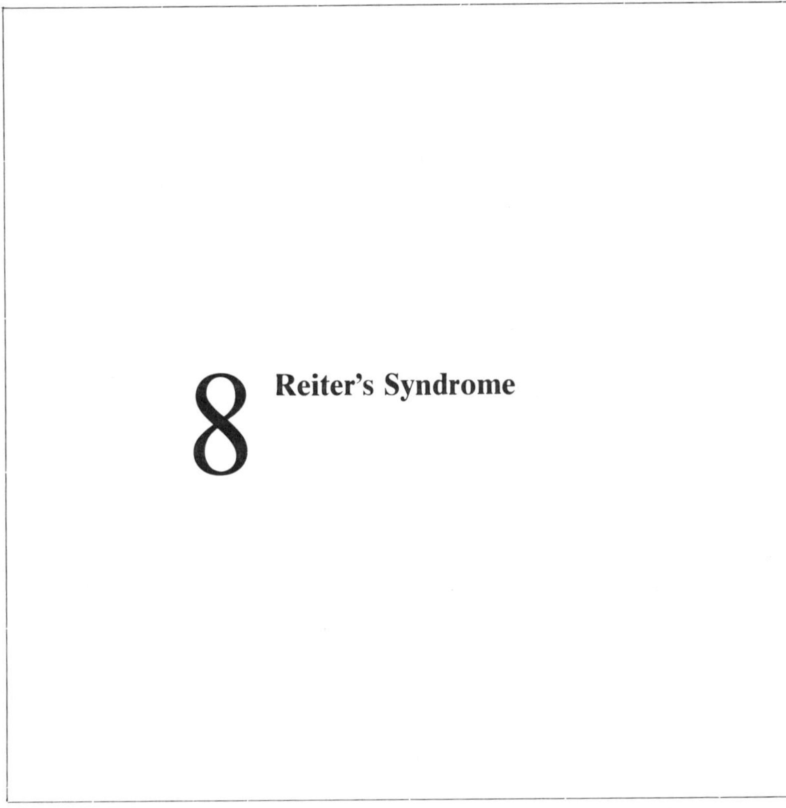

8 Reiter's Syndrome

HISTORICAL ASPECTS

Since the early 1960s there has been speculation that chlamydiae may play an etiological role in Reiter's syndrome (RS). Hans Reiter (1916) published a case history of a young German soldier who developed what is now known as the classical triad — urethritis, conjunctivitis, and arthritis. The syndrome was named after Reiter on the basis of this report, although Sir Benjamin Brodie (1836) had clearly described the condition in the early nineteenth century. In the literature, there are a number of synonymous terms. The most common are "oculourethrosynovial syndrome," and, in the French literature, "Syndrome du Fiessinger-Leroy-Reiter." The latter name recognizes that Fiessinger and Leroy (1916) observed the triad in a French soldier. Ironically, their case and Reiter's occurred in soldiers on opposite sides of the same battle. Both followed outbreaks of dysentery. Reiter's syndrome is essentially a disease of young men, since there is a very marked preponderance of male cases to female cases.

142

CLINICAL DESCRIPTION

Although RS is generally considered a triad, it is quite reasonable to consider it a tetrad, because mucocutaneous lesions represent a significant part of the syndrome (Engleman and Weber, 1968). Although not pathognomonic, the mucocutaneous lesions may be the most specific. Oral lesions are usually asymptomatic, but may be commonly found during examination. They are relatively superficial erythematous ulcerations. The skin lesions (keratodermia blennorrhagica) are most often found on the soles of the feet, occasionally on the palms of the hand or the limbs, and least often on the trunk. Superficially these lesions may resemble those of psoriasis. Initially macular, they may develop into confluent nodules with a hyperkeratotic, crusted appearance. Nails that are involved may fall off. Balanitis, often circinate, is also common. Despite the severe appearance of these lesions, there is usually complete regression.

The urethritis in RS may be quite variable. It is usually nongonococcal or postgonococcal. Discharge may be scant and serous, or mucopurulent. Dysuria is common, as is prostatitis. Urinalysis should be performed on patients suspected of having RS but lacking genitourinary symptoms. In such cases the urinalysis or urethral scrapings may show significant numbers of leukocytes, indicating asymptomatic urethritis.

The arthritis of RS is generally asymmetric. Though large joints, such as the knee, are commonly involved, the hip is usually spared. Small distal joints may be involved, either singly or as a few joints. When a few close distal interphalangeal joints are involved, a "sausage toe" may develop. Sacroileitis is common, but often asymptomatic (particularly in initial episodes of RS) and discovered only after X-ray of the lower back. A common complaint of patients with RS is heel pain which is associated with plantar fasciitis and Achilles tendonitis.

Patients with RS may have constitutional symptoms. They may feel weak, be febrile, and suffer weight loss. Some patients have cardiac involvement, and a severe aortic insufficiency may be the most serious clinical complication. Laboratory tests are usually not helpful. Sedimentation rates are elevated and rheumatoid factor is not found. Joint fluid tends to contain many inflammatory cells. The predominant cell type is the polymorphonuclear leukocyte, although macrophages, many of them filled with phagocytosed cells and debris, are commonly seen. These latter cells are grossly similar to the Leber cells of trachoma. Joint fluids in RS often show elevated complement levels.

Eye involvement in Reiter's syndrome affects the conjunctiva, cornea, and anterior uveal tract. The conjunctivitis is characteristically a smooth, intensely hyperemic infiltration of the mucosa without giant papillae or lymphoid follicles, although rare cases of Reiter's syndrome have followed a follicular conjunctivitis (Fig. 1, Plate 7) (Dawson et al. 1970b; Ostler et al., 1971). The corneal disease takes many forms with punctate epithelial erosions, epithelial erosions, or stromal infiltrates (Dawson et al., 1970b; Ostler et al., 1971; Vergnani and Smith, 1974; Mills and Kalina, 1972). The uveal involvement is characterized by increased protein in the aqueous (the "flare" seen by slit lamp) and fine cells in the aqueous, on the corneal endothelium, and occasionally in the anterior vitreous (Fig. 2, Plate 7) (Ostler et al., 1971). Adhesions may form between the iris and lens (posterior synechiae), but can be prevented by vigorous treatment. Recurrent bouts of iritis can occur along or in conjunction with joint and urethral disease.

Even in those patients shown to have chlamydial infection, treatment with systemic tetracycline does not abort the attack or reduce the risk of recurrent bouts of disease. The iritis responds to treatment with topical corticosteroids, which must be given in doses sufficient to suppress the inflammatory signs, and with mydriatics to prevent the formation of posterior synechiae. Salicylates and phenylbutazone can be effective in treating the joint disease, and might be considered as adjuncts to treatment of the iritis (Engleman and Weber, 1968).

The disease occurs in two epidemiologic forms. Some cases, representing the epidemic, or postdysenteric form, are seen following outbreaks of shigellosis (Paronen, 1948; Noer, 1966). The sporadic venereal form, currently more common in developed countries, appears to follow sexual activity and may be associated with pre-existing venereal disease (particularly gonococcal or nongonococcal urethritis). In some cases there may be considerable difficulty in differentiating between gonococcal arthritis and RS. The RS may not always appear as a full triad, and incomplete forms or a forme fruste is recognized. Such patients usually have urethritis and arthritis, or occasionally ocular manifestations and arthritis. In the majority of cases the symptoms are coincident. However, in many cases there may be a spread of weeks or even months between onset of the different components. The urethritis generally precedes the development of the other symptoms.

RS is usually considered self-limited, and of variable duration, but chronicity and recurrences are common. In Finland, a 20-year follow-up of postdysenteric RS revealed that 42% of the patients had permanent disability (Sairanen, Paronen, and Mähönen, 1969). The spinal disease may become severe and chronic and can present a problem in differential diagnosis with ankylosing spondylitis, especially in those patients who have severe uveitis and severe sacroileitis.

EVIDENCE FOR CHLAMYDIAL INVOLVEMENT

There are many reasons to consider chlamydiae as potential causes of RS. It is well established that chlamydiae cause arthritis in sheep and cattle (Storz, 1971). Infections in these animals are systemic; genital tract and ocular symptoms may also be observed. The infectious agents are often carried in the intestinal tract. They may be recovered from feces of apparently healthy animals and from blood, joints, conjunctiva, and semen of diseased animals. The parallel between the organ systems involved in these animals and those involved in patients with RS is obvious.

Lymphogranuloma venereum is sometimes complicated by arthritis, urethritis, and dermatologic and ocular manifestations (Koteen, 1945). The TRIC agents whose very names are associated with the eye diseases discussed earlier, are also significant as genital tract pathogens. They can cause cervicitis in women and are a major cause of nongonococcal urethritis (NGU) (Dunlop et al., 1972 a,b; Kuo et al., 1972; Oriel et al., 1972; Richmond, Hilton, and Clarke, 1972). Some workers consider RS a complication of nongonococcal urethritis, with an estimated rate of 1% of cases developing arthritis (Morton, 1972). In fact, the first reports linking chlamydiae and RS were those showing typical TRIC agent inclusions in the urethral epithelium of men with RS and NGU (Siboulet and Galistin, 1962; Amor, Coste, and Delbarre, 1967; Zhodzishskii, 1966). These observations, in sum, led several workers to undertake projects assessing the possible role of *Chlamydia* in RS.

STUDIES AT THE UNIVERSITY OF CALIFORNIA, SAN FRANCISCO

Most of our studies were performed from 1964 through 1968. During those years a concerted effort was made to study all available patients with RS. Since 1969 we have studied patients with RS on an irregular basis and have isolated chlamydiae from urethras, conjunctivae, and (rarely) synovia of a proportion of those tested. Approximately one-third of the patients have yielded isolates, the great majority being from the urethra. The later results are not presented because the series was small, patients may have been selected, and changes in laboratory methods and clinical follow-up prevent direct comparison with the earlier results. The techniques used in the earlier studies have been published (Schachter et al., 1970). Briefly, they include isolation attempts performed in the yolk sac of embryonated hens' eggs; complement fixation (CF) tests with chlamydial group antigen; and attempts to demonstrate chlamydial inclusions using Giemsa and fluorescent antibody (FA) stains. The rheumatologic studies were performed under the direction of E.P. Engleman, M.D.

ISOLATION ATTEMPTS

Table 1 summarizes the results of chlamydial isolation attempts and CF tests. In the first two years of this study, eight patients with RS were available for laboratory studies (Schachter et al., 1966). Evidence of active chlamydial infection was found in five, and chlamydiae were isolated from four of five synovial biopsy specimens tested. From 1966 on, partially as a result of these preliminary results, more RS patients were referred, and although some were infected with chlamydiae, the percentage of positive results decreased as the number of patients increased (Schachter, 1967b). Every year from 1964 through 1967, at least one patient with RS yielded a *Chlamydia* from synovial specimens, as did two patients with other forms of arthritis. Both of the latter had positive CF titers. One was diagnosed as having rheumatoid arthritis. The other patient had atypical (seronegative) arthritis and developed prostatitis a year later (chlamydiae were also isolated from prostatic fluid), concurrent with arthritis. We therefore retrospectively considered him to have had RS.

Table 1
**Chlamydial Isolation and Complement Fixation Tests
in 89 Patients with Reiter's Syndrome**

Test	No. Positive/No. Tested
Isolation Attempts	
Synovial Membrane	5/29 (17.2%)
Synovial Fluid	4/34 (11.8%)
Urethra	12/81 (14.8%)
Conjunctiva	3/33 (9.1%)
CF ($\geq 1{:}16$)	20/89 (22.5%)

Of the 89 RS cases tested over the five years, 25 (28.1%) had isolation attempts or CF tests positive for chlamydiae (Table 1). Of these 25 patients, 10 were CF-positive and isolate-negative; 5 were isolate-positive and CF-negative; and 10 were positive in both tests. The greatest number of isolates was derived from urethral scrapings, with 12 of the 81 patients so tested yielding isolates. Chlamydiae were recovered from 10 synovial specimens collected from 6 patients. Five of 29 patients tested yielded isolates from synovial membrane, and

4 of 34 patients tested yielded isolates from synovial fluid. Of these, 3 patients yielded isolates from both synovial fluid and membrane, while 3 were positive in one but negative in the other. Three conjunctival specimens from the 33 patients tested yielded isolates.

As controls for the isolation studies, specimens from more than 125 patients with negative CF titers and arthropathies other than RS were tested. Isolation attempts on 129 synovial, 32 genital, and 28 conjunctival specimens were negative. These specimens were handled in parallel with those from patients with RS, and diagnosis for both groups was made available only after laboratory results were reported.

This control group included 12 patients with ankylosing spondylitis, which, like RS, may affect the eye and genital tract as well as the joints. No chlamydiae were isolated, and only 1 of 12 patients had a CF of 1:16. Results were uniformly negative for patients with psoriasis or psoriatic arthritis.

CYTOLOGIC STUDIES

Attempts to detect typical chlamydial inclusions in specimens from the genital tract and synovia of patients with RS have not been performed systematically and have met with only sporadic success. Inclusions have been seen twice in Giemsa-stained smears of synovial specimens (one yielded an isolate) and five times in urethral scrapings (three being isolate-positive and CF-positive, two being isolate-negative and CF-positive). Results are not complete for attempts by means of fluorescent antibody techniques. The FA method had been fruitful with urethral and conjunctival specimens, showing a higher rate of positive results than Giemsa staining (Dawson et al., 1970b; Schachter et al., 1970). Technical difficulties have limited the usefulness of the test with synovial tissues. In some patients with RS (but not in controls), mononuclear cells in synovial preparations fluoresce, but the fluorescence is throughout the cells' cytoplasm and may be nonspecific, since discrete intracellular inclusions are not found. In many synovial specimens, background fluorescence made the slides impossible to read, regardless of diagnosis.

STUDIES PERFORMED IN OTHER LABORATORIES

Conflicting results have been obtained in chlamydial isolation studies performed in different parts of the world (Table 2). Thus, in France, Amor, Coste, and Delbarre find most of their RS patients have chlamydial infections (Amor, 1969; Amor, Coste, and Delbarre,

Table 2
Recovery of Chlamydiae from Patients with Reiter's Syndrome

Worker	No. Positive/ No. Tested	Anatomic Site
Ford	0/38	
Gordon	1/16	Conjunctiva and urethra
Dunlop	3/10	Urethra — no treatment
	0/19	Urethra—previous treatment
Amor	80% have inclusions	

1967; Amor, Delbarre, and Coste, 1965), while in Canada none of Ford's 38 patients have yielded chlamydiae (Ford, 1968; Ford and McCandlish, 1969; Ford and McCandlish, 1971). Gordon found only 1 of 16 RS patients yielding chlamydiae, the agent being recovered from the patient's urethra and conjunctiva (Gordon et al., 1973). Vaughan-Jackson found that 3 of 10 RS patients had urethral chlamydial infections, while none of the 19 RS patients who had previously been treated with antibiotics yielded any agent (Vaughan-Jackson et al., 1972). This observation emphasizes a problem in chlamydial isolation attempts: tests are often negative if the patient has been treated, and the true infection rate is almost certainly higher than laboratory results indicate.

Mordhorst, studying TRIC agent infections in Denmark, observed that 2 of 12 fathers of infants with inclusion blennorrhea had RS (Mordhorst and Dawson, 1971). We have also observed this juxtaposition of diseases, having studied a couple where one partner had inclusion conjunctivitis while the other had RS (Dawson et al., 1970b). Russian workers have reported recovery of chlamydiae from synovium of a patient with RS (Shatkin et al., 1973).

IMMUNOLOGIC RESPONSE TO CHLAMYDIAE IN REITER'S SYNDROME

In our laboratory we have used the complement fixation test for chlamydial group antigen to study the antibody response in RS. Approximately 22% (Table 1) of the patients with Reiter's syndrome had CF antibody titers of $\geq 1:16$. Several other workers have used the same test and have found no difference between the CF reactor rates (at $\geq 1:16$) in patients with Reiter's syndrome and selected patients attending VD clinics (Table 3) (Ford, 1968; Kinsella, Norton, and Ziff, 1968; Sharp, Lidsky, and Riley, 1968). We have compared the CF response in 77 patients with RS and in controls (matched for age, sex, and race) with gonorrhea (GC) and nongonococcal urethritis

148

Table 3
Serologic Tests for Chlamydiae
in Patients with Reiter's Syndrome

Serologic Test	Reiter's (%)	VD Patients (%)
Ford — CF	20	17
Kinsella — CF	12.5	14.9
Sharp — CF	14.3	30
Dunlop — FA	80	?

(Schachter, 1971). The differences in CF rates between RS (28.4%) and NGU (5.2%) or GC (9.1%) were statistically significant. In addition, the CF titers in 10% of the RS patients were at the very high levels often seen in LGV (a systemic chlamydial infection) and much higher than those ever obtained in men with TRIC agent urethritis (a localized chlamydial infection). Using a microimmunofluorescent method, English workers have found high rates (80%) of antibodies to chlamydiae in patients with RS (Vaughan-Jackson et al., 1972). We have also used this test and find the background rate in sexually active individuals to be very high. The differences observed between RS cases and controls with venereal disease in the CF test are not found. More data on controls must be forthcoming from the English studies before they can be assessed.

In France, approximately 75% of patients with Reiter's syndrome show lymphoblastic transformation when their cultured lymphocytes are exposed to chlamydial antigen (Amor et al., 1972; Doury, Pattin, and Durosoir, 1973) (Table 4). With a small number of patients, we have found that both lymphocyte transformation and leukocyte migration inhibition tests give essentially the same results as the other microbiologic tests for chlamydial infection. Alepa found that only clinically inactive RS patients had positive transformation reactions (Alepa, 1968).

Table 4
Lymphocyte Transformation Tests with Chlamydial
Antigen in Reiter's Syndrome

	Reiter's (%)	Normals
Alepa	82 inactives only	0
Amor	76	0
Doury	75	0

EXPERIMENTAL STUDIES

Some chlamydiae isolated from patients with RS have been tested for their ability to produce arthritis or eye disease in experimentally infected rabbits and subhuman primates. We have found that both invariably develop an acute arthritis after direct inoculation of the organism into the joint (Smith et al., 1973). In monkeys the arthritis is self-limited; in rabbits the arthritis becomes chronic. Inoculation of the agent into the anterior chamber of the rabbit's eye produces a severe uveitis (Ostler, Schachter, and Dawson, 1970). Both arthritis and ocular responses are dose dependent and relatively small numbers of organisms produce the disease. Viable multiplying organisms are necessary, because inactivated organisms or control fluids do not produce inflammatory responses. Of considerable interest is the observation that approximately 15% to 20% of the rabbits develop systemic manifestations — for example, animals inoculated in the eye may develop arthritis several weeks later, while animals inoculated in the joint may develop iritis several weeks later.

The arthritis in rabbits is amenable to chemotherapy, and early, adequate administration of tetracycline will prevent or reverse the arthritic process. However, once the arthritis is well established (between one and two weeks) tetracycline has no effect, and a chronic phase persists for periods of longer than one year (Gilbert et al., 1973).

DIAGNOSIS OF REITER'S SYNDROME

The studies on the role of chlamydiae in RS have led to several questions regarding diagnosis of RS. It is clear that a patient appearing with nongonococcal urethritis, certain types of joint involvement, conjunctivitis and/or iritis, and mucocutaneous lesions has classical Reiter's syndrome. The diagnosis is more difficult when these symptoms do not occur at the same time or if the patient develops only two of the symptoms in the complex. We have attempted to correlate evidence of chlamydial infection with clinical findings (Table 5). Chlamydiae are more often recovered from patients *lacking* the classical triad or tetrad. The highest rate of recovery has been from patients having what is called the forme fruste or incomplete RS — nongonococcal urethritis and seronegative polyarthritis. This difference has been statistically significant; the other differences observed in this study were not, although several were suggestive (for example, patients with mucocutaneous lesions tended not to have chlamydial

150

Table 5
Characteristics of Patients with Reiter's Syndrome
Related to Chlamydial Positivity

Clinical Feature (number)	Present	Absent	X^2
Urethritis and arthritis only (84)	9/19*	14/65	4.93
Triad (84)	12/46	10/38	0.04
Tetrad (84)	2/12	21/72	0.81
Mucocutaneous lesions (84)	2/23	21/61	5.56?
Uveitis (84)	5/10	18/74	2.92
Previous treatment (52)	8/28	12/24	2.51

* No. *Chlamydia* positive/No. tested.

infections). These findings may indicate subclassifications within RS or perhaps that several etiologically distinct (but clinically similar) entities are lumped into RS.

THE ROLE OF CHLAMYDIAE IN REITER'S SYNDROME

Could Chlamydiae Be the Sole Cause for RS?   The finding that in France virtually all patients with RS have chlamydial infection while in the United States some patients and in Canada none of the patients with RS have chlamydial infection indicates that chlamydiae cannot be the sole cause. In addition, the lack of response to antibiotics indicates that RS is not caused by a simple, direct, infectious process due to chlamydiae. If a superficial chlamydial infection were to become systemic and the patient were to develop disease in the infected sites, one would expect the chlamydial disease to respond to rapid chemotherapy. The course of RS is so variable that it is difficult to assess chemotherapeutic results, but all evidence indicates that at least the arthritic process and iritis, even when treated early, are not responsive to chemotherapy. It is, therefore, unlikely that chlamydiae are the sole cause of RS.

Could Chlamydiae Be Passengers with an Epidemiologic Pattern Similar to That of the True Etiologic Agent? Obviously, this is a possibility one must consider, but it is impossible to discuss this likelihood meaningfully until a candidate is proposed. It is true that much of the chlamydial infection in RS could reflect the high prevalence of TRIC agent genital tract infections in sexually active individuals. However, RS patients with chlamydial infections have a wider age range and less sexual exposure than most patients with chlamydial oculogenital infections (Dawson et al., 1970b).

Do Chlamydiae Cause Part of the Clinical Complex of RS? This is clearly true. RS is a symptom complex — a syndrome — and many patients with RS have nongonococcal urethritis. Chlamydiae are certainly a major cause of nongonococcal urethritis and it is equally certain that they cause nongonococcal urethritis in some patients with RS. Despite difficulties in assessment due to spontaneous recovery in some patients, it has been observed that the urethritis in RS may disappear promptly upon administration of tetracycline. This would suggest that in at least some patients with RS, chlamydiae cause the urethritis. This poses a nosologic problem: if the patient is diagnosed as having RS because he has urethritis and the other symptoms, and if the urethritis is caused by one identifiable agent while the other symptoms are not, we are then left with a patient who does not have RS (as a discrete clinical entity) but simply has arthritis (and possible ocular manifestations) of unknown etiology. This suggests the possibility that RS may be a mixed infectious disease or, as will be discussed below, may be a syndrome, some of whose manifestations are caused by host response and not by direct infection.

Could Chlamydiae Be One of Many Causes of Reiter's Syndrome? This is an attractive hypothesis. It is obvious that RS can occur in a sporadic endemic or venereal form as well as in an epidemic form following an outbreak of shigellosis. In some areas chlamydiae are recovered with regularity from patients with RS, in some areas they are recovered from a proportion of patients with RS, and in some areas they are never recovered. It is possible that there are multiple causes of RS, and that chlamydiae may be one of them (and not simply a venereally transmitted background contaminant). In this case one would suspect that something other than simple infection and response to infection is involved in the etiology of the diseases. This of course leads to another possibility.

Does the Patient Select for His Disease Response? Although purely hypothetical, this question presents an intriguing possible approach to the etiology of RS. In other words, a patient may have the genetic capability to develop RS as a form of hyperreactivity or altered reactivity to certain infectious or antigenic stimuli. In fact, it is possible this preprogramming may allow the patient to develop either RS or another disease in response to a simple stimulus. A very exciting and pertinent observation has been the very high association of a single histocompatibility antigen (HLA B27) with ankylosing spondylitis and also with RS (Brewerton et al., 1973; Morris et al., 1974; Schlosstein et al., 1973). Some studies have indicated a somewhat heightened reactivity to microbial antigens in patients with RS. Our studies in California have shown that while 22% of patients with RS have antibodies to chlamydiae, half of these patients have the CF antibody level that one would expect from a simple TRIC agent urethritis while the other half have the much higher titers characteristic of such systemic infections as LGV. Phillips and Christian (1970) have found heightened reactivity to some viral antigens and French workers have found high levels of cellular immune responses to chlamydial antigens in patients with RS. If one assumes that chlamydial antigens are quite common and that there is a high background of sexually transmitted chlamydial infection, one could conceive of RS as being an altered or impaired abnormal host response to a very common infection. Some of the immunologic evidence suggests this may be true. The very striking association of the HLA B27 antigen with RS provides a possible mechanism for this. This antigen is not a common one, being found in approximately 4% to 8% of the population (depending on racial group). If one assumes that roughly 30% or 40% of men with NGU have TRIC agent infection and 4% to 8% of these men will have HLA B27 antigen (and that this antigen is an indicator of a genetically determined, altered response to specific types of environmental insults), one could assume that between 1% and 3% of patients with nongonococcal urethritis would be predisposed to develop RS after being exposed to this common venereally transmitted organism. This prediction is not very far from the observed figure of approximately 1% of NGU cases who develop RS. Thus, one would hypothesize a preprogrammed, susceptible patient developing RS, while others infected with the same agent have a normal response to this antigen (agent) and develop only a minor form of urethritis. While purely speculative at present, this analogy seems to offer a reasonable explanation of the potential role of chlamydiae in human arthritic disease. One could also assume that a susceptible patient might respond to other antigens, or other infections or insults, by developing RS. Thus, a similar, relatively small proportion of patients with shigellosis could develop RS. This hypothetical schema is obviously an oversimplification. The conditions with high HLA B27 prevalence (RS, ankylosing spondylitis, and almost predictably psoriatic arthritis, and some of the difficult-to-categorize arthropathies associated with uveitis) appear to have common pathologic characteristics. If they are mediated by immune responses, one would have to postulate "immune response" genes linked to the HLA B27 locus. These genes would control the immunologic response, while the HLA B27 association would indicate the clinical response. Thus, some of the studies on chlamydiae may indicate a pathogenetic mechanism or a pathway for the development of a disease rather than a straightforward infectious disease response. The evidence indicates that chlamydiae do not (except perhaps rarely) cause RS by invasiveness, but possibly they, along with other infections, play the roles of initiators.

9   The Role of Chlamydiae Derived from Lower Mammals in Human Disease

PROVEN HUMAN INFECTIONS

Chlamydiae are virtually ubiquitous parasites of lower mammals (Storz, 1971) and they produce a variety of diseases. They commonly parasitize mucous membranes and the intestinal tract, and great numbers of infectious chlamydiae may be excreted in discharges or feces. But, even though the possibility for environmental contamination and subsequent human exposure is great, there is no convincing proof that these chlamydiae are significant human parasites.

Some of these chlamydiae are capable of infecting humans. Laboratory infections have been reported (Barwell, 1955; Meyer, 1965). A single case report has suggested that the *Chlamydia* causing enzootic abortion of ewes might have been involved in a human abortion (Roberts, Grist, and Giroud, 1967). Other French workers have referred to human infections with neorickettsial organisms, but, as mentioned in Chapter 1, the identity of all these organisms is not clear; however, it is possible that some of the infectious chains they hypothesize have involved human-lower mammal-*Chlamydia*

154

interaction, with associated human disease (Giroud, 1969; Jadin and Giroud, 1963). Enright and Sadler (1954), in a serologic survey of slaughterhouse workers, found a high rate of chlamydial sero-reactors and suggested that these might reflect infections with chlamydiae derived from sheep or cattle.

Chlamydiae have been recovered from human spontaneous abortion tissue (Schachter, 1967b), but since most of these organisms could not be differentiated from the TRIC agents, and since the specimens obviously passed through potentially infected cervices, it is difficult to hypothesize an etiologic role for the chlamydiae in the abortions. However, at least one of the chlamydiae recovered from human abortions had the biological characteristics commonly associated with mammalian chlamydiae; it would have been designated a *Chlamydia psittaci* agent. Experimental infection of cattle with this isolate resulted in placentitis and abortion (Page and Smith, 1974).

The agent of feline pneumonitis is capable of infecting man. We have observed two human infections (both involving conjunctivitis, see Chapter 5, Fig. 12) resulting from close association with cats that had active feline pneumonitis and conjunctivitis. The conjunctivitis in these animals was most marked, and both ocular and nasal discharges were heavily infected with chlamydiae. The conjunctiva of the two patients was most likely the portal of entry (Schachter, Ostler, and Meyer, 1969).

Thus, the potential for human infection with mammalian chlamydiae seems reasonably clear. However, it is likely that these organisms are not highly invasive and do not, as yet, present a known significant health hazard to human beings.

CAT-SCRATCH DISEASE

Cat-scratch disease (CSD), or nonbacterial lymphadenitis, was first described by Foshay in 1932 (Daniels and MacMurray, 1952). Case reports published in the early 1950s suggested that this relatively benign lymphadenitis, associated with a scratch or contact with healthy cats, was rare. However, since then, reports of several large series of patients have been published showing that cat-scratch disease may be relatively common. The cat is presumed to be a healthy carrier for an agent causing the disease in man. However, the cat is not the only host for this putative agent; exposure to dogs, monkeys, and occasionally scratches from inanimate objects, have caused this condition (Margileth, 1968).

Cat-scratch disease is relatively benign and usually self-limiting, and, although it may be considered in the differential diagnosis, it is often not proved because of inadequate diagnostic tools. There is a skin test to confirm the diagnosis. The antigen is derived from pus of a patient with a positive skin test. Some evidence suggests that there are differences in the reactivity of antigen preparations taken from different patients. Because the antigen is of human origin and is prepared for use by being heated at 60° C for varying periods (up to three days depending on the technique used), many physicians prefer not to use it because of the possible danger of transmitting heat-stable human viruses, such as hepatitis.

In 1951, Mollaret et al. described inclusion bodies similar to those observed in psittacosis infections and presented evidence of the presence of antichlamydial antibodies in the sera of patients with CSD. Other workers have confirmed and extended these serologic observations. The speculation that CSD is caused by a chlamydia has been based largely on positive CF results in these patients. In New Zealand, Manning and Reid (1958) have shown that of 35 CSD patients with positive skin tests, 23% had CF titers of 1:8 or higher compared to only 2% of normal blood donors. In the United States, Armstrong and associates (1956) had a slightly higher rate of reactors in patients with CSD (20%) than in controls (11.3%). Kalter (1961) found that 25.8% of 170 patients had CF reactions compared to 3% of controls.

Other evidence often cited in support of a possible chlamydial etiology of CSD includes the obvious similarity of some of the clinical features of CSD to those of lymphogranuloma venereum; healthy cats may carry a chlamydial agent that can cause pneumonitis and conjunctivitis in felines and has been shown capable of infecting man. On the other hand, several features of these studies suggest that chlamydiae do not directly cause cat-scratch disease. For example, the delayed hypersensitivity reaction associated with chlamydial infections is group-specific, and the cat-scratch and Frei-test antigens do not give cross-reacting results. In addition, chemotherapy with broad-spectrum antibiotics such as tetracyclines is not useful in treatment of CSD (Margileth, 1968) although a response is usually expected with chlamydial diseases. Rising titers to chlamydial group antigen would be expected in at least some patients if this disease were caused by chlamydiae, but this has not been shown. Most of the CF titers observed in patients with CSD are low, while those of systemic chlamydial infections are high.

In the past 10 years, we have attempted to isolate chlamydiae from 20 patients with a presumed diagnosis of CSD. Most of the specimens tested were aspirates from suppurative lymph nodes, although some conjunctival scrapings from patients with Parinaud's oculoglandular syndrome following cat scratch were also tested. No chlamydiae were recovered in yolk sac or tissue culture. Richard Emmons, M.D., of the California State Department of Health, Epidemiology Division, has accumulated sera from 69 patients with cat-scratch fever. We have tested these sera (19 paired) with the CF test and fluorescent antibody tests against several chlamydiae, including a feline pneumonitis agent recovered from an infected human. In addition to Emmons' sera, those from 40 other CSD patients were submitted for testing. We observed many low-grade CF titers (15%) together with a few high titers (1:256), but no changes were seen when paired sera were tested. The more sensitive indirect fluorescent antibody test had higher reactor rates but no rising titers. In addition, IgM antibodies were not detected; their presence might have been expected if the patients had had acute or active chlamydial infections.

Obviously, evidence for chlamydial infection as the cause of CSD does not withstand close inspection. Appropriately controlled studies have never been performed. It is true that the chlamydiae causing feline pneumonitis can infect man; this might explain some of the complement-fixing antibodies in the sera of people exposed to cats. An appropriate control population would have to be people with similar exposure to cats who have not developed cat-scratch fever. Although patients with CSD do have a high rate of exposure to chlamydiae, there is no convincing evidence to support an etiologic role for these agents in this disease.

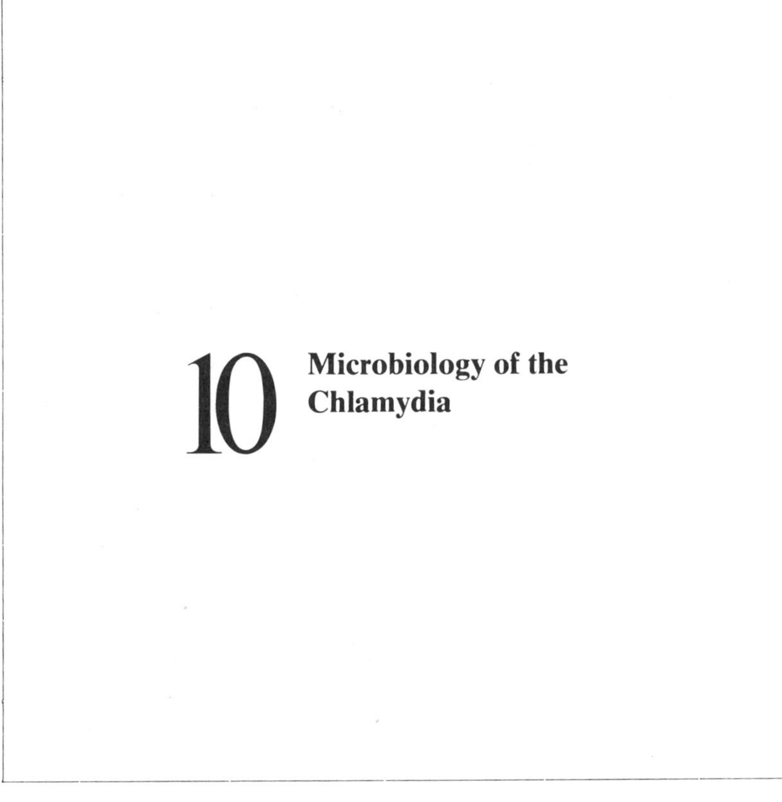

10   Microbiology of the Chlamydia

MORPHOLOGIC CHARACTERISTICS

The chlamydiae generally present two types of particles. The smaller, infectious forms are electron-dense particles which appear to be spherical and in electron microscopic studies seem to have a relatively loose outer membrane which gives purified particles a "derby hat" appearance. These particles are between 200 and 400 millimicrons in diameter and are slightly basophilic in their staining reactions. The second form of particle is less electron-dense and seems to have a relatively flat outer structure. These particles (initial bodies) are noninfectious, occur earlier in the developmental cycle as precursors of the infectious elementary bodies, and may range in diameter up to 1 micron (Figs. 1–4). These particles are more basophilic than the elementary bodies. Both particles seem to be gram-negative, although they do not stain well by this technique. The larger reticulate forms appear to have a trilaminate cell wall (Anderson et al., 1965).

158

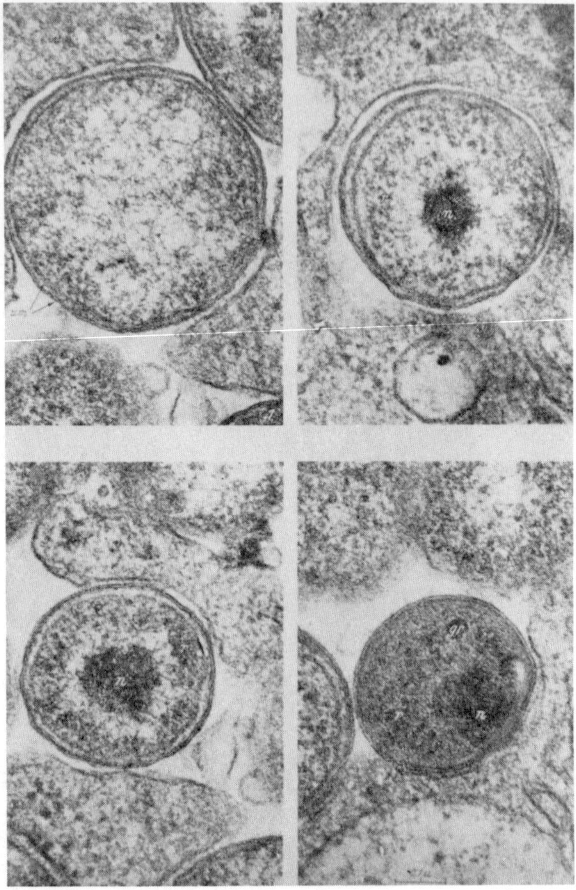

Fig. 1. Development stages of ornithosis agent (upper left and three elementary body forms) showing the presence of two bilaminar membranes. Glutaraldehyde fixation. (From Lepinay et al., 1971)

BACTERIAL NATURE

It has been apparent from virtually the first sophisticated studies on the psittacosis agents that these are not, in fact, viruses. For example, Bedson and Bland (1934), in their elegant studies on the growth cycle of the organism, recognized the morphologic integrity of the infectious particles. On this basis they stated that the psittacosis agent is a microorganism with bacterial affinities. Meyer (1942), on the basis of morphology, staining reaction, and site of multiplication, suggested that the psittacosis agents belonged with the bacteria rather than with the true viruses. The major problem was that the definitions of virus and bacteria were not yet very precise. It only required the

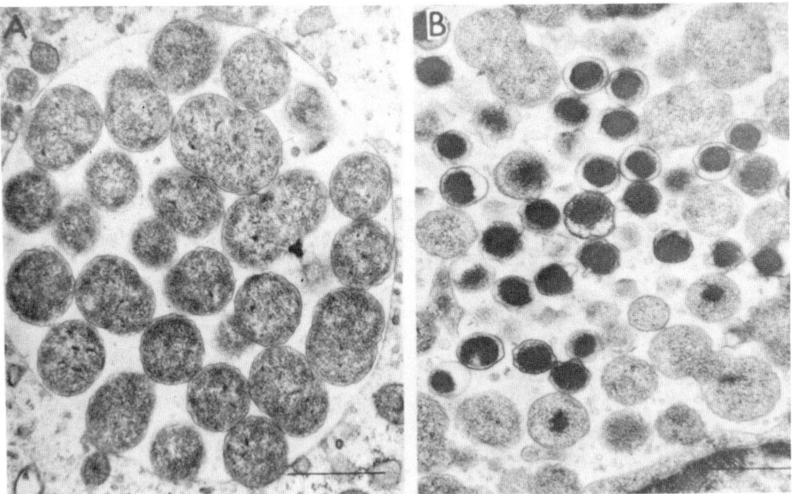

Fig. 2. *Chlamydia psittaci* growing in L cells.
A. Inclusion 24 hours after infection showing initial or reticulate bodies, some of which appear to be undergoing binary fission (16,000X).
B. An inclusion 48 hours after infection with many elementary bodies, initial bodies, and intermediate forms. (From Matsumoto and Manire, 1970a)

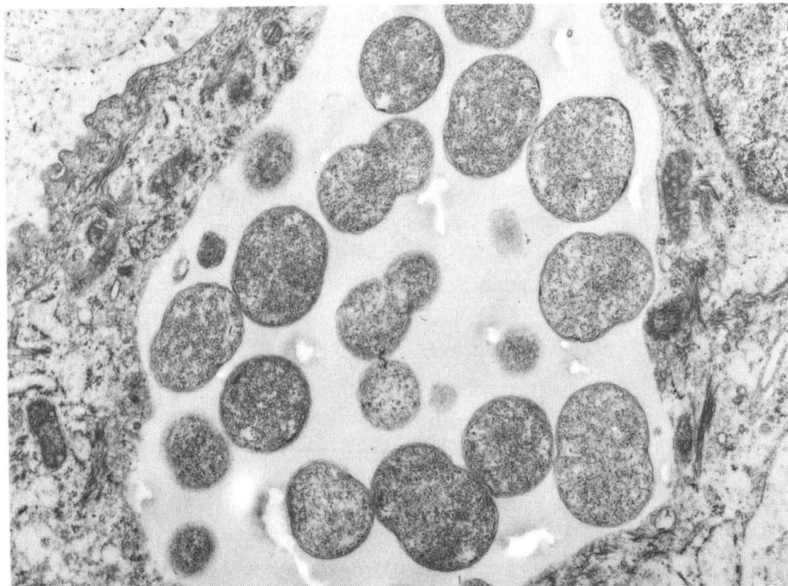

Fig. 3. An initial body inclusion in a conjunctival epithelial scraping from a patient with endemic trachoma in Tunisia. Even though a vesicle membrane cannot be well distinguished, the chlamydial organisms appear to lie in a well-defined vacuole clearly separated from epithelial cell cytoplasm.

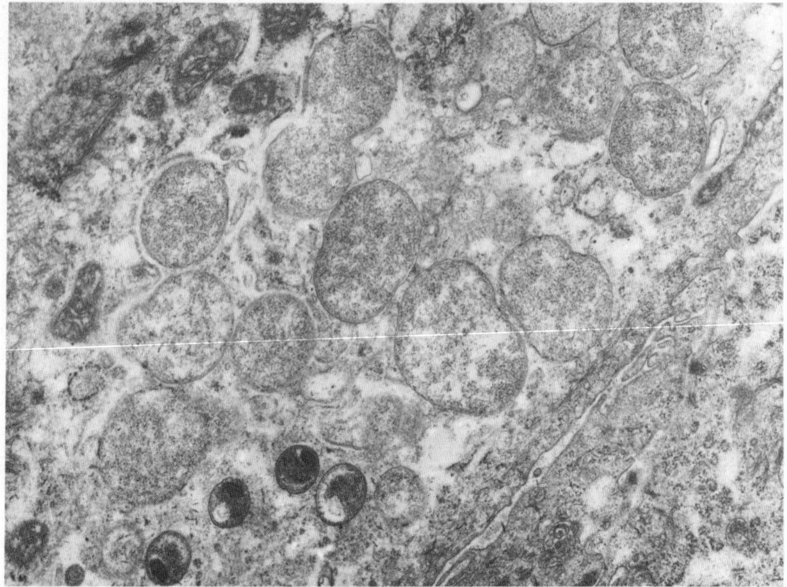

Fig. 4. Elementary and initial body forms in an epithelial cell from a patient with endemic trachoma in Tunisia. The cell vacuole is not well defined in this instance.

development of suitable biochemical tests and the studies of Lwoff (1957) and Stanier (1964) to define these two major groups and to allow the proper recognition of the chlamydiae as bacteria, with a few superficial similarities to the viruses.

Although much of the evidence had accumulated over the years, Moulder (1962a,b, 1964, 1966) presented the most compelling arguments for acknowledging the bacterial nature of the chlamydiae. The unique nature of these organisms' developmental cycle has been stressed (Terskikh et al., 1969) and was used by Storz and Page (1971) as the basis for a proposal that the chlamydiae be placed in a new order, Chlamydiales.

The properties of chlamydiae may be compared to those of bacteria and viruses (Table 1). The only similarities between chlamydiae and viruses lie in the obligatory intracellular nature of their parasitism and their mutual lack of independent energy production. Chlamydiae share many properties in common with bacteria: most important, in practical terms, is their sensitivity to antibiotics.

DEVELOPMENTAL CYCLE

The developmental cycle of the chlamydial organisms is apparently unique to the chlamydiae and serves to differentiate them

Table 1
Properties of Chlamydiae, Viruses, and Bacteria

	Chlamydiae	Viruses	Bacteria
Size (nm)	Ca 350	15-350	300-3,000
Shape	Coccoid	Symmetrical	Varied
Obligatory intracellular parasites	+	+	−
Nucleic acids	2	1	2
Complex cell wall	+	−	+
Muramic acid	−	−	+
Reproductive mode	Complicated cycle and fission	Eclipse-synthesis-assembly	Fission
Sensitivity to sulfonamides or antibiotics	+	−	+
Ribosomes	+	−	+
Metabolic enzymes	+	−	+
Energy production	−	−	+

from all other known microorganisms. It has formed the basis for separation of these organisms into their own order. It is very complex and as yet not clearly understood. However, in the simplest terms, it may be described as follows: The first step is the attachment of an infectious elementary body onto the surface of a susceptible cell. The cell then actively phagocytizes the attached particle into a phagocytic vesicle; this is the agent's mode of penetration and it may be selective or enhanced. The chlamydial particle remains intact and undergoes some sort of reorganization so that within 6 or 8 hours it has changed from an elementary body to an initial body (reticulate particle). These particles are metabolically active, synthesize material, and multiply actively until approximately 18 hours postinfection (Figs. 2A, 3). During this time only the initial bodies are seen. (Early in the cycle some giant forms are also occasionally seen, but their role in the cycle is not yet understood.)

At approximately 18 to 24 hours postinfection, the initial bodies which had been multiplying by binary fission stop multiplying and undergo another reorganization, during which they become elementary bodies on approximately a one-to-one ratio (Figs. 2B, 4). The elementary bodies are then released from the inclusion and from the cell to infect other cells.

The initial bodies are highly labile and do not survive well outside the cell; the elementary bodies are relatively stable and persist well in an extracellular milieu. These forms probably represent evolutionary adaptation to an intracellular or extracellular environment. This developmental cycle was observed by light microscopy by Bedson and Bland (1932) with psittacosis agents, by Thygeson (1934) with inclusion conjunctivitis agent, and by Findlay, Mackenzie, and Mac-Callum (1938) and Rake and Jones (1942) with LGV agent. Many

162

studies have been performed with electron microscopy; these studies have further defined the fine structure of the chlamydial particles and have provided convincing evidence of binary fission (Fig. 2). (Further information on metabolic properties during the cycle has been elucidated in biochemical studies and is discussed later in this chapter.)

The internal cell membranes of the host cell appear to be altered and possibly destroyed during infection by *C. psittaci* (Stokes, 1973). It is possible that this reflects the observation that the cellular or subcellular structure of the host is deranged (Lepinay et al., 1971; Friis, 1972). Possibly this results from the activation of lysosomal enzymes (Kordová, Wilt, and Sadiq, 1971). It appears that the ultimate destruction of the cell is mediated by breakdown of lysosomes, which occurs relatively late in the chlamydial developmental cycle. Earlier fusion of the lysosome with the phagosome appears to be specifically inhibited (Friis, 1972). Identification of this inhibitor would be most important, for if it were antigenic it would offer hope of a vaccine against a virulence antigen. It should be noted that the chlamydial inclusion is at all times, until the virtual death of the cell, surrounded by a membrane of host cell origin (Figs. 2A, 3). It is possible that some of these membranes are modified (Stokes, 1974), but it would appear that much of the inclusion's limiting membrane consists of the cell's outer membrane. The mode of expansion of the inclusion membrane is not known, although obviously it enlarges considerably from the small vacuole surrounding the infecting elementary body to the very large membrane surrounding an inclusion or a colony of chlamydial particles, which may occupy most of cell's cytoplasmic space.

EFFECT OF PENICILLINS

Penicillins are active in killing bacteria by interfering with cell-wall synthesis. The specific action of the antibiotic involves blocking the incorporation of UDP-muramic acid peptide into the cell wall. In the presence of penicillin, replication of the chlamydiae results in bizarre giant forms (Fig. 5), apparently analogous to the bacterial forms produced under the influence of this drug (Weiss, 1950; Hurst et al., 1953; Kramer and Gordon, 1971).

Thus, grossly, it appears that the action of penicillins is essentially the same with chlamydiae as with other bacteria. The report that at least traces of muramic acid were present in chlamydial cell walls (Jenkin, 1960; Allison and Perkins, 1960) gave further support to this viewpoint. Moulder and associates (1955) and Gordon, Andrew, and Wagner (1957) had shown that a *C. psittaci* strain could develop

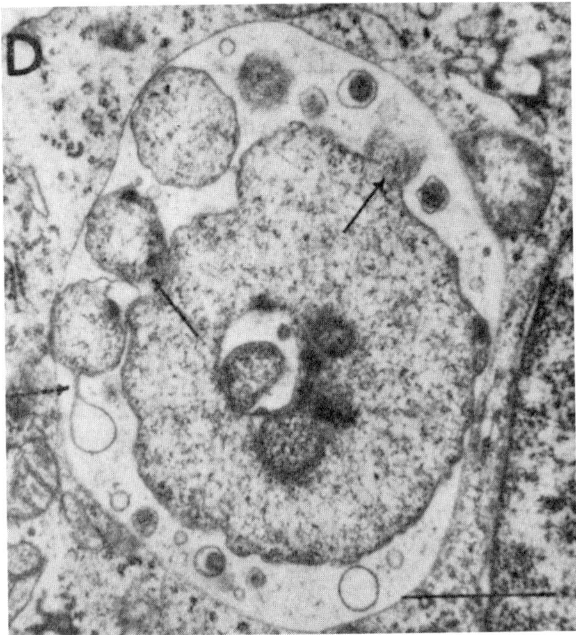

Fig. 5. *Chlamydia psittaci* in an L cell following incubation with penicillin. The formation of small reticulate bodies from the single, large abnormal form is shown by the solid arrows; the broken arrow indicates an empty vesicle or bleb attached to a small reticulate body. (From Matsumoto and Manire, 1970a)

penicillin resistance. The penicillin-resistant derivative was not neutralized by antiserum prepared against the parent; thus it was assumed that the cell wall structure had been changed when resistance to penicillin developed (Moulder et al., 1958; Woodroffe and Moulder, 1960).

It should be noted, however, that there is some controversy concerning the presence of muramic acid in the chlamydial particle and cell wall. The most recent results, using sensitive techniques, have been unable to confirm the presence of this taxonomically significant sugar (Garrett, Harrison, and Manire, 1974). At the very least the amount of muramic acid is far less than is found in bacterial cells. Thus, it appears that the mode of action of penicillin on these organisms, although grossly similar in that it interferes with cell wall synthesis, is very different at the molecular level than with eubacteria.

CHEMICAL COMPOSITION

Of the common amino acids only arginine and histidine appear to be missing from the meningopneumonitis agent (Gogolak and Ross,

164

1955; Jenkin, 1960). Both RNA and DNA are present (Moulder, 1966). Some workers could not find RNA in their preparations and this at one time was assumed to provide supporting evidence for the chlamydiae's classification as viruses, but these results are now recognized to represent artifacts of the purification techniques which allowed the RNA present in the particles to leak out (Moulder, 1962b).

The chlamydiae are as chemically complex as the bacteria. The dry weights are approximately 35% protein, with a lipid content approximately 40% to 50%. Nucleic acids are present (both RNA and DNA) in both elementary bodies and initial or reticulate forms, although the latter have higher quantities of RNA. The protein content of the particles is approximately 33% in both intact particles and cell walls. The carbohydrate content is between 1% and 2%, the RNA content ranges from 2% to 7%, and the DNA from 3% to 4% (total nucleic acid content of the elementary body is approximately 6%).

The cell walls of the elementary bodies (Fig. 6) are quite anal-

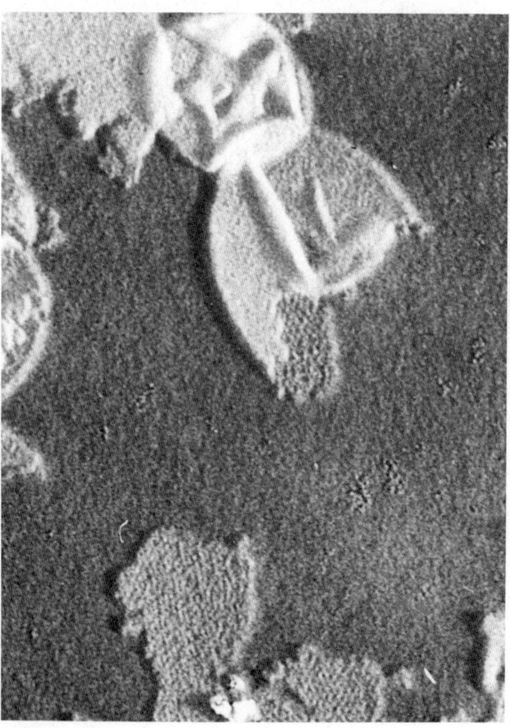

Fig. 6. Fine structure of cell wall of meningopneumonitis organism. Shadowed preparation showing regular geometric arrangement of subunits approximately 20 nm in diameter, approximately 75,000X. (From Matsumoto and Manire, 1970b)

ogous in structure to the cell walls of gram-negative bacteria (Manire and Tamura, 1967). There are very slight differences in amino acid content between chlamydial cell walls and *E. coli* cell walls, while there are very marked differences from those of gram-positive bacteria.

NUTRITIONAL REQUIREMENTS

The only in-depth study on nutritional requirements of this group of organisms has been performed by Morgan and associates (Bader and Morgan, 1961; Morgan, 1952a,b, 1956; Morgan and Bader, 1954, 1957). In a series of papers they exploited the finding that a psittacosis strain (6 BC) could be used to infect L cells, and that once the infection had taken place, replacement of the tissue culture medium with a minimum maintenance medium prevented replication of the chlamydiae. Although not replicating, the chlamydiae persisted in a viable state, and when growth medium was used to replace the maintenance medium, the agents would multiply. It was, therefore, possible to utilize synthetic media which were capable of supporting the propagation of the agent and, by varying the constituents of the synthetic media, to determine the nutritional requirements of the organism. The organism did not require any components which were not required for the growth of the host cell, thus supporting the inference that a metabolically active, functioning cell is required for multiplication of this obligatory intracellular parasite. Arginine and histidine were not required for the growth of the 6 BC agent (these two amino acids have been found to be missing in preparations of the meningopneumonitis strain). The psittacosis agents did not require glutamate or glutamine. They apparently can synthesize their own lysine by decarboxylation of diaminopimelic acid (Moulder, 1962a,b). They did not require the presence of folic acid or riboflavin; of course, sulfa-sensitive organisms possess the ability to synthesize folic acids, while resistant ones convert them (Colón, 1962).

METABOLISM

It must be noted here that most of the metabolic studies performed on purified chlamydiae have utilized the wrong developmental stage of the organism. This has been largely dictated by technical considerations, since the stable infectious elementary body is the particle easiest to purify and to obtain in large quantities. Unfortunately the elementary body is probably the least metabolically active morphologic form of chlamydiae. If a difference in metabolic capabilities of chlamydiae were to exist, it would probably be the initial bodies (i.e., those

166

particles that are predominant at approximately 8 to 20 hours after infection) which would have the greatest metabolic capabilities. It is possible that the chlamydiae have some form of sequential metabolic capabilities which would allow certain enzymes to be detected only at certain developmental stages (although this might require an extreme enzyme lability).

Some evidence has been obtained that the chlamydial particles may utilize certain host enzymes in preparing substrates for their own enzyme activities (for example, they lack hexokinase but utilize the products of host hexokinase reactions to produce glucose phosphate for their own reactions). Vender and Moulder (1967) demonstrated that the initial steps in chlamydial glucose catabolism are dependent upon host cell hexokinase. Therefore, the chlamydiae may enter into the citric acid cycle by producing α ketoglutarate and succinate from glutamate but proceed no further, so that no fumarate or malate have been demonstrated (Weiss, 1967). However, this may not be indicative of a defective citric acid cycle resulting in no net energy, but may simply reflect the increased needs of the organism for the product of that reaction. It is possible that the chlamydiae are such efficient parasites that their limited metabolic capabilities are very specifically directed to supply only those precursors or building blocks that the organism may require in greater quantities than will be produced by the host cell. Weiss and Wilson (1969) have demonstrated that exogenous ATP is needed for the synthesis of lipids by the chlamydiae. Thus, there is further evidence for this organism's requirements for host ATP, and indirect evidence that the limited metabolic capabilities of this parasite may not be directed toward energy production as are those of other organisms.

Moulder (1964, 1966) has emphasized that chlamydial particles in their growth cycle are essentially energy parasites, and that many of their metabolic activities occur independently of the host cell's biosynthetic activities. Gill and Stewart (1970a) showed that infected L cells increased their oxygen and glucose consumption approximately two fold following infection with the psittacosis agent. The end product of glucose catabolism was lactic acid. The glucose concentration affected the yield of psittacosis agents. Thus, it would appear that chlamydial infection directly or indirectly caused the cell's energy-producing activities to be stimulated, with peak stimulation occurring between 12 and 24 hours (the time of greatest metabolic activity of the chlamydial particles). Oxygen consumption by infected cells also increased, with a peak at approximately 27 hours after infection (Gill and Stewart, 1970b).

Further support for the chlamydial particles' dependence on host cell ATP was shown by Gill and Stewart (1970c), who treated infected cells with antimycin, which blocks the utilization of the cyto-chrome system (which is not complete or active in chlamydiae), and thereby reduces the cells' ATP production. The presence of the drug prevented the multiplication of the chlamydial particles, but when the drug was removed the particles multiplied. The effect was essentially the same as that observed by restricting the glucose in the medium. In addition, it was noted that the effect of antimycin on the growth of psittacosis organisms diminished after 24 hours. In other words, the organism was most sensitive to this inhibitor of cell energy production in the early parts of its growth cycle.

With the obvious exception of folic acid synthesis, there does not appear to be any marked difference in metabolic activity of *C. psittaci* and *C. trachomatis*.

PROTEIN SYNTHESIS

The proper experimental system to allow chlamydial particles to produce proteins extracellularly has not yet been developed. Therefore, in order to study protein synthesis it is necessary to study the metabolism of chlamydiae in the infected cell. Unfortunately, the chlamydial component of the metabolic activity of the infected cell is much smaller than that of the cell itself. It is, therefore, extremely difficult to segregate the cell's contributions from the parasite's contributions. A number of studies have been performed using cell fractionation procedures (Schechter, 1966), which allowed certain information to be obtained showing that protein synthesis begins approximately 10 to 15 hours after infection, when multiplication of chlamydial particles begins. A major technical contribution was made by utilization of differential metabolic inhibition. In other words, chemical agents were used which would specifically inhibit the metabolic activities of either the parasite or the host cell. Alexander (1968, 1969) made extremely good use of this principle, utilizing cyclohexi-mide to inhibit specifically the synthetic capabilities of the host cell and chloramphenicol to inhibit specifically protein synthesis of the chlamydial particles. Thus, in this system it became possible to separate the net production of proteins or nucleic acids by the parasite alone at different time periods. These experiments conclusively showed that the chlamydial organisms possess an independent protein synthetic capability which is not dependent upon the host's synthetic abilities. Schechter (1966) found that L cells after infection showed decreased rates of RNA and DNA synthesis, but no apparent change in protein synthesis. The meningopneumonitis agent's DNA, RNA, and protein synthesis were clearly evident at 15 to 20 hours after infection, in other words, in the period of highest agent multiplication. These rates of synthesis increased for a short period and then decreased. The logarithmic phase lasted for approximately 10 hours. Alexander (1968) also showed that host protein synthesis was not inhibited by infection with the meningopneumonitis agent. In further studies, Alexander (1969) compared chlamydial infection in logarithmically growing cells and stationary phase cultures and found that both host-specific DNA and protein synthesis were inhibited in the infected L cell. This was apparently due to the restriction in the growth of the cell. Metabolic capabilities of the agent and host together were equal to the metabolic capabilities of logarithmically growing host cells alone. This latter experiment clearly showed the difference in the rates of synthesis of proteins caused by the infection.

Becker and Asher (1972) used emetine to inhibit protein synthesis by the host cell and demonstrated that a *C. trachomatis* strain could develop essentially as it did in untreated cells, indicating that the synthesis of host cell proteins was not required for development of *C. trachomatis*. In fact, in these studies there was a stimulation in that the yield of agent was higher than in controls, suggesting the possibility that there may have been some competition between the protein-synthesizing systems of the organism and those of the host cell.

DNA SYNTHESIS

Pelc and Crocker (1961) showed that chlamydiae could not incorporate added thymidine into their DNA. Tribby and Moulder (1966) confirmed and extended this observation to show that other nucleosides could be incorporated. Since the chlamydiae do synthesize DNA, it became important to determine how thymidine (or the thymine of DNA) was synthesized and incorporated. The common pathway involves the enzyme thymidine kinase acting on thymidine. This enzyme is usually present in mammalian cells and is very seldom lacking in microorganisms. Those viruses capable of infecting cells that do not have thymidine kinase induce the synthesis of an enzyme which has characteristics genetically determined by the virus.

Lin (1968) found that thymidine kinase was absent in both the meningopneumonitis agent and in cells infected with this strain, which suggests that an alternate pathway might be involved (uridine monophosphate as a precursor of deoxyuridine monophosphate acted on by thymidylate synthetase to produce thymidine monophosphate). It appears that the chlamydial strains, upon infecting the cell, turn off the cell's DNA replicating capacity by preventing, either directly or indirectly (this is not yet known), the production of the enzyme thymidine kinase.

Thymidine kinase is a labile enzyme which is continually produced by the uninfected cell. This enzyme is not active by the time chlamydial DNA synthesis can be measured. The DNA synthesis of the organisms apparently begins approximately 10 to 15 hours after cell infection and reaches a peak approximately 25 hours after infection.

Lin (1968) showed that the nucleic acids of the L cell are not degraded at an accelerated rate following infection with meningopneumonitis agent. It thus appears that the chlamydiae's nucleic acids are synthesized from the cytoplasmic pool of the host cell, and not from nucleic acid components of the host cell. The parasite effectively utilizes the cell's ability to produce DNA precursors, for its rate of DNA production is never higher than the total DNA production of rapidly multiplying, uninfected cells. The infecting particle essentially turns off the multiplying features of the host cell and utilizes the cell's freed biosynthetic capabilities. Crocker et al. (1965) discussed the possibility that chlamydiae could inhibit the initiation of cellular DNA replication which is required for cell multiplication. The ability to prevent multiplication of the host cell is apparently dependent upon the stage of the cell's developmental cycle at which infection takes place. Officer and Brown (1960) have shown that infected host cells could replicate, and that daughter cells in the division either might contain an inclusion or not. In other words, an infected mother cell could divide to yield an infected daughter cell and a normal daughter cell. Thus, it becomes obvious that infection at a certain stage of the cell's life cycle will not terminate the cell's ability to multiply. Therefore, it would appear that there is a crucial stage during which mitosis and division of the cell are inhibited and the cell's metabolic capabilities are effectively parasitized.

Schechter (1966) used several clones of L cells and showed that the more rapid the dividing time of the host cell, the earlier the onset of inhibition of DNA synthesis. The specific inhibiting effect probably occurs at the same biochemical event in different cells regardless of differences in generation time.

RNA synthesis begins shortly before development of multiplying chlamydial particles, and inhibition of RNA synthesis (with actinomycin D) effectively inhibits the multiplication of infectious particles up to 20 hours after infection (Tamura and Iwanaga, 1965). It would thus seem that new RNA is no longer required by the chlamydial particles during the time when the so-called reorganization into infectious elementary bodies takes place.

DNA HOMOLOGY

In DNA homology studies, one measures the degree of binding between two purified DNA preparations. The binding that is observed apparently reflects the complementarity of the DNA molecules. This is an indication of polynucleotide sequences and thus presumably measures genetic relatedness.

Kingsbury and Weiss (1968) compared the DNA homology among *Chlamydia psittaci, C. trachomatis,* and several *Neisseria* species. Two strains of *C. psittaci* demonstrated reactions of identity, while all three *C. trachomatis* strains reacted almost completely with each other. However, the *C. psittaci* and *C. trachomatis* strains did not react significantly with each other. In fact, their degree of relatedness was of the same order of magnitude as seen between the chlamydiae and the three *Neisseria* species. On the basis of these homology studies the relatedness of these chlamydial strains was further support for their separate speciation. It is of interest to note that part of the *Chlamydia-Neisseria* reaction was thermostable, indicating related sequencing.

Weiss et al. (1970) compared the polynucleotide sequence relationships of four strains of *C. trachomatis*. Three of the strains of human origin gave DNA duplexing of virtually homologous nature. The single strain of murine origin (the mouse pneumonitis strain), although it had essentially the same base ratio (approximately 42.5% guanine plus cytosine), reassociated at only a 30% to 60% level. The single *C. psittaci* strain (meningopneumonitis) showed virtually no binding with the *C. trachomatis* DNA. In addition, these workers compared the glucose metabolism as indicated by carbon dioxide production and found minimal differences in CO_2 production between *C. trachomatis* and one *C. psittaci*.

Gerloff, Ritter, and Watson had earlier shown (1966) that there was considerable DNA homology (ranging from 51.5% to 63.8%) between meningopneumonitis strain DNA and the DNA obtained from four other chlamydiae. One of the strains they tested was a lymphogranuloma venereum strain (Squibb strain). It is difficult to reconcile the discrepancy between these results and those obtained by Kingsbury and Weiss, who showed no DNA homology between the meningopneumonitis strain and the DNA of an LGV isolate. A possible explanation is that the LGV strain tested by Gerloff et al. was in fact a *C. psittaci* strain (as has been shown for a number of old laboratory strains bearing the label LGV). Kingsbury and Weiss (1968) showed that two *C. psittaci* strains had guanine + cytosine (G + C) base compositions of approximately 41% while three *C. trachomatis* strains had guanine + cytosine percents of approximately

45%. They felt these differences were significantly different, possibly reflecting the difference between the species. However, Gerloff, Ritter, and Watson (1970), testing a larger number of strains, showed that the G + C percentage presented a spectrum of values ranging from 41% to 44%. Thus, there were some differences at either end of this particular spectrum that might be of taxonomic significance, but the overlap was such as to render it minimally useful.

Kingsbury (1969) compared the genome size of a number of bacterial species. The chlamydiae had the smallest genome (6 to 8.5×10^5 pairs) and had DNA approximately one-half the size of neisserial or rickettsial DNA. *Escherichia coli* had the largest DNA content (4.5×10^6 pairs), while a virus (bacteriophage T4) had only 2×10^5 pairs.

LIPID SYNTHESIS

Jenkin (1960) showed that a large portion of the chlamydial particle was lipid. While part of this content was specifically associated with the cell wall, much of it was associated with the group antigen, which could be solubilized. Gogolak and Ross (1955) had shown that the hemagglutinin activity could be associated with phospholipid. Jenkin and colleagues (1970) pointed out that phosphatidyl choline and phosphatidyl ethanolamine fraction were the major lipid classes of the phospholipids, with considerable difference in branched-chain fatty acids. The actual structure of the hemagglutinin is as yet unknown, and these authors pointed out that the structure is considerably more complicated than may have been previously discerned. Jenkin (1967) showed that different chlamydial isolates had fatty acids which differed from those found in the host material and from other isolates. The synthesis of lipids within the cell was shown by Gaugler et al. (1969) and Makino et al. (1970) to include lipids which do not exist in the host cells used for the propagation of the chlamydiae. For example, the 6 BC strain lipid was 15% phosphatidyl glycerol, which was not found in the host MK-2 cells. Thus, in this one particular instance there has been no problem with host contaminants for those few lipids that are uniquely chlamydial.

SYNTHESIS OF POLYSACCHARIDES

From the results of Jenkin and Fan (1971), one may assume that the production of polysaccharide in the inclusion is directed by the organism. Although the product coprecipitated with shellfish glycogen, it was shown that ADP glucose was preferentially utilized by the infected cells and UDP glucose by the normal HeLa cell.

Fan and Jenkin (1970) showed that the TW-3 strain of *C. trachomatis* had a marked increase in glycogen accumulation approximately 48 to 60 hours after infection. On the other hand, the cells infected with meningopneumonitis agent (*C. psittaci*) had much lower levels (by at least 50%) than those infected with TW-3. It is not completely clear whether differences in synthesis or in accumulation (different rates of breakdown?) of glycogen are responsible for the glycogen-staining inclusion that helps to define the species.

GROWTH IN CELL CULTURE

Chlamydial strains vary considerably in their infectivity for cell cultures and other laboratory hosts. The general rule of thumb for microbiologists has been that trachoma and inclusion conjunctivitis (TRIC) strains grow well only in the nonselective medium of the embryonated hen's egg. The only experimental animal system involves conjunctival infection of man or subhuman primates. TRIC agents grow very poorly in cell cultures, although some have been adapted to serial growth in cell culture (Mitsui et al., 1964; Mitsui, Kitamuro, and Fujimoto, 1967). The so-called fast TRIC strains, which are now recognized as being biologically identical to LGV agents (Wang and Grayston, 1971b), grow well in eggs and tissue culture systems and are infective for mice by the intracerebral and intranasal routes. Although heavy inocula of some TRIC strains have been shown capable of multiplying in the mouse lung (Graham, 1965), this has not been a widely accepted experimental system.

With *C. psittaci* strains there is considerable variation in infectivity for laboratory animals, but most of these strains grow quite well in cell cultures. Differences in virulence for laboratory animals include variation by different routes of inoculation as well as varying virulence for different animals. Thus, some isolates may kill mice (by any route of inoculation) and guinea pigs; other isolates may kill mice (by any route of inoculation) but are innocuous to guinea pigs; still other isolates may be lethal for mice after intracerebral infection but not after intraperitoneal infection. This variability appears to be relatively systematic and has been utilized in the past in identifying isolates on a crude basis by the use of pathogenicity patterns, pathogenicity indices, or pathotypes (Meyer and Eddie, 1952; Page 1959a, 1967).

Tissue culture systems have been used for growth of psittacosis isolates for many years, going back to the 1930s when organ explant cultures were shown to support the growth of these agents and allowed studies on the growth cycles, antigen preparation, and biologic properties of the organism (Bedson and Bland, 1934; Meyer, Eddie, and Yanamura, 1939).

From the work of Gordon and Quan (1965b) and Weiss and Dressler (1960), it appeared that the major limitation in the ability of TRIC agents to infect cells was the efficiency of their attachment and penetration into the host cell. Utilization of centrifugation to enhance the contact between the parasite and the cell increased the infectivity of a number of chlamydial isolates in both species. Although this technique was originally applied to normal cells, Gordon obtained better results centrifuging TRIC agents into irradiated McCoy cells. This system evolved into the first generally applicable tissue culture method for isolation of these agents. The refinements that have been made in the system have been reviewed (Darougar et al., 1972). Alternate methods, such as use of iododeoxyuridine treatment as a substitute for irradiation (Wentworth and Alexander, 1974), have also been developed. The routinely useful methods of cultivation of chlamydiae are discussed in greater detail in Chapter 11, dealing with diagnostic methods.

Harrison (1970) used pretreatment of cells with DEAE-dextran to enhance the infectivity of an ovine chlamydial strain. DEAE-dextran is a positively charged macromolecule which has been shown to enhance the infectivity and transforming ability of a number of lytic and nonlytic viruses. It would appear that the key aspect of this pretreatment involves changing the surface charge of the cell to allow for greater attachment of the elementary body to the cell membrane. Presumably this attachment is simply electrostatic. Becker, Hochberg, and Zakay-Rones (1969) have shown that treatment of elementary bodies already absorbed onto the cell membrane with heparin (a negatively charged polysaccharide) results in very marked elution of a *C. trachomatis* agent from the cell surface, resulting in decreasing infectivity. The enhancing effect of DEAE-dextran has been utilized in isolation procedures for trachoma-inclusion conjunctivitis agents. Thus, Rota and Nichols (1971) and Kuo et al. (1972) found that DEAE pretreatment of tissue cultures resulted in enhanced inclusion counts when the infecting inoculum was centrifuged into either McCoy or HeLa cells. Although DEAE-dextran enhanced the infectivity of the TRIC agents, it was apparent from the results of Rota and Nichols (1973) that centrifugation of inoculum is the most important single step to be utilized to increase infectivity, and that centrifugation at approximately 33° C represents the optimal system for inclusion production.

Kuo, Wang, and Grayston (1973) further investigated the effect of polycations, polyanions, and neuraminidase on the infectivity of

TRIC agents and LGV organisms. These workers found that TRIC agents and LGV organisms differed significantly in the response to DEAE-dextran and neuraminidase in that the LGV organisms were not affected, while infectivity of the TRIC agents was enhanced by the DEAE-dextran treatment and inhibited by neuraminidase treatment. Thus, the authors considered that there may well be different receptor sites or points of attachment of LGV and TRIC agents. Further evidence was obtained for this viewpoint when they found that the TRIC agents' attachment could be specifically blocked by pretreatment of the cells with heat-inactivated TRIC organisms, but not by utilization of heat-inactivated LGV strains or influenza virus. The authors, therefore, concluded that with respect to these two modes of cell treatment it was possible that there might be three groups of chlamydiae: the TRIC strains enhanced by DEAE-dextran and inhibited by neuraminidase, the LGV isolates unaffected by either, and the single strain of psittacosis agent that was enhanced by DEAE-dextran pretreatment but unaffected by neuraminidase.

C. psittaci strains have been shown capable of infecting and completing the developmental cycle in tissue culture prepared from cold-blooded animals such as the tortoise (Shindarov, Runevski, and Vassileva, 1971). The length of the growth cycle appears to be dependent on the temperature of incubation, being shorter at higher temperatures.

In our laboratory we have demonstrated that a number of chlamydial strains of avian or bovine origin can multiply in tissue culture lines derived from mosquito, tick, or moth cells.

Psittacosis strains have been shown to grow in a variety of cells. Their growth in mouse L cells, Chang's human liver cells, fetal mouse lung cell cultures, and human diploid cells seems to be quite similar (Officer and Brown, 1960; Pearson et al., 1965). Officer and Brown (1960) studied psittacosis agents' growth in tissue culture. They used the 6 BC and Borg strains in Chang's human liver cells, Chang's human conjunctival cells, and a fetal mouse lung cell line. They found that fetal mouse lung and Chang's human liver strains supported the growth of the Borg strain at essentially the same level, but that the 6 BC strain was much more invasive for the liver line than the fetal mouse lung line. They observed that attachment between the agent and the cell was a highly inefficient process, and it required a high multiplicity of infection in order to initiate an observable reaction. Chlamydial absorption was the same at temperatures ranging from 22° to 37° C and at pH values between 6.0 and 8.0. The morphologic development of the 6 BC strain and the Borg strain was the same in both cells but differed between agents.

The forms of the inclusions produced by the 6 BC strain and by the Borg strain in Chang's human liver cells differ so greatly that the terms "diffuse" and "rigid" in determining inclusion types are mean-ingless for taxonomic purposes. In our opinion, it would be very easy to call the 6 BC inclusions rigid or compact and the Borg inclusions diffuse, yet both of these strains are in the same species, *C. psittaci.*

Chlamydiae may not only be grown in cells in monolayers; they can be grown in suspended cells in spinner culture (Schechter, 1966). Also, growth of the meningopneumonitis strain in L cells supported by a defined medium in spinner cultures has been reported (Morrison and Jenkin, 1972). For chlamydial strains capable of continued multiplication in tissue culture, plaquing systems have been developed. Higashi and Tamura (1960) used L cells, and Piraino and Abel (1964) used chick fibroblasts. Banks et al. (1970a), using L-929 cells, developed a highly sensitive, reproducible method which has proven effective in assaying plaque-forming infectivity of a wide variety of *C. psittaci* isolates of avian and mammalian origin, and with LGV strains. This assay has been utilized in the development of a plaque reduction system to measure neutralizing antibodies. This sys-tem has allowed a relatively crude serotyping of chlamydial strains of avian and mammalian origin (Banks et al., 1970b; Schachter et al., 1974, 1975b).

Harrison (1972) found that absorption of chlamydiae (ovine origin) onto Hep-2 cells is more efficient at 37° C than at 30° C. The smaller the volume, the more efficient the inoculum's absorption. In the studies of Banks et al. (1907b), it was found that the efficiency of absorption had to be carefully counterbalanced against the inacti-vation of the agent. Longer periods of contact between inoculum and agent may, in some systems, yield higher plaque counts, but in other systems the titers fell because of the thermolability of the agent. In some systems it was found that serum expected to contain neutralizing antibody actually enhanced the titers of infecting agent. Further studies showed that this enhancement was due to the protective effect of the serum protein. When dilutions were made in normal serum or with addition of a protein diluent, the titers stabilized and the effect of immune serum in reducing plaque counts could be shown.

LATENT INFECTIONS IN VITRO

Since Meyer's early studies on psittacosis in the 1930s, it has been recognized that latent or inapparent infections of the animal host are a hallmark of chlamydial infections. This host-parasite rela-tionship holds true for many of the chlamydial infections of domestic mammals (Storz, 1971) and is equally true for trachoma-inclusion conjunctivitis infections of man (Jawetz et al., 1967). In some systems it has been possible to establish latent infections in cell cultures. Bader and Morgan (1961) simulated a latent infection by nutritional depletion of the media. Enzyme antagonism mediated by aminopterin (Pollard and Sharon, 1963) resulted in latent infection in McCoy cells.

Manire and Galasso (1959) found that the HeLa cell clone S3 could be persistently infected with meningopneumonitis agent; this persistent infection was the result of a balance in cytopathic effect. Cell multiplication and chlamydial replication were in fine adjustment. The agent was produced continually, although the number of inclusion-containing cells varied from time to time. The persistent infection was established by inoculation of cells in maintenance medium, with actual production of agent being shown when complete medium was added. Once the system was established, it was possible for the authors to maintain their cells in infected state with complete medium for two years. Galasso and Manire (1961) then showed that antiserum prepared in rabbits had no effect on persistence of the agent, and that penicillin, although suppressing agent multiplication when included in the medium at 500 units per ml for 100 days, did not eradicate chlamydial infection. After removal of the penicillin the yields of infective agent rapidly rose to levels obtained in the untreated control. Tetracycline was highly effective in eradicating the persistent infection state, with 10 μg of tetracycline/ml for 14 days sufficing to clear infection.

Officer and Brown (1961) pursued studies on chronic infection of 6 BC agent in Chang's human liver cells and determined that several passages of the infected cells resulted in selection for an enhanced virulence on the part of the agent. However, continued passage of the surviving cells and organisms resulted in the appearance of a more resistant cell line. Thus, the isolated chlamydial agent selected from the 10th passage was much more virulent than the original parent, and the cells isolated after surviving the chlamydial infection were more resistant to the variant strain of agent. This system allowed persistence of infection in these cells for over a year. The chronically infected state developed from the mutual adaptation of both chlamydiae and host cells, with selection of the population allowing survival of both. It may be noted that variations in inclusion morphology were noted in the types of inclusions formed by the Borg strain in two different clones of human liver cells, wherein the same inoculum yielded diffuse inclusions in one clone and compact inclusions in the other, again indicating that part of the morphology of the inclusion may be a function of the host cell and not exclusively determined by the infecting agent.

Schoenholz (1968) established latent infections in rabbit cornea cell culture systems. He was able to do this by infecting with small inocula of a *Chlamydia* of avian origin. The latent infection could be activated by modifying the environment (reducing pH or heating the cultures to 39.3° C). These observations were extended to latent infections in macrophages obtained from infected mice (Schoenholz, 1970). In this system, normal macrophages and those obtained from infected animals had the same survival time in vitro unless the temperature was raised. Higher temperature led to rapid deterioration of the infected cells. Their complete destruction within five days was accompanied by increased chlamydial infectivity in the supernate. Addition of lymphocytes obtained from immune mice (but not those obtained from normal mice) protected the macrophages from the temperature-induced activation of infection. Thus, evidence was obtained in vitro that latency was dependent on an immune mechanism. The protective effect of the immune lymphocytes could be abolished by the addition of antilymphocyte serum. If extrapolation back to the intact host is possible, the chlamydiae presumably multiply and persist at a low level in macrophages, with their level checked by the interaction of immune lymphocytes and macrophages.

STABILITY OF CHLAMYDIAE

The chlamydiae have unjustly received reputations for being extremely labile organisms. A number of studies have shown that *C. psittaci* strains will survive for relatively long periods. Page (1959b) showed that viable chlamydiae could persist in the tissues of naturally infected turkeys for at least a year when frozen at −20° C. In fact, some of these tissues yielded isolates for several years (Meyer and Eddie, unpublished). The chlamydiae will persist in dry litter or feces from avian species for months (Eddie et al., 1962; Stiller, thesis, 1973). Page (1971) has pointed out that the heat lability of chlamydiae may be a function of their natural host's body temperature. Isolates from small birds with naturally higher body temperatures are more thermostable than isolates from larger hosts. In the laboratory, it seems that the major protective components of solutions for maintenance of chlamydiae are proteins, and Moulder (1962b) added serum albumin to the diluents. For many years we have used simple nutrient broth with highly satisfactory results.

Usually the *C. trachomatis* strains are more labile than the *C. psittaci* strains. The general experience seems to be that most strains lose infectivity in approximately 48 hours at 35° to 37° C. In unpublished studies at the World Health Organization Reference Centre, we have tested isolates for long-term storage and have

178

confirmed the lability at 37° C and have found that the major component in maintaining stability of the *C. trachomatis* strains is the yolk sac tissue and not the diluent. In the refrigerator (4° C), concentrated yolk sac suspensions maintain titer for a matter of weeks and when frozen at −60° C will maintain titer for approximately 5 years. When stored in liquid nitrogen, the isolates appear to maintain titer for longer periods (at least 10 years). With the use of tissue culture media, some workers have recommended addition of yolk or yolk sac before storage of chlamydial strains in order to maintain their infectivity. Weiss and Dressler (1962) found that the commonly used rickettsial diluent could be improved for chlamydiae by using a diluent of 0.4 M sucrose in 0.02 M sodium phosphate buffer (pH 7-7.4). We have recently recovered *C. psittaci* from lyophilized or frozen suspensions that have been stored in excess of 30 years.

Chlamydiae are relatively heat labile; they can be inactivated in a matter of minutes at 56° C, and can be inactivated by a variety of common disinfectants such as formalin or phenol. The suspensions must, as usual, be free of large clumped material to allow penetration of the disinfecting chemical, otherwise the chlamydiae will survive at much higher concentrations than the 0.1% to 0.25% formalin that is normally used.

Nabli and Tarizzo (1967) found that chlamydiae could persist for 2 to 3 days in tap water.

CHLAMYDIAL ANTIGENS

The major antigenic component of all chlamydiae is a heat-stable, group-specific antigen. This appears to be associated with the cell wall and can be detected throughout the growth cycle of the organisms (Reeve and Taverne, 1962). This antigen is heat-stable and ether-soluble, and it may be extracted or partially solubilized from chlamydial particles by boiling or treating with acid, alkali, deoxycholate, or ether. The antigen is inactivated by periodate. It may be precipitated with acetone. There appear to be separable components within the group antigen (Benedict and O'Brien, 1956; Benedict, Tips, and Eddy, 1955), but it is not known whether this is a reflection of physical state or actual chemical structure. It appears that lecithin may be a carrier, since some of the purified antigens were inactive in the CF test until lecithin was added.

Dhir and colleagues (1972) have further studied the antigen, purified the active moiety, and identified it as a 2-keto-3-deoxyoctanoic acid.

SPECIFIC ANTIGENS

Although indications of specific antigens had been obtained as far back as 1936 by Bedson, it was not until 1949 that he and his colleagues were able to identify species-specific chlamydial antigens. They accomplished this by utilizing the heat lability of the specific antigen and the heat stability of the group antigen. They absorbed the immune sera with heated antigen, and showed that reactivity was maintained for crude unheated suspensions. Other workers have demonstrated specific antigens in cell walls and have shown that both toxin-neutralizing and infectivity-neutralizing antibodies could be absorbed by cell wall suspensions (Jenkin, Ross, and Moulder, 1961; Ross and Jenkin, 1962). The neutralization of infectivity with specific hyperimmune sera was accomplished by Hilleman (1945) in a highly tedious system involving hyperimmunization of roosters and the scoring of lung lesions in intranasally infected mice. Unfortunately no good source of neutralizing antibody has been found, and most workers utilizing this technique have been forced to use hyperimmune rooster antiserum which is very difficult to produce. This system has been applied to studies involving neutralization of egg infectivity and plaque reduction tests (Moulder et al., 1958; Piraino, 1965).

The chlamydiae also possess a murine toxin which is capable of killing mice within a few to 24 hours following intravenous inoculation. Antiserum has been shown to prevent this, and was utilized by Manire and Meyer (1950) to differentiate a variety of *C. psittaci* strains. In addition, the mice may be immunized, and this mouse-toxicity prevention test (Bell et al., 1959) has been used as the basis for differentiating *C. trachomatis* strains (Alexander, Wang, and Grayston, 1967).

There is no readily useful technique for differentiating *C. psittaci* strains on the basis of antigenic structure. Workers at the Hooper Foundation have tried to develop a serologic system for classification, and the results suggest that isolates of avian origin seem to have an antigenic pattern which reflects the species in which they naturally occur. Those isolates obtained from domestic mammals seem to be more restricted in antigenic structure, with the same general serotypes being recovered from sheep, cattle, and other mammals (Banks et al., 1970b; Schachter et al., 1974, 1975a).

The *Chlamydia trachomatis* strains may be immunotyped with much greater ease. This is largely owing to the efforts of Wang and associates in applying the microimmunofluorescence test. This test, developed in 1970 by Wang and Grayston, has allowed identification of a number of related serotypes of trachoma-inclusion conjunctivitis

180

and lymphogranuloma venereum strains.* At this writing, trachoma-inclusion conjunctivitis types (designated with letters) are recognized from A through K, and three serotypes of lymphogranuloma venereum strains (L-1, L-2, and L-3) are also recognized. These antigens appear to be shared to some degree, with serotypes reacting to a greater or lesser degree in a manner reminiscent of the senior-junior antigenic evolution of the influenza viruses. None of these antigens has been identified biochemically. This test has not yet been applied systematically to the *C. psittaci* strains but shows promise in this application, as well.

HEMAGGLUTINATION REACTIONS

The chlamydiae produce a hemagglutinin during their growth cycle. This hemagglutinin appears to be related to the group antigen in both activity and physical properties (Gogolak, 1954). It was first described in infective allantoic fluids and reacts with murine erythrocytes (Hilleman, Haig, and Helmold, 1951). It will also agglutinate red blood cells from hamsters and chicken erythrocytes if the latter cells are susceptible to agglutination by vaccinia virus (Barron, Zakay-Rones, and Bernkopf, 1965). These hemagglutination reactions can be inhibited by antichlamydial antibodies, but this is not a useful diagnostic test.

CROSS-REACTIONS WITH OTHER ORGANISMS

The chlamydiae do not share antigens with any other organism. One-way cross-reactions have been reported between chlamydial group antigen and an organism known as *Bacterium antitratum* (Volkert and Matthiesen, 1956) and *Herrellea* species (Shimizu and Bankowski, 1963). These bacterial antigens react with chlamydial antibodies, but antibodies against these bacterial antigens do not react with chlamydial antigens; therefore, there is no known cross-reaction which would interfere with serologic diagnosis of chlamydial infections.

---

* The test is presented in detail in Chapter 11, dealing with diagnostic procedures, and is discussed in the chapters referring to the specific diseases where it has been used as an epidemiologic tool.

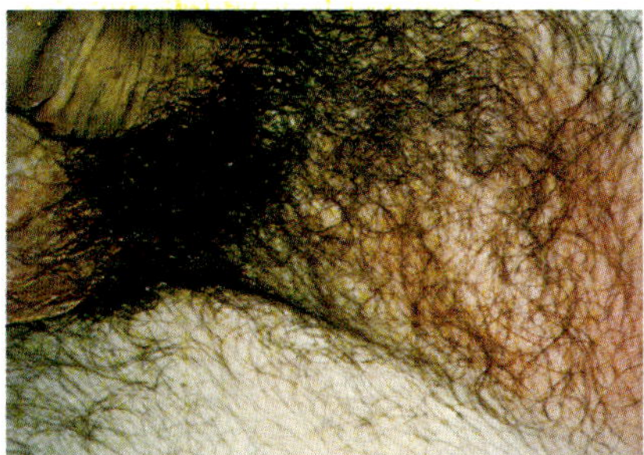

Fig. 1. Lymphadenitis with marked erythematous zone. Note primary lesion on frenulum. (Courtesy of Dr. Axel Hoke)

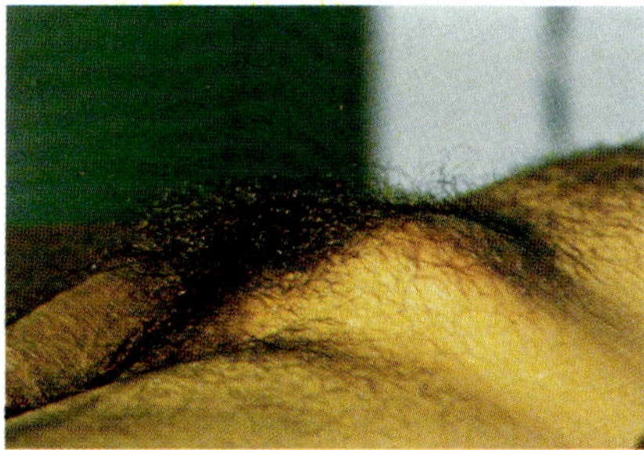

Fig. 2. Typical presentation of inguinal bubo. (Courtesy of Dr. Axel Hoke)

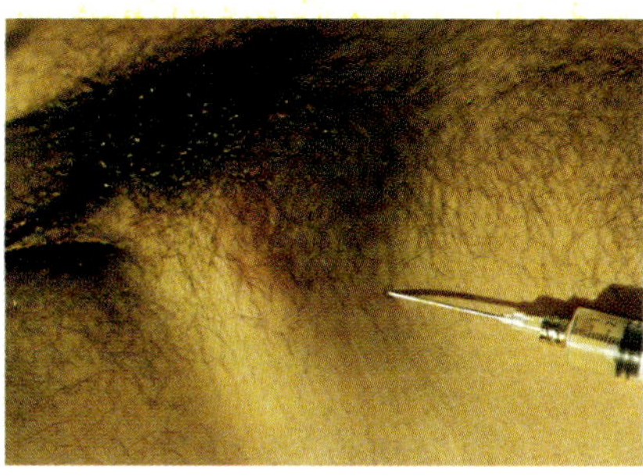

Fig. 3. Preferred method for aspiration of bubo. Note that the node is approached through healthy adjacent tissue. Frank pus is being withdrawn into this syringe. (Courtesy of Dr. Axel Hoke)

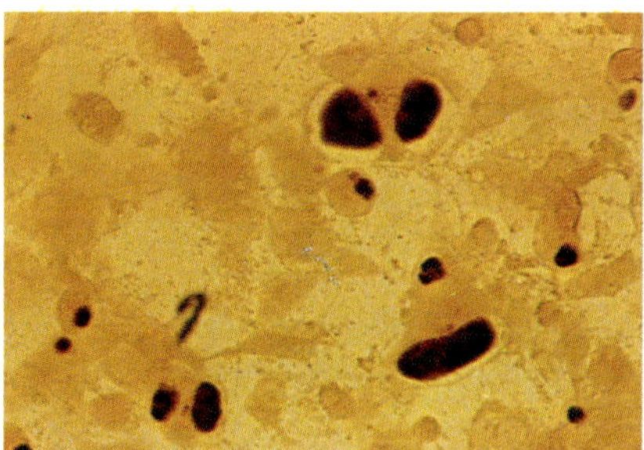

Fig. 4. Typical iodine-staining chlamydial inclusions in tissue culture 65 hours after inoculation of a 10^{-2} dilution of the material collected in Fig. 3.

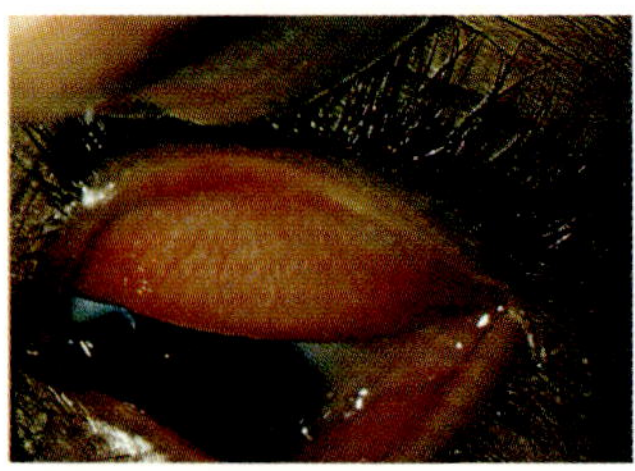

Fig. 1. Mild trachoma with lymphoid follicles (clear white spots) and papillary hypertrophy (punctate red dots). The normal conjunctival vessels extend upward on the everted tarsal plate. (Clinical scoring: follicles [F] 2; papillae [P] 1; scarring [C] 0; intensity mild; MacCallan stage I)

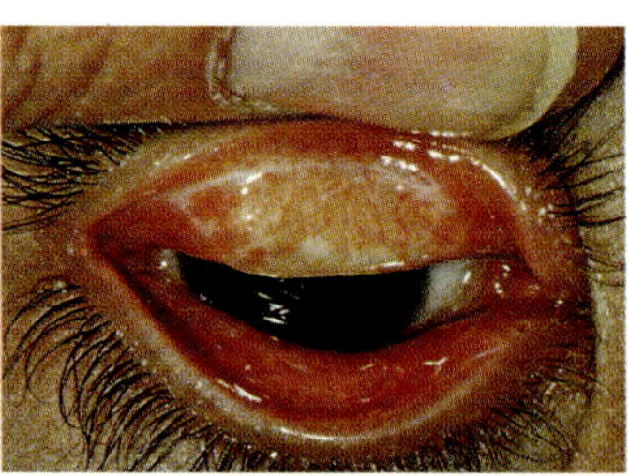

Fig. 2. Conjunctival scarring in mild trachoma with a linear white scar parallel to the margin of the upper lid and a few lymphoid follicles on the tarsal plate indicative of some degree of disease activity. (Clinical scoring: F2; P1; C3; intensity mild; stage III)

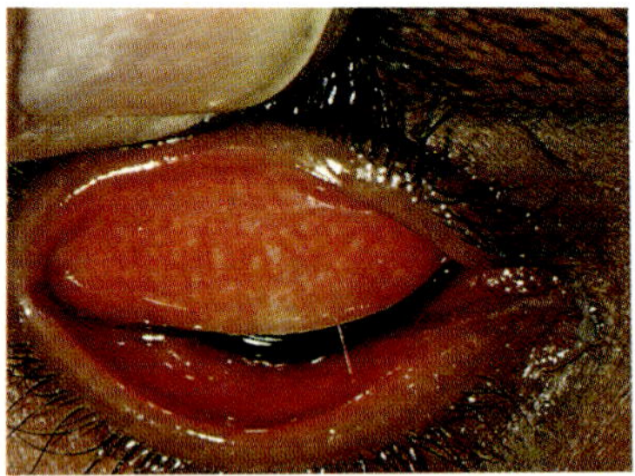

Fig. 3. Moderate intensity trachoma with lymphoid follicles, partially obscured vessels on the tarsal conjunctiva, and moderate conjunctival scarring. (Clinical scoring: F3, large; P2; C2; intensity moderate; stage III)

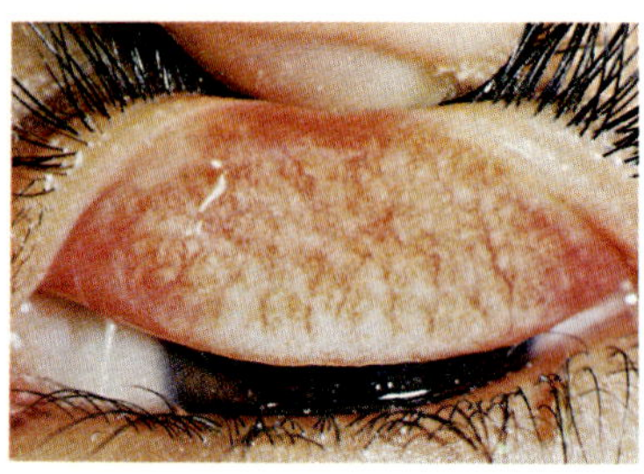

Fig. 4. Moderate to mild trachoma intensity with conjunctival scarring. Follicles appear to merge with scars and there is moderate papillary hypertrophy. (Clinical scoring: F3, small; P2; C2; intensity mild; stage III)

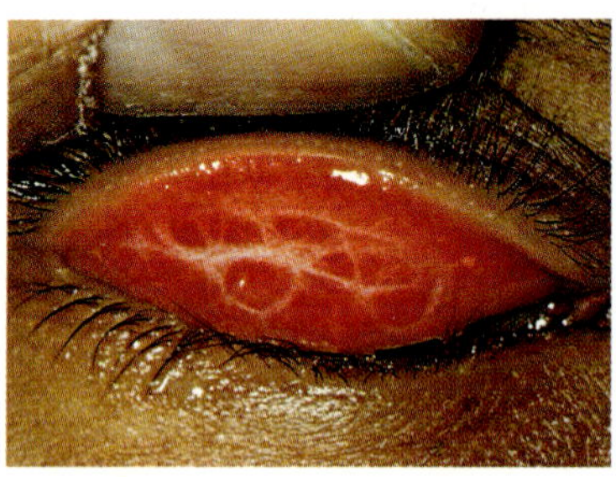

Fig. 5. Severe conjunctival scarring with active inflammation. The lid is distorted by dense conjunctival scars. Marked papillary hypertrophy and buried follicles are on the unscarred conjunctival surface. (Clinical scoring: F3, small; P3; C3; intensity severe; stage III)

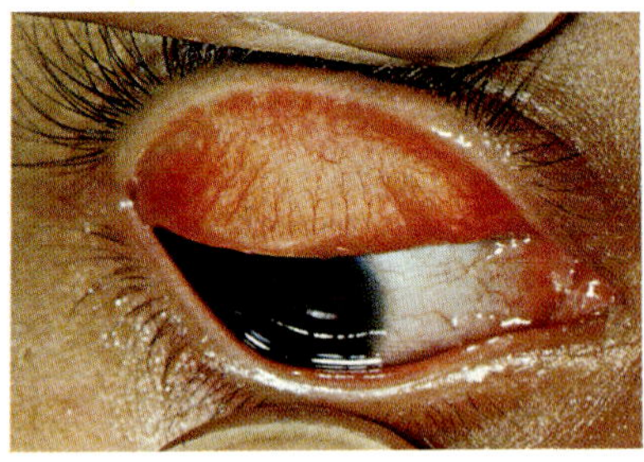

Fig. 6. Healed trachoma with small conjunctival scars and a few follicles along the retrotarsal lid margin. (Clinical scoring: F1; P1; C1; intensity inactive; stage IV)

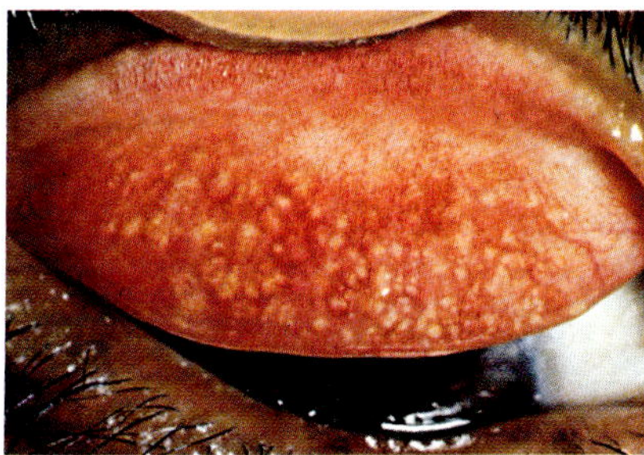

Fig. 7. Secondary conjunctival changes with trachomatous scarring ("post trachomatous degeneration"). The yellow spots are epithelial cysts due to scarring and contain a greasy material. (Clinical scoring: F1; P2; C3; intensity inactive; stage IV)

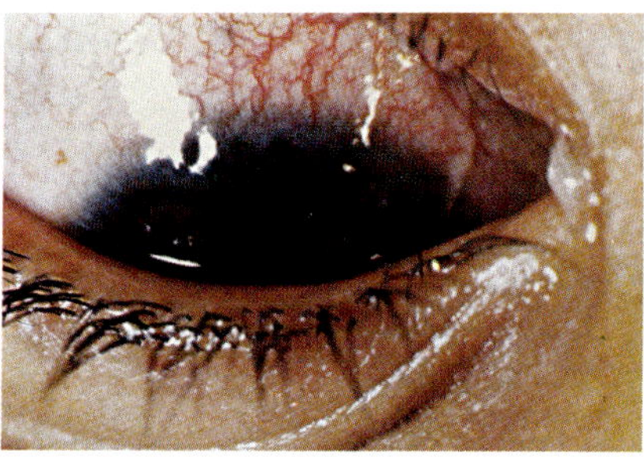

Fig. 10. Corneal infiltrates and blood vessels in active trachoma. The round, clear areas at the edge of the sclera are Herbert's peripheral pits, the site of lymphoid follicles. (Clinical scoring: Corneal vascularization [V] 2; corneal infiltration 1)

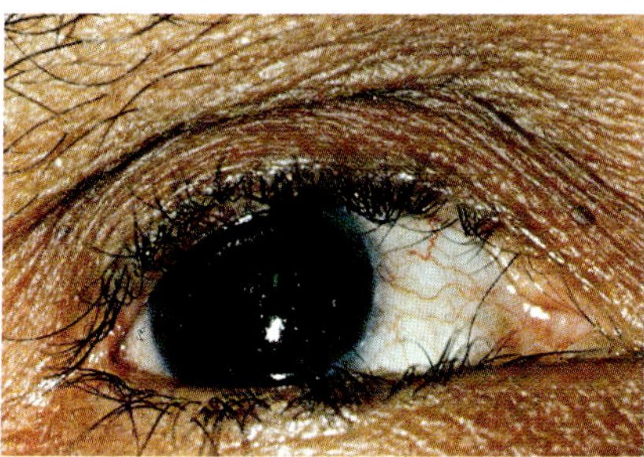

Fig. 8. Trichiasis (inturned eyelashes). The conjunctival scarring has caused misdirection of the eyelashes. The constant abrasion leads to ulceration and scarring of the cornea. (Clinical scoring: trichiasis/entropion [T/E] 3)

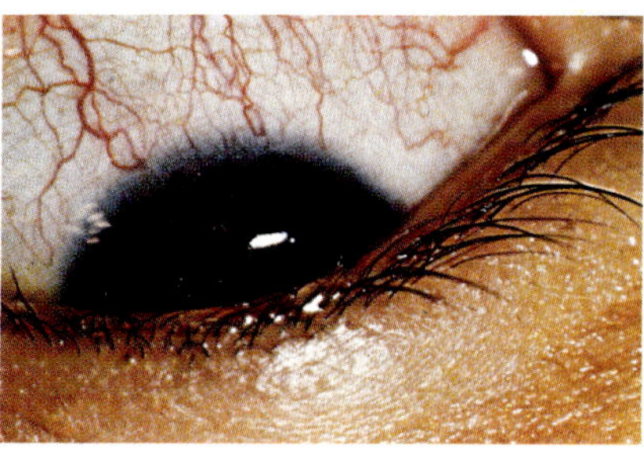

Fig. 11. Herbert's pits and corneal vascularization. These signs persist for the life of the individual.

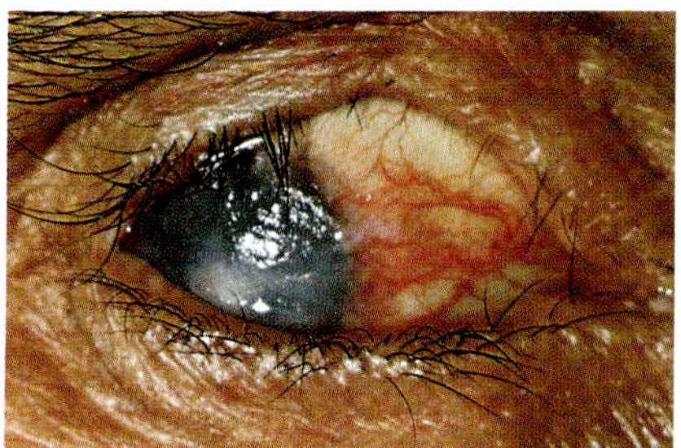

Fig. 9. Total corneal scarring and partial loss of the upper lid following surgery by a practitioner of "traditional medicine." (Clinical scoring: T/E 3; corneal scarring [CC] 3)

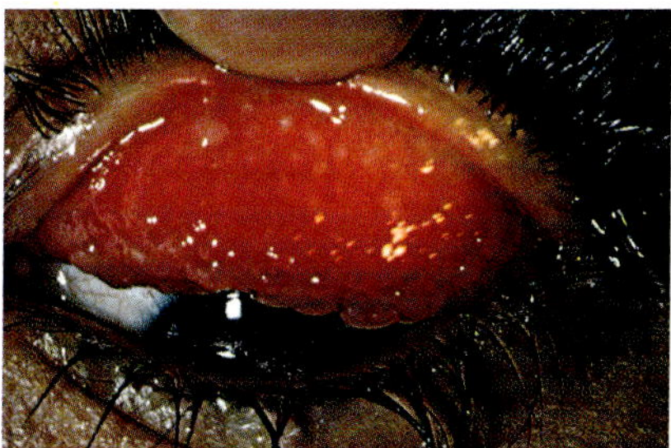

Fig. 12. Severe intensity trachoma with large follicles. Papillary hypertrophy completely obscures the normal vascular pattern. (Clinical scoring: F3, large; P3; CO; intensity severe; stage IIB)

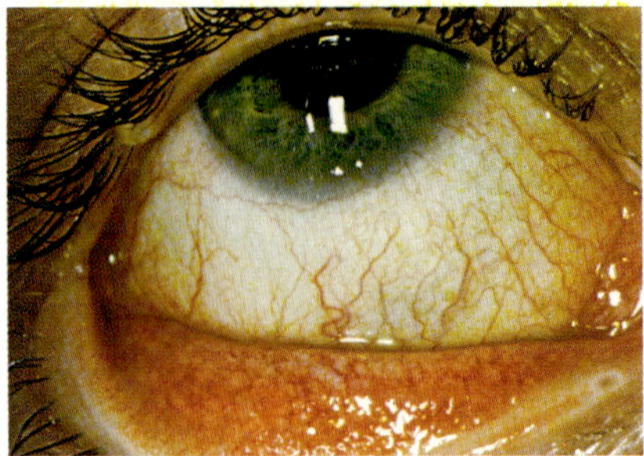

Fig. 13. Pseudo-trachoma with molluscum contagiosum of the lid margin. This is sometimes accompanied by conjunctival scarring and corneal pannus.

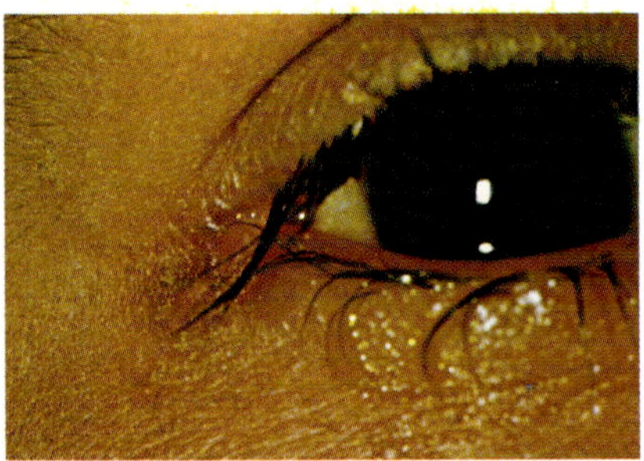

Fig. 14. Angular blepharitis with macerated skin and exudate at the temporal and nasal angles of the lids. It is commonly caused by mixed infection with *Moraxella* species (*M. lacunata*) and *Staphylococcus aureus*.

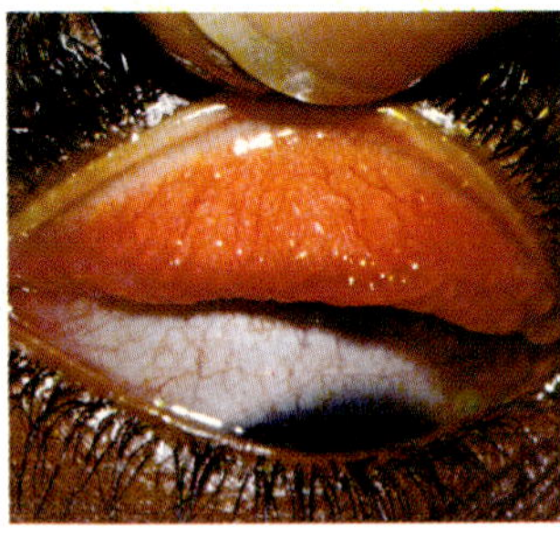

Fig. 15. Severe folliculosis or Axenfeld's chronic follicular conjunctivitis in a 14-year-old girl; this exuberant follicular hypertrophy was not associated with *Chlamydia* infection.

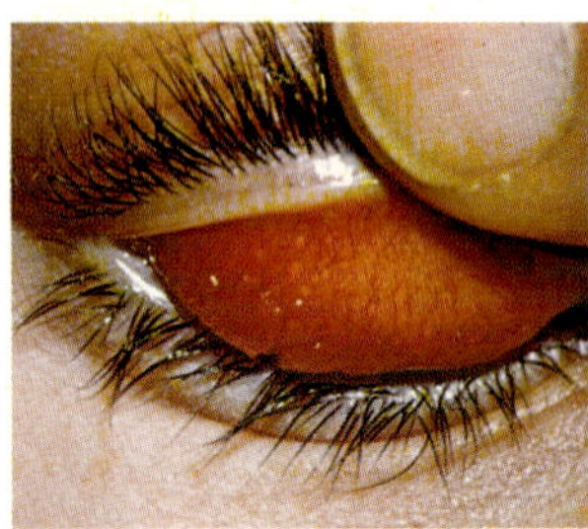

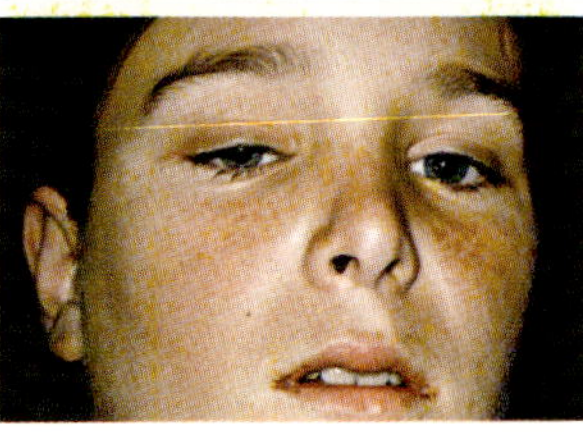

Fig. 16A. Parinaud's oculoglandular syndrome. A focal conjunctival lesion with follicles around a dense yellow area of infiltration consisting of granulomas. **B.** Massive enlargement of the preauricular node on the side of the affected eye.

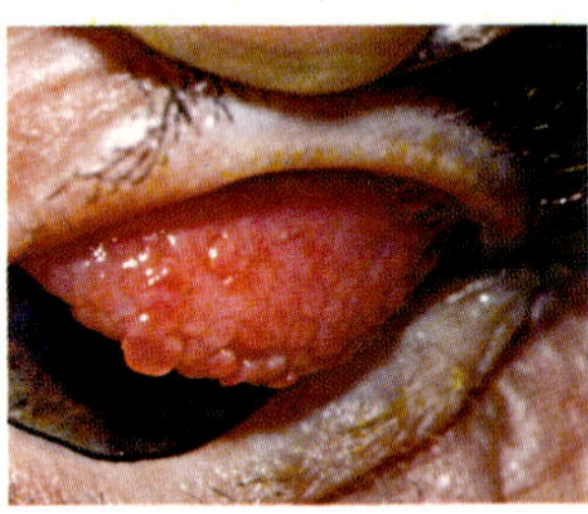

Fig. 17. Giant or "cobblestone" papillae on the tarsal conjunctiva that occur in vernal (spring) catarrh and atopic keratoconjunctivitis.

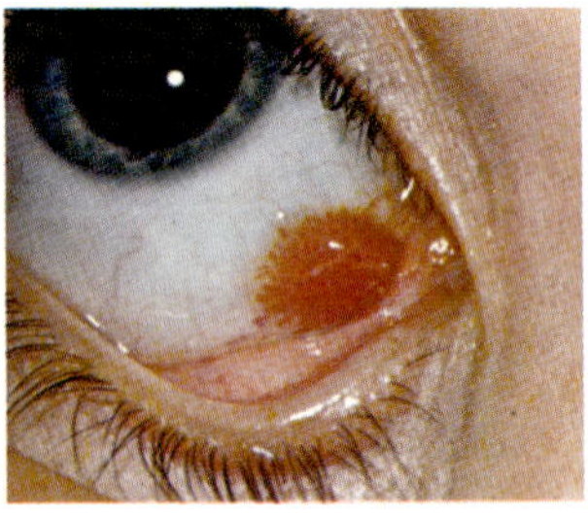

Fig. 18. Conjunctival papilloma. In some cases these lesions may be infectious.

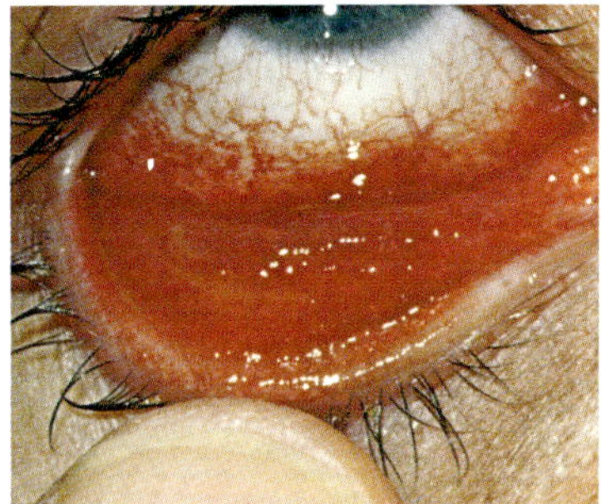

Fig. 1. Acute inclusion conjunctivitis of 2 weeks' duration with large conjunctival follicles in the inferior fornix surrounded by inflammatory infiltration.

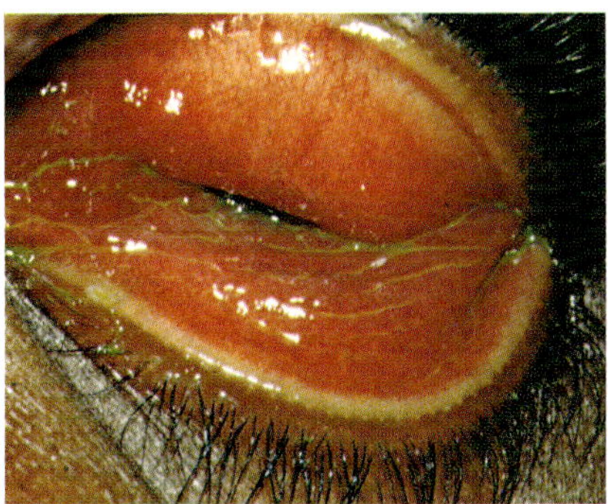

Fig. 2. Adult inclusion conjunctivitis of 3 weeks' duration with follicles in the lower fornix, and a few follicles and papillary hypertrophy on the everted tarsal plate.

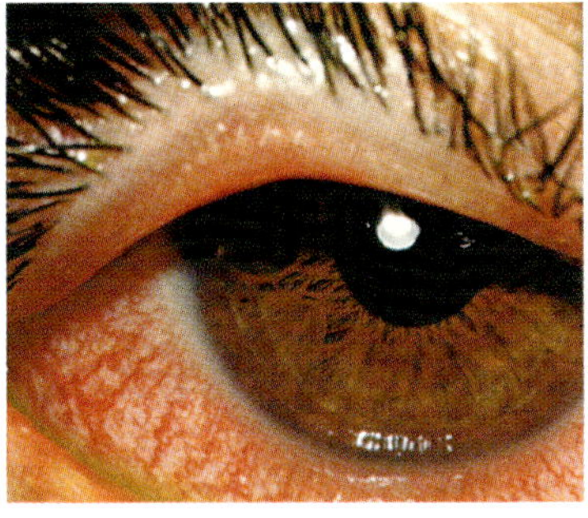

Fig. 3. Corneal infiltrate in a case of inclusion conjunctivitis (white spot at 9 o'clock in the cornea just below the lid margin).

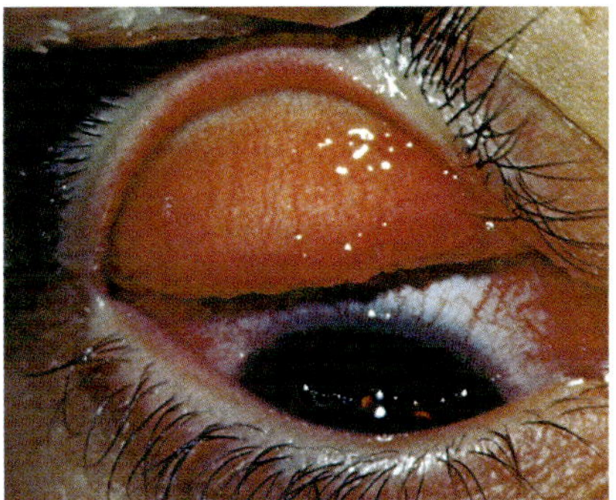

Fig. 4. Adult inclusion conjunctivitis of 3 months' duration with minimal papillary hypertrophy and lymphoid follicles at the edge of the tarsal plate. Conjunctival blood vessels have extended onto the corneal surface (pannus formation).

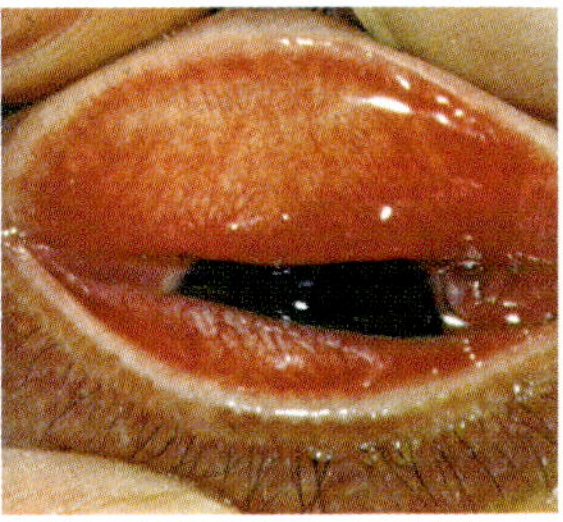

Fig. 5. Acute adenovirus conjunctivitis (epidemic keratoconjunctivitis). In the first week of illness there is usually a marked, watery discharge and inflammation of the conjunctiva, but follicle formation is not marked.

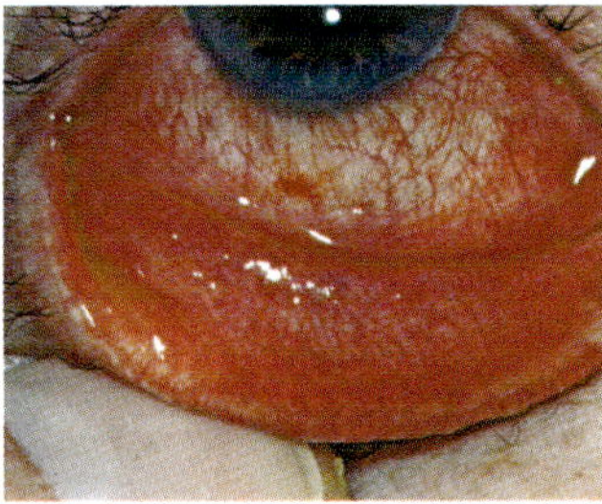

Fig. 6. Acute adenovirus infection. This acute eye infection usually runs its course in 2 weeks or less and subconjunctival hemorrhages are common. Follicle formation is not usually as florid as in adult inclusion conjunctivitis.

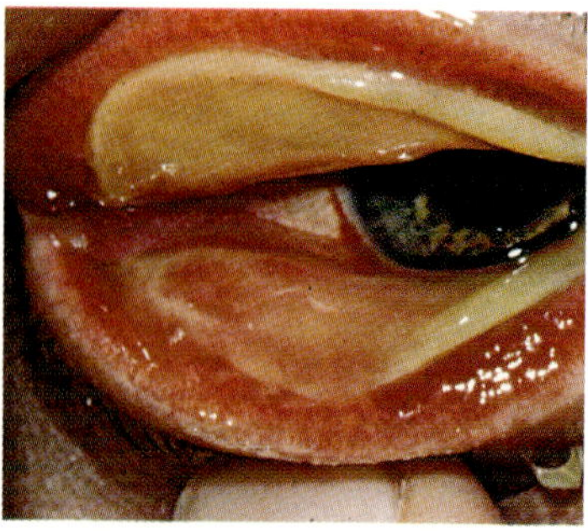

Fig. 7. Membrane formation in an acute adenovirus type 8 infection (epidemic keratoconjunctivitis), with a subconjunctival hemorrhage next to the cornea.

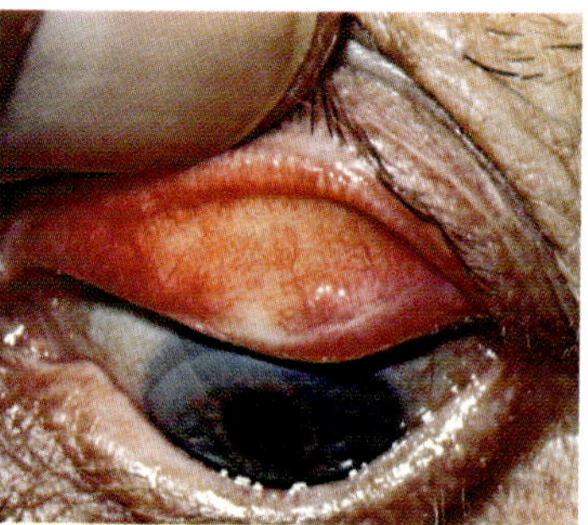

Fig. 8. Linear conjunctival scarring following membranous conjunctivitis due to adenovirus. This sign is not associated with any lid deformity.

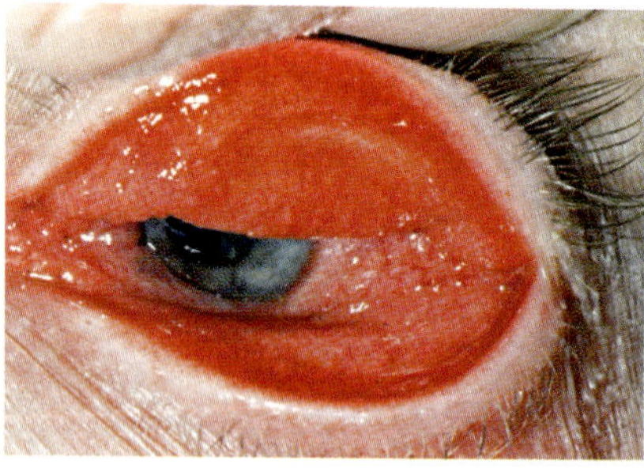

Fig. 9. Acute follicular conjunctivitis due to herpes simplex virus. This patient has a corneal ulceration (opacity in the pupillary area), but herpetic conjunctivitis is not always accompanied by corneal involvement.

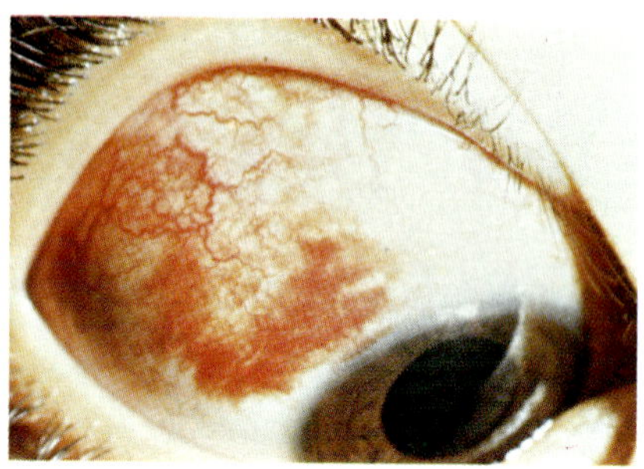

Fig. 10. Acute hemorrhagic conjunctivitis. This syndrome has an acute onset with marked subconjunctival hemorrhages during the first 24 hours and limited follicle formation. The disease subsides in 4 to 5 days.

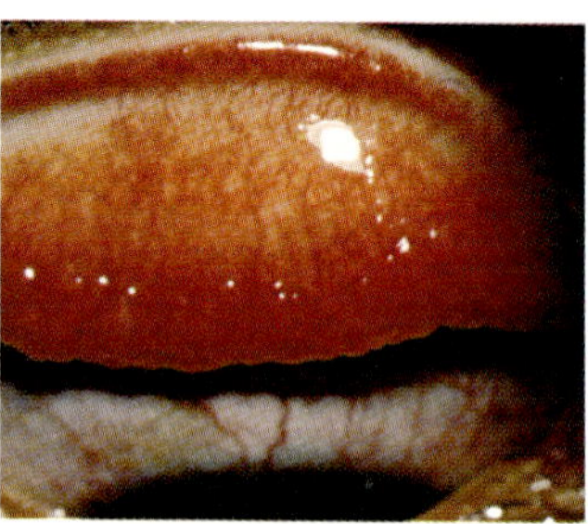

Fig. 11. Chronic follicular conjunctivitis due to psittacosis agent with follicle formation at the end of the everted tarsal plate and moderate infiltration. There was only a minor corneal involvement in this case.

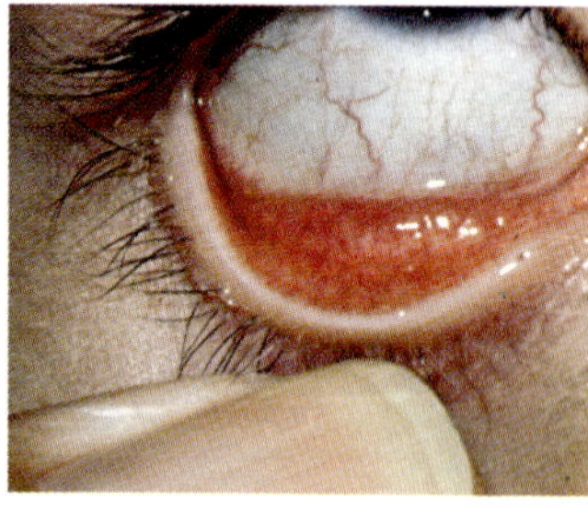

Fig. 12. Feline pneumonitis infection presenting as a chronic follicular conjunctivitis in a 7-year-old girl. There is a moderate amount of follicular hypertrophy and conjunctival inflammation but no corneal involvement.

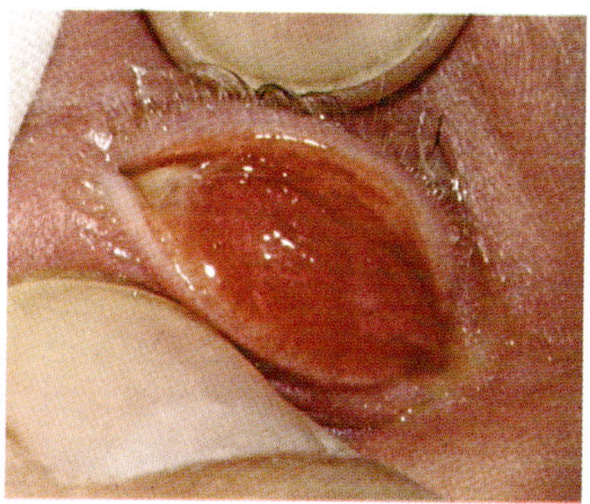

Fig. 1. Acute eye infection in a newborn at 3 weeks of age with onset at 8 days. There is hyperemia, engorgement of the conjunctiva, and a mucopurulent discharge. The cornea is not affected.

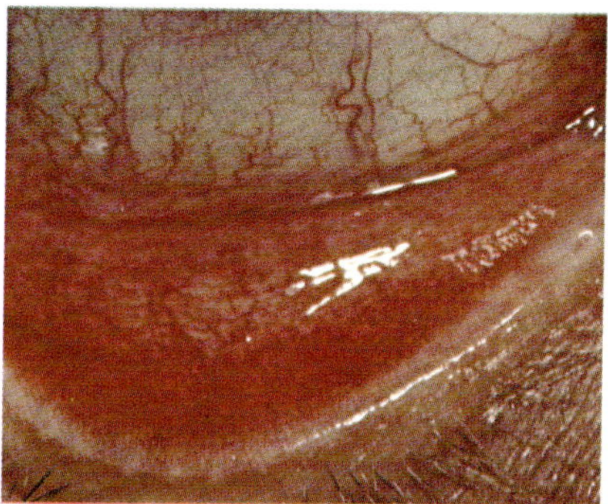

Fig. 1. Papillary conjunctivitis in a patient with Reiter's syndrome. In most cases there is a smooth infiltration of the conjunctiva and a watery discharge; follicles are entirely absent. Occasionally, patients with Reiter's syndrome present with a conjunctivitis identical to that found with adult inclusion conjunctivitis associated with large follicle formation.

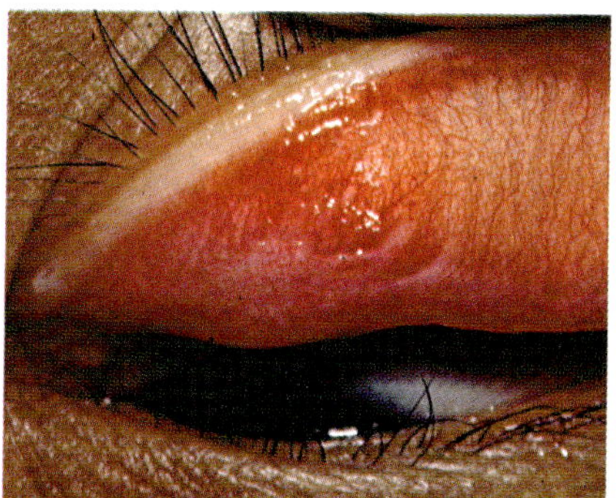

Fig. 2. Sheet scarring in an 11-year-old child who had neonatal inclusion conjunctivitis proven by laboratory diagnosis. There were no symptoms from the scarring.

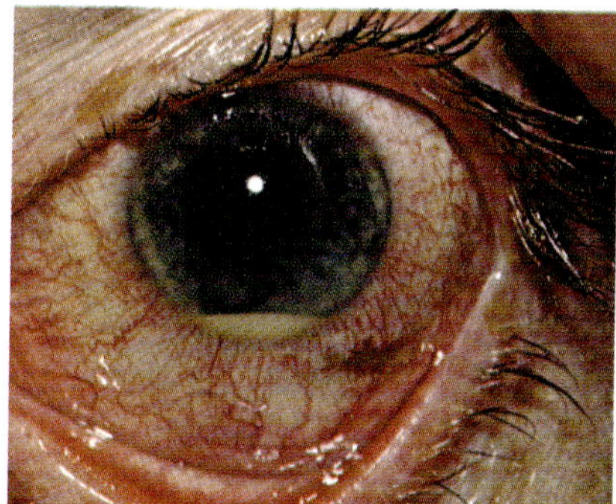

Fig. 2. Acute anterior iritis in Reiter's syndrome. This patient had previously had genital involvement and urethritis. The acute inflammation in the anterior segment of the eye has produced a collection of inflammatory cells which are seen as the level, white mass filling the anterior chamber below the pupil. This patient had several simultaneous recurrences of eye and joint disease. Chlamydial agent had been demonstrated in his urethra, and he had been treated with tetracycline, but this did not prevent recurrent disease.

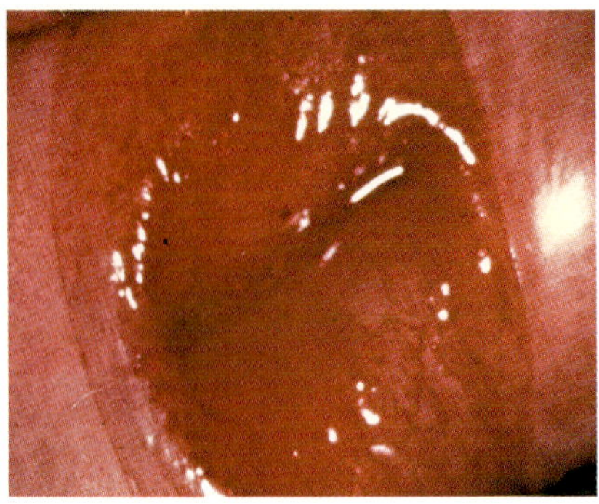

Fig. 1. Chlamydial urethritis showing marked papillary congestion and mucopurulent discharge. (From Dunlop et al., 1966a)

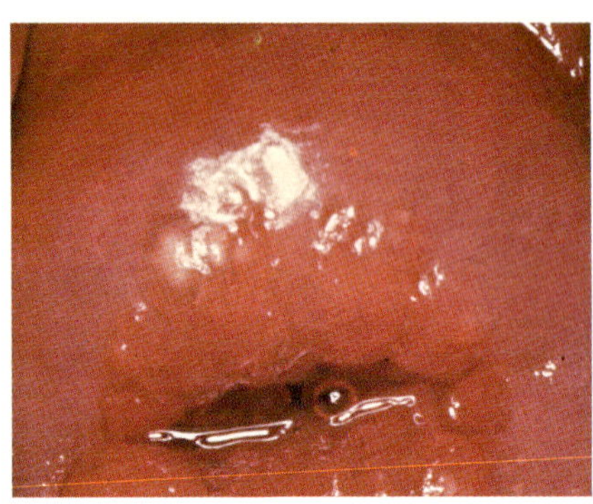

Fig. 3. Chlamydial cervicitis with "follicular" appearance. (From Dunlop et al., 1964)

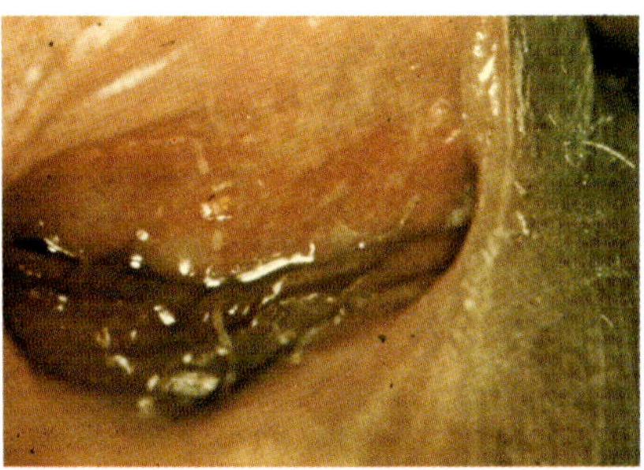

Fig. 2. Chronic chlamydial urethritis in father of an infant with inclusion conjunctivitis. Note the "follicle-like" intraurethral findings. (From Dunlop et al., 1966a)

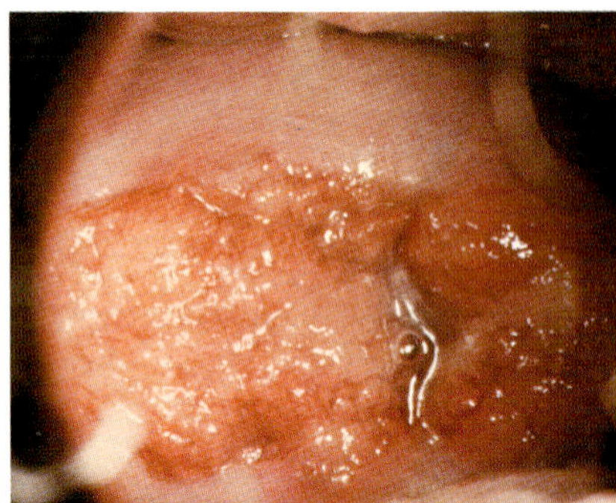

Fig. 4. Severe, progressive cervicitis associated with chlamydial infection.

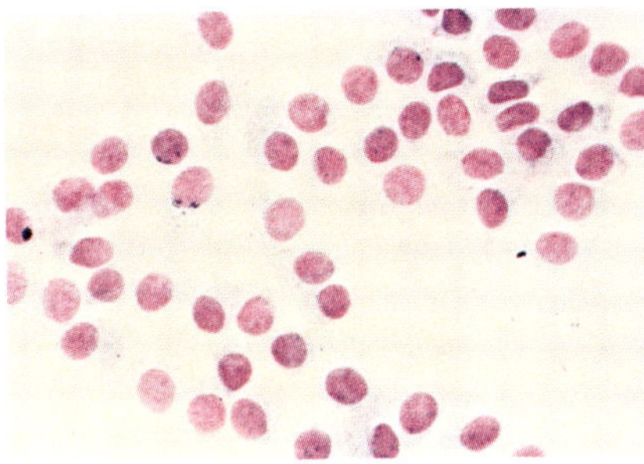

Fig. 1. A Giemsa-stained conjunctival scraping from a patient without inflammatory disease. These epithelial cells are present as a continuous layer. The dark particles of the cell cytoplasm are melanin granules.

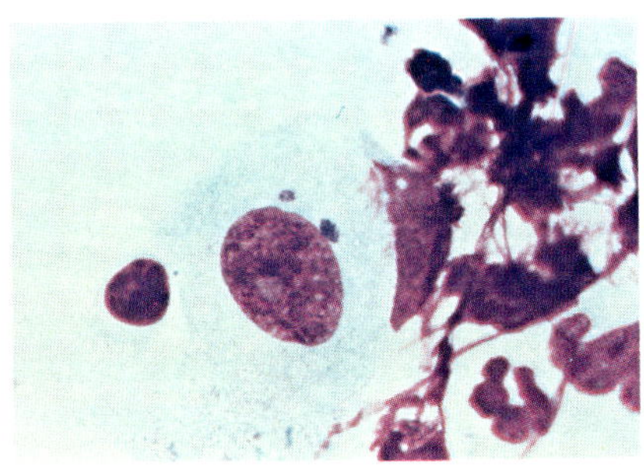

Fig. 2. Two initial body inclusions in a conjunctival epithelial cell from a Tunisian child with endemic trachoma.

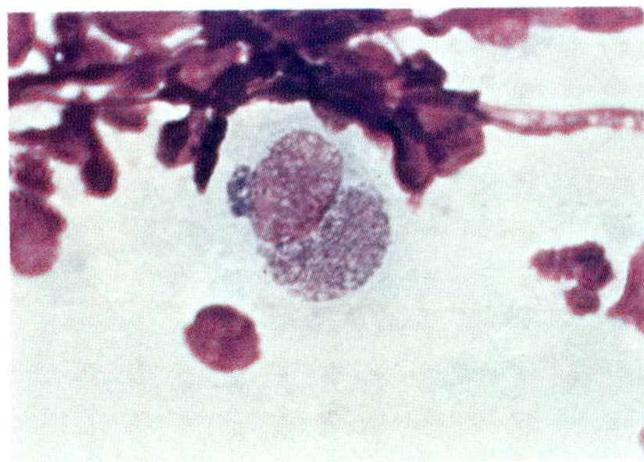

Fig. 3A. A Giemsa-stained conjunctival smear showing an initial body inclusion and an elementary body inclusion in a single cell from a case of endemic trachoma.

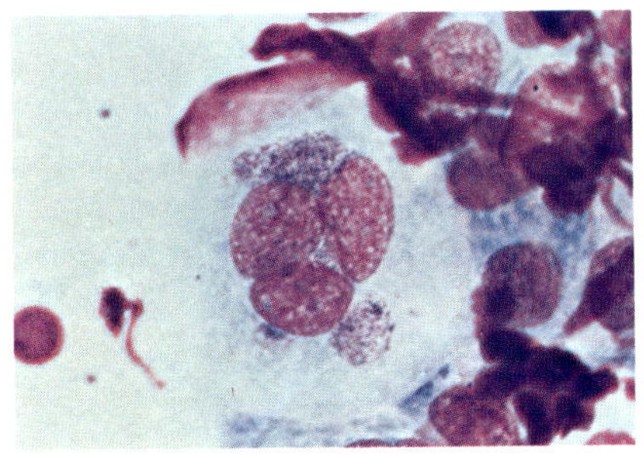

Fig. 3B. Giant cell with multiple elementary body inclusions.

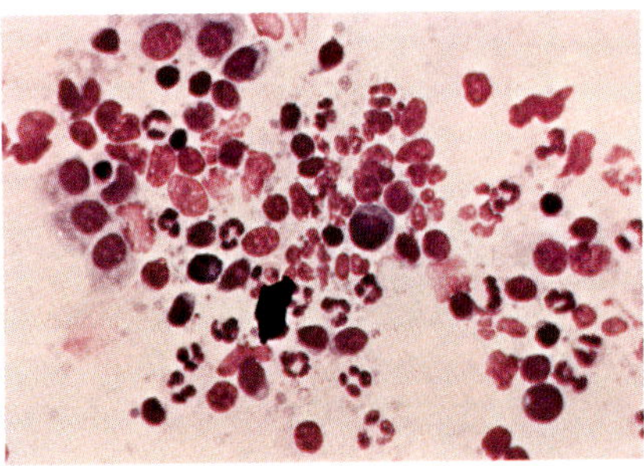

Fig. 4. Typical trachoma cytology showing separated epithelial cells, many polymorphonuclear leukocytes with mononuclear elements, lymphocytes, and occasional plasma cells or other elements.

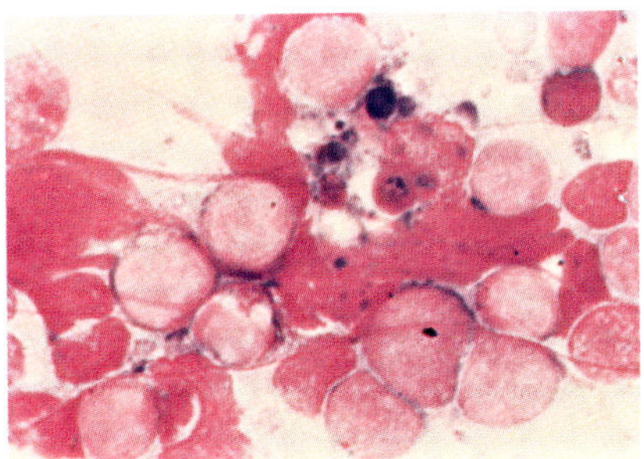

Fig. 5. A follicular expression from the conjunctiva in a patient with chronic trachoma showing numerous immature lymphocytic cells, a macrophage, and other elements.

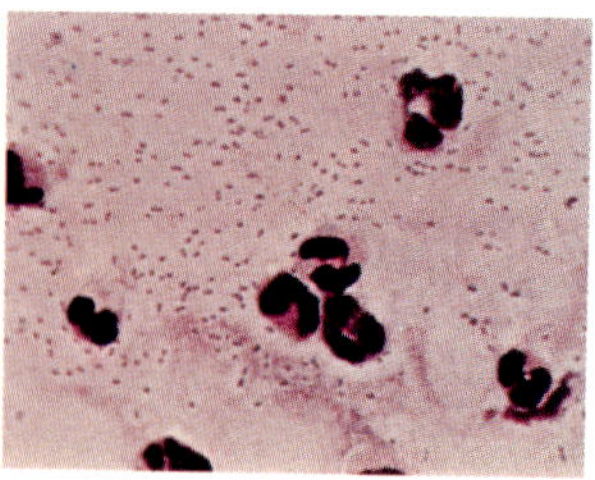

Fig. 6. Giemsa-stained conjunctival preparation showing diplococci, probably pneumococcus. This ocular pathogen occurs more frequently in winter months in trachoma endemic areas. (From Yoneda et al., 1975)

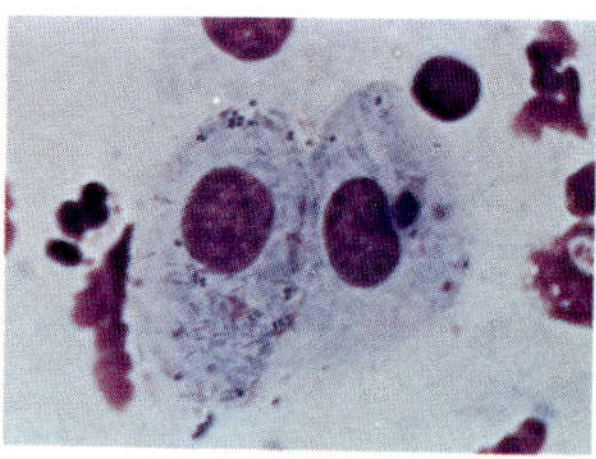

Fig. 7. Giemsa-stained conjunctival scraping from an Egyptian child with chronic trachoma and purulent conjunctivitis. Dense staining diplococcus, probably *Neisseria* species (an outbreak of *Neisseria* conjunctivitis was occurring in this community at the time and both *N. meningitidis* and *N. gonorrhoeae* have been identified from ocular specimens). In addition there are faint staining rods (probably *Haemophilus aegyptius* or Koch-Weeks bacillus) on this epithelial cell.

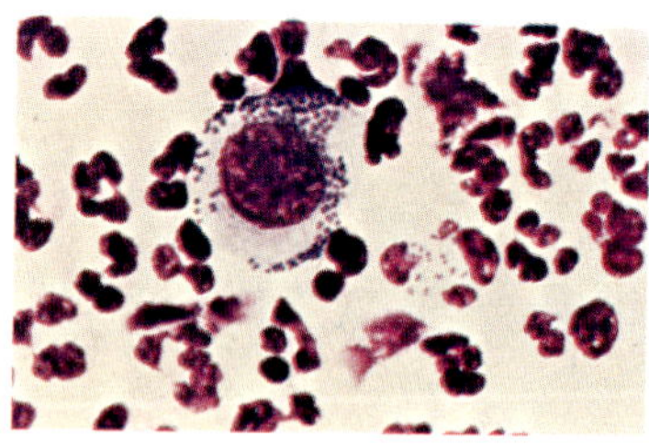

Fig. 8. *Neisseria*-like diplococci in a polymorphonuclear leukocyte and, as is more common in conjunctival scraping, coating an epithelial cell from the eye of a child with purulent conjunctivitis. (From Yoneda et al., 1975)

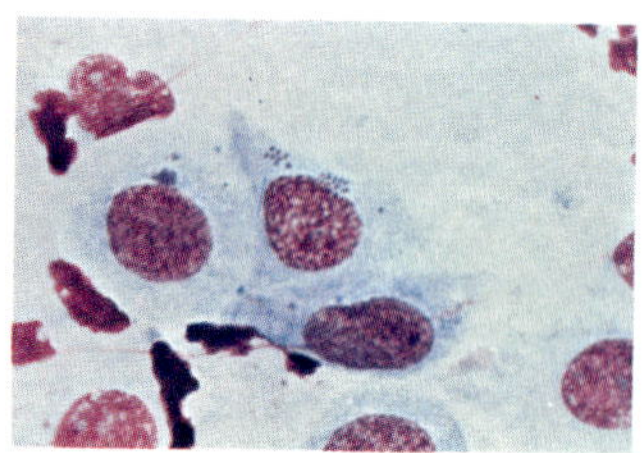

Fig. 9. *Neisseria*-like forms in or on a conjunctival epithelial cell; these diplococci are very regular in size and shape. In the cell to the left there are two initial body inclusions with similar tinctorial properties but with less regular staining characteristics and varying in particle size.

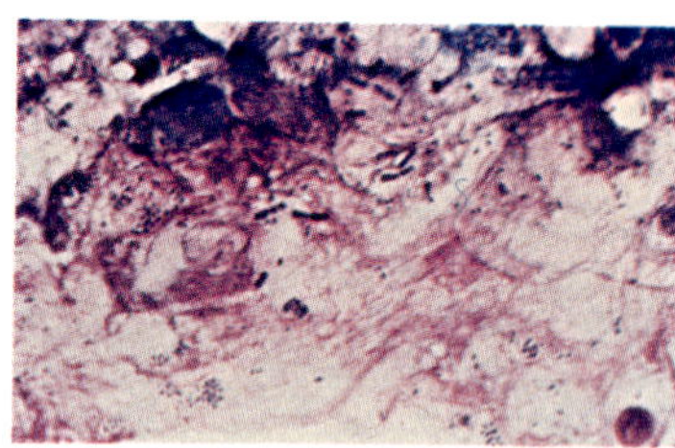

Fig. 10. Conjunctival smear showing Giemsa-stained diplobacilli (*Moraxella* species). Some small coccal forms are also present in this smear, probably pneumococcus. Note the difference in size between the *Moraxella* and the presumed pneumococcal forms.

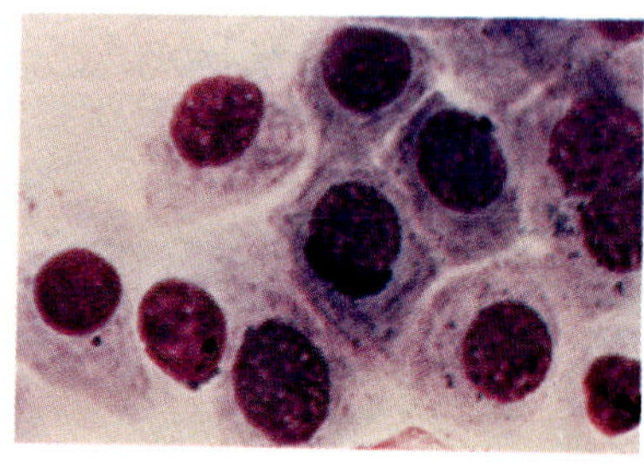

Fig. 11. Melanin granules in a conjunctival epithelial cell forming a cap over the nucleus suggestive of a chlamydial inclusion. Melanin can be distinguished by its green-black color on Giemsa-stained preparations and by the presence of individual granules scattered throughout the cytoplasm of adjacent cells. (From Yoneda et al., 1975)

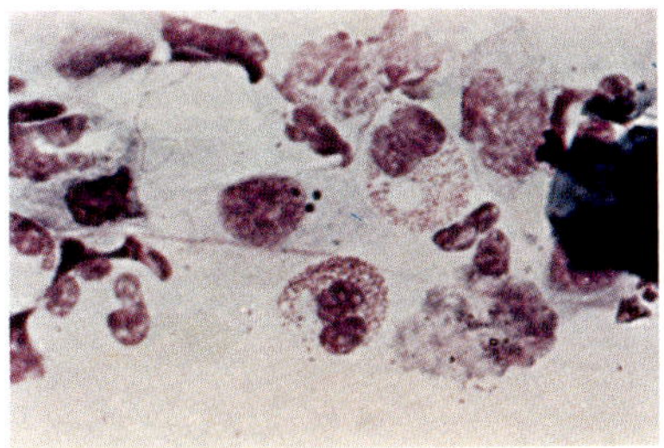

Fig. 12. Eosinophilic polymorphonuclear leukocytes and free eosinophilic granules. The distinctive red color and presence of the leukocytes distinguish these granules from elementary bodies and inclusions. Both eosinophilic leukocytes and free granules occur in large numbers of patients with atopic conjunctival reactions. (From Yoneda et al., 1975)

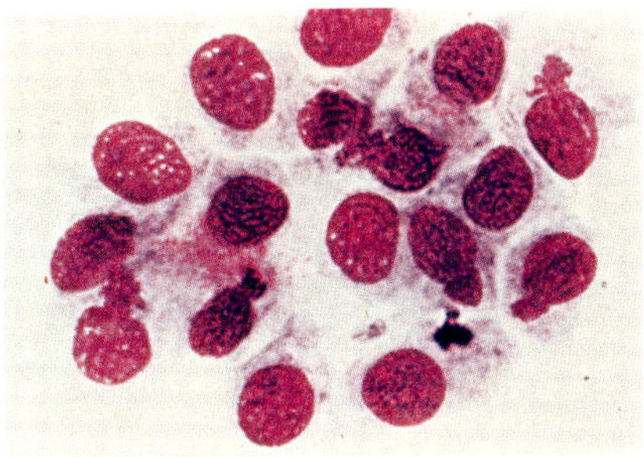

Fig. 13. A Giemsa-stained conjunctival scraping showing nuclear extrusions of the cytoplasma of epithelial cells. These extrusions are usually attached to, and have the same color and consistency as, the nucleus.

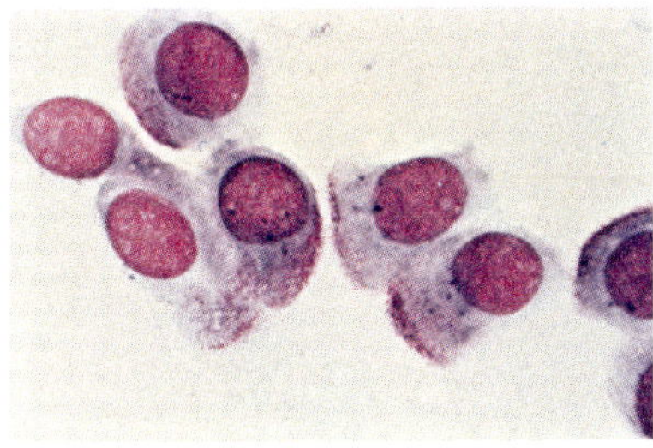

Fig. 14. Granular cytoplasm may be an artifact of fixation or may be found in goblet cells.

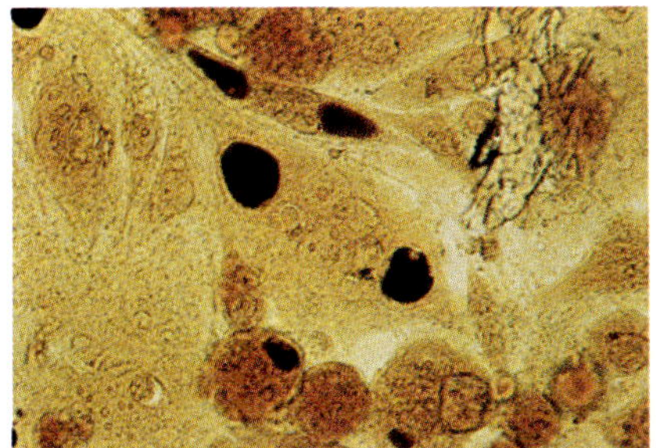

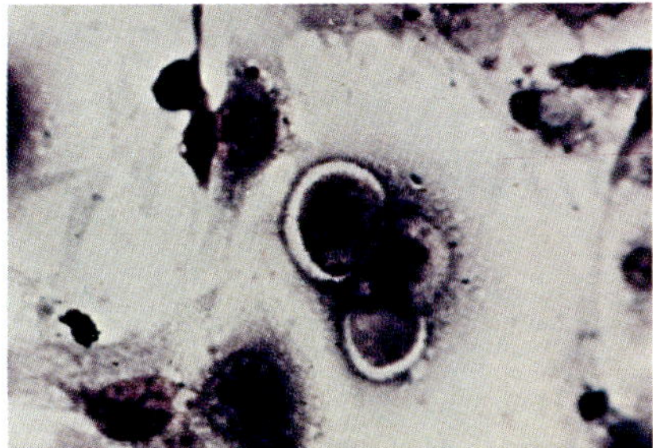

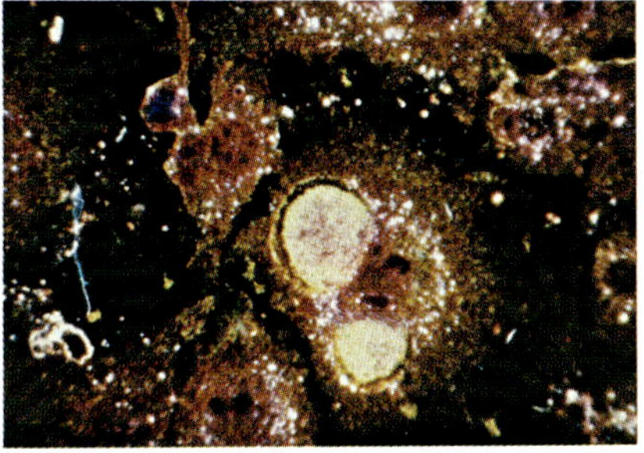

Fig. 15. Visualization of *C. trachomatis* inclusions in irradiated McCoy cells. **A.** Iodine-stained. **B.** Giemsa-stained—bright field illumination. (Courtesy of Dr. S. Darougar) **C.** Same preparation as in B visualized by dark field illumination. (Courtesy of Dr. S. Darougar)

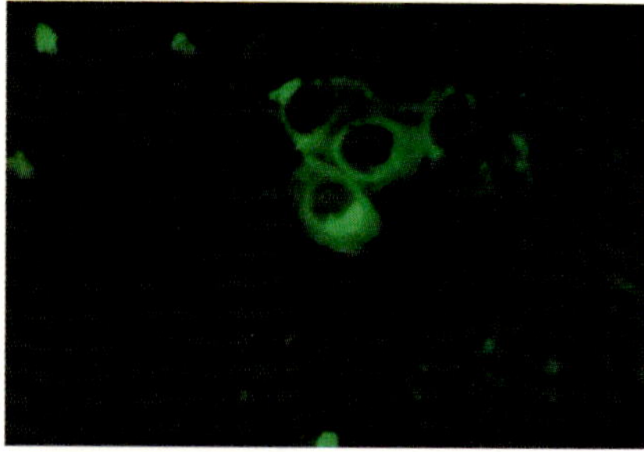

Fig. 16. Fluorescent antibody-stained inclusion in conjunctival scraping from patient with trachoma.

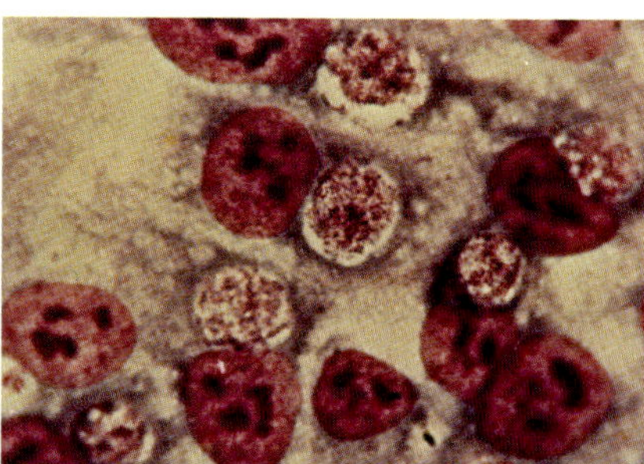

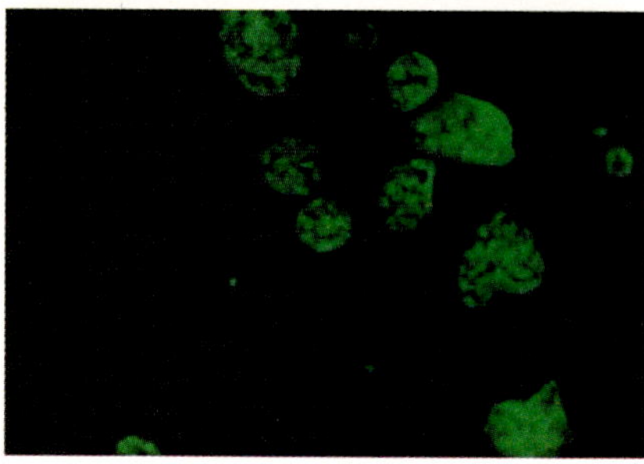

Fig. 17. Lymphogranuloma venereum agent in HeLa cells. Inclusion shown by: **A.** Giemsa stain **B.** fluorescent antibody.

Fig. 18. See Chapter 11.

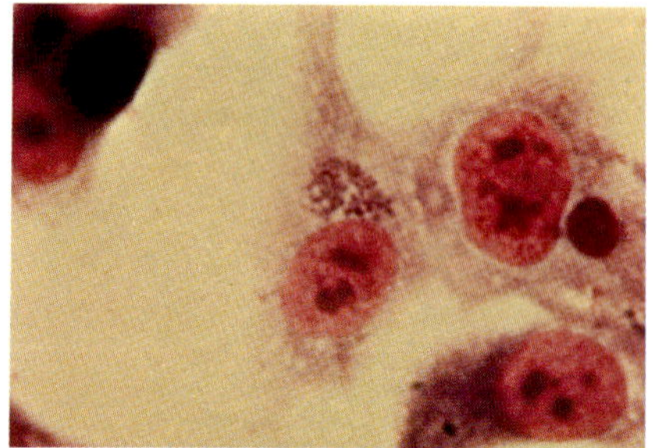

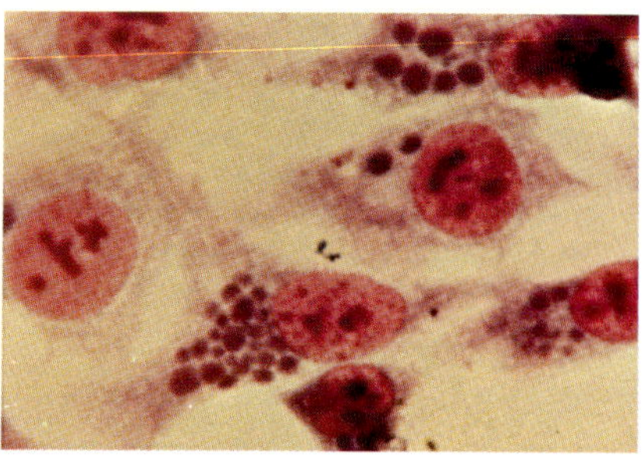

Fig. 19. Psittacosis agent in HeLa cells. **A.** An initial body inclusion (particulate) and an elementary body inclusion. The elementary bodies are often packed so tightly that individual particles are difficult to visualize. **B.** Multiple inclusions are commonly found in single cells. Note absence of vacuoles found with *C. trachomatis* infection.

11 Laboratory Diagnosis

Laboratory diagnosis of human chlamydial infections may be achieved by three general methods: (1) cytologic, in which the typical intracytoplasmic inclusions are demonstrated in the patient's cells; (2) isolation,* in which the infection is proven by recovery of chlamydiae from the patient's tissues; and (3) serologic, in which antichlamydial antibodies are measured.

In the present chapter we shall neither review the evolution of these diagnostic tests nor try to present a complete inventory of the techniques and technical variations that have been published, except for those cases where much recent progress has been made. Rather, we shall try to focus on the tests we use regularly and to present technical details and a critical evaluation of results.

Unfortunately, the different human diseases (psittacosis, lymphogranuloma venereum, trachoma, inclusion conjunctivitis, and the

---

* Isolation of psittacosis agents should not be undertaken by laboratories lacking suitable isolation or containment facilities. These are highly infectious human pathogens, and laboratory infections are common among even the most experienced laboratory workers.

181

genital tract infections) differ sufficiently in the hosts' responses and the biologic properties of the infecting chlamydiae to usually require different diagnostic tests. Even when the same test can be used for more than one disease, the interpretations may differ. It is partially because of problems in interpretation of laboratory results, and the effects of other chlamydial infections on interpretation of serologic results, that we have elected to discuss diagnostic methodology and interpretation separately. We shall discuss in detail the diagnostic tests mentioned briefly in previous chapters dealing with specific diseases.

The selection of the most suitable tests may vary with different conditions. For example, countries with severe endemic trachoma may lack sophisticated laboratory equipment or expertise, so the choice of tests may differ from those used in diagnosing sporadic infections occurring in industrialized countries.

CYTOLOGIC TECHNIQUES

Human psittacosis can rarely be diagnosed on cytologic grounds. Occasionally inclusions can be demonstrated in touch preparations and, in rare instances, in sections from involved sites studied at autopsy. The impression smears may be stained by the Giemsa, Giminez, or Macchiavello techniques described below. These techniques are highly successful in experimental systemic chlamydial infections. For example, psittacosis agents inoculated intraperitoneally into mice will yield spleen and liver smears rich in inclusions. Stained impression smears are occasionally helpful in detecting chlamydial infection in the tissues of infected birds (studied as sources of human disease).

Our experience with examining sections has shown that the thickness of the section is of paramount importance. Sections should be cut at $<4\mu$ (preferably 2μ) from tissues that have been fixed in Zenker's, Bouin's, Carnoy's, or Schaudinn's fixative. The recommended stains include Wolbach's Giemsa and Noble's stain; the reader should consult standard histopathology books for procedures (or see Meyer and Eddie, 1964). Use of newer embedding materials (such as epon) may improve results, but the search for inclusions is rarely rewarded, in part due to sampling problems. Histopathology is generally applied in experimental work. We never use this technique in routine diagnostic work, and use it only for retrospective testing when fixed tissue is available and a suggestion of chlamydial infection is made too late for other tests to be used.

Fluorescent antibody (FA) procedures have been described for the diagnosis of *Chlamydia psittaci* infections in birds and experimental hosts (Buckley, Whitney, and Rapp, 1955; Donaldson et al., 1958; Lewis, Thacker, and Cacciapuoti, 1973). We do not find these techniques helpful in experimental systems, and they currently play no role in diagnosing human psittacosis.

It is rarely worth the effort to search for inclusions in pus aspirated from the buboes of LGV. Although chlamydial developmental forms have occasionally been shown, it is very difficult to recognize chlamydiae against the background of cell detritus and active phagocytosis in frank pus. Rarely, inclusions can be demonstrated in biopsy or necropsy material from late lesions of LGV, but none of these procedures can be recommended.

Collection of the Specimen

For cytologic studies, the goal of specimen collection is to obtain an adequate amount of material (at least 1,000 epithelial cells) and to distribute it on the slide in a manner that will facilitate microscopic examination. The specimen should be spread in a manner that minimizes heaping of cells and allows visualization of single cells (Fig. 1, Plate 9). The scrapings, usually collected after topical anesthesia with a spatula (usually blunt, although some workers prefer sharp edges), are spread on the slide. Specimens are usually collected from the upper fornix in the case of trachoma and lower conjunctiva in inclusion conjunctivitis. Genital tract specimens can be collected with spatulas (the Jones-Dunlop curettes are excellent) and are usually collected from 3 to 6 cm down the male urethra and from the transitional zone of the cervical epithelium.

If follicular expressions are particularly sought, the follicles can be removed with a curette or ring forceps, and the collected material spread on the slide.

The Giemsa Stain

It is in the diagnosis of the ocular chlamydial infections, trachoma and inclusion conjunctivitis, that cytology has been most important. Visualization of the typical intracytoplasmic inclusion has been the classical method of diagnosis (Figs. 2, 3, Plate 9). The Giemsa stain has been the time-honored method to which all new techniques must be compared. The essential epidemiology of ocular and genital tract TRIC agent infections was elucidated by this technique long before the agents were isolated.

Each of the three generally accepted methods for demonstrating TRIC agent inclusions in clinical specimens offers certain advantages depending on the specific situation. The Giemsa stain provides permanent preparations and allows the observer an assessment of the patient's inflammatory cell response; it can also help to identify secondary bacterial infections. The inflammatory cells may be particularly helpful in the diagnosis of sporadic cases of adult inclusion conjunctivitis. With these cases there may be a problem in differential diagnosis with other forms of acute follicular conjunctivitis (primarily adenovirus and occasionally herpesvirus infections). Presumptive differentiation may be made on the basis of cell response, for the viral infections have a predominantly lymphocytic response while the chlamydial infection is typified by a mixture of polymorphonuclear leukocytes (PMN), lymphocytes, and other cells (Yoneda et al., 1975); atopic conjunctivitis and vernal catarrh, which are sometimes confused with trachoma, may be recognized by the presence of eosinophilic leukocytes and free granules in smears.

The cell response in active trachoma may also be characterized (Yoneda et al., 1975). In addition to the PMNs, there are also lymphocytes and macrophages (Fig. 4, Plate 9). In active cases, with mature follicles, there may be many immature lymphoid cells and plasma cells together with necrotic material (Fig. 5, Plate 9). Leber cells, or giant macrophages containing phagocytosed material, may be present. Inclusions (found in epithelial cells) may or may not accompany the typical cell population. Because inclusions are difficult to find, some workers, notably Thygeson (1946) and Hardy et al. (1967), have advocated using the cytologic response to establish a presumptive diagnosis of chlamydial infection. Although sympathetic to such efforts, we feel strongly that the sole cytologic laboratory proof is the visualization of an inclusion. While the cellular response in trachoma may be characteristic, none of the components is pathognomonic, except for inclusions. Clearly, the typical cellular response should heighten the microscopist's suspicion and lead to a thorough search for inclusions. Yoneda et al. (1975) evaluated Giemsa-stained conjunctival scrapings taken from Tunisian children with trachoma, and found inclusions only on slides showing many separated epithelial cells and many PMNs, although only 3% of smears with these two elements alone had inclusions. When numerous lymphocytes were also present, 25% of smears were inclusion positive. When the other cellular elements (Leber cells, plasma cells, immature lymphocytes) were also seen, 70% of smears had inclusions (Table 1). The conclusion of this study was that the microscopist should use the cellular response to screen and to select those slides which might reward intense scrutiny. Experience has shown that slides with intact sheets of epithelial cells and few inflammatory cells do not reward long scrutiny. Moreover, severe trachoma is often complicated by secondary infections with bacteria which may also be indentified by the Giemsa methods (Figs. 6–10, Plate 10).

Table 1
Association of Cytologic Features and Identification
of Inclusions in 927 Giemsa-Stained Smears
from the Conjunctivas of Trachoma Cases

Cytologic Features				No. Inclusion Positive/ Total Number (% positive)
Separated Cell Sheets (>50%)	PMNs 3+	Lymphocytes 3+	Other*	
—	—	—	—	0/155
+	—	—	—	0/27
—	+	—	—	0/320
+	+	—	—	6/233 (3)
—	+	+	—	0/3
+	+	+	—	24/97 (25)
+	+	+	+	64/92 (70)

* Plasma cells, blastoid and stem cells, Leber cells, and multinucleated epithelial cells.

The necessity for close examination of slides is one of the drawbacks of the Giemsa stain. Scanning of slides is best left to only the most experienced microscopists. If slides are not examined under oil immersion (at 400X to 1,000X), many inclusions can be missed. It is common to spend 30 minutes to an hour or more in examination of a single slide. Obviously this is an arduous procedure for surveys. Another potential drawback to the use of this staining procedure is the presence of artifacts and cellular structures which may be confused with inclusions. The literature is replete with articles on trachoma or other chlamydial infections ostensibly proven by demonstrating inclusions; upon examination, these "inclusions" prove to be keratin, pigment granules, or bacteria. As an aid to the microscopist, we have an annotated series of photographs (Figs. 11–14, Plates 10, 11) of typical chlamydial inclusions, together with the most common intracellular structure with which they are confused (see also Yoneda et al., 1975). Typical cellular responses and the most frequently found bacterial infections are also depicted.

It should be noted that the above description applies to the use of Giemsa stain in areas where severe trachoma is endemic. In areas where trachoma is very mild, or disappearing (such as among American Indians), chlamydial inclusions are found only rarely in Giemsa-stained smears (Schachter et al., 1971). In highly endemic areas, inclusions are seldom found in patients with mild trachoma, whereas they may be found in 10% to 30% of scrapings collected from patients with active trachoma.

In neonates with inclusion conjunctivitis who produce copious amounts of agent, Giemsa stain is as good as any technique for establishing the diagnosis — but virtually all tests will be positive. In the adult form, inclusions are found in approximately 50% of those who can be proven infected by any means. In proven genital tract infections, approximately 50% of the cervical scrapings and 15% of the urethral scrapings will show inclusions (Schachter et al., 1970). Other workers have had greater success using the Giemsa method to study genital tract infections. Sompolinsky et al. (1973) found that 34% of cervical scrapings and 51% of urethral scrapings collected from their test population contained inclusions. These figures are comparable to or greater than the Giemsa-positive rates we have observed in patients with proven infections.

Naib (1970) reviewed the cytology of TRIC agent infections in the eyes of newborn infants and in the genital tracts of the mothers. He found typical diagnostic intracytoplasmic inclusions in 99 of 120 conjunctival scrapings so studied. Fifty-four of the mothers had had cervical scrapings and 33 (61%) had similar diagnostic clusters of intracytoplasmic inclusions in the endocervical and squamous parabasal cells. Of interest is the finding that 40% of the women in this group had cervical atypia. These results were obtained with the Papanicolaou staining. In addition to inclusions, much cellular material similar to that seen in lymphoid follicles was found in the conjunctiva. The author claimed that Papanicolaou stain seemed to be superior to the iodine or Giemsa stain usually used to demonstrate inclusions. While we do not dispute the fact that an experienced cytologist could recognize chlamydial inclusions in a Papanicolaou stain, our experience does not agree with that of Naib. We have never seen inclusions in squamous cells (they are not known to support the growth of chlamydiae). We would not recognize or accept many of the pictures published in Naib's paper as inclusions, and we do not often find follicular cells in conjunctival scrapings from neonates. We have attempted a direct comparison of Giemsa and Papanicolaou staining of highly inclusion-positive clinical material and infected cell cultures and have found the "Pap" stain to be specifically unrewarding and of little help in demonstration of the inclusions. We still feel the Giemsa method is the best stain in inclusion blennorrhea.

From our experience, we cannot recommend routine use of Giemsa stain for genital tract specimens, since it is relatively insensitive and time-consuming. Cervical scrapings, in particular, are difficult to read because bacteria may obscure cells and appear intracellularly in forms that could be confused with inclusions. We must conclude that isolation in tissue culture is the diagnostic method of choice for the chlamydial genital tract infections.

The Giemsa stain is also used to demonstrate inclusions in histological sections, impression smears, and tissue cultures. For *C. trachomatis* isolates, this technique has been used to identify the inclusions in tissue culture isolation systems (Fig. 15B, Plate 11). This method is more time-consuming than the iodine or FA stains. The screening of the coverslips may be speeded up by using dark field illumination of the Giemsa-stained monolayers (Darougar et al., 1972). The inclusions appear as lemon-yellow particles within a vacuole (Figs. 15B, 15C, Plate 11). Unfortunately this technique prohibits the use of swabs that produce particulate material (alginate). There also appears to be some degree of variability in results with different batches of stain.

Giemsa-Staining Method This method gives excellent permanent preparations if a reliable brand of stain is used (for example, National Aniline and Chemical Company, Incorporated, New York, or Gradwohl Laboratories, St. Louis).

As the stain is being prepared for use, dilutions can be made with neutral distilled water (orange with neutral red, or purple with hematoxylin), but buffered water solution is more reliable.

Buffered water:
1. Prepare M/15 Na_2HPO_4 using 9.5 gm of the anhydrous salt in 1 liter of distilled water.
2. Prepare M/15 NaH_2PO_4 by dissolving 9.2 gm of the salt in 1 liter of distilled water.

To make buffered water of pH 7.2, mix 72 ml of (1) with 28 ml of (2) and 900 ml of distilled water.

Commercial cytologic buffers may also be used. Any pH between 6.8 and 7.2 is acceptable (although the more basic side may be preferable) as long as it is kept constant to minimize tinctorial variation.

Giemsa stain is prepared by dissolving 0.5 gm of powder in 33 ml of acetone-free, absolute methanol. The solution is mixed thoroughly, allowed to sediment, and stored at room temperature for use as stock. Dilutions of this stock stain are made with neutral distilled water or buffered water, in a ratio of 1 part of stock Giemsa solution to 40 or 50 parts of diluent. There is some variability in currently available, prepared stock Giemsa solutions, and these commercial products should be screened before being accepted for routine use.

The smear is air dried, fixed with absolute methanol for at least 5 minutes, and again dried. It is then covered with the diluted Giemsa stain (freshly prepared the same day) for 1 hour. The slide is then rinsed rapidly in 95% ethyl alcohol to remove excess dye and to enhance differentiation; it is then dried and examined microscopically. Longer staining periods (1.5 hours) may be preferable with heavy tissue culture monolayers. Elementary bodies stain reddish purple (Figs. 2, 3, Plate 9). The initial bodies are more basophilic (Figs. 2, 9, Plates 9, 10), staining bluish, as do most bacteria (Figs. 6–10, Plate 10).

On balance, we feel the Giemsa stain still has much to offer, and we recommend that all workers starting research on chlamydiae should familiarize themselves with the inclusions stained by Giemsa's method. Since microscopists can be trained by experienced workers and since the method is not complicated (requiring only access to the patient, specimen collection, staining reagents, and the microscope), the Giemsa stain is probably the method of choice in areas with severe endemic trachoma. In endemic areas the Giemsa test provides an effective tool to detect chlamydial inclusions, gives an estimate of the prevalence of bacterial infection, and is by far the least expensive in terms of laboratory costs and trained personnel.

Fluorescent Antibody (FA) Staining of Smears

The FA technique has been most successfully applied to the diagnosis of trachoma (Fig. 16, Plate 12). The major proponents of this method have been the groups at the Harvard School of Public Health and the Department of Microbiology, University of California, San Francisco. The Harvard group, in studies of severe endemic trachoma in Saudi Arabia, has shown that FA was more sensitive than Giemsa staining and egg isolation (Nichols et al., 1963), and has applied the technique extensively in epidemiologic studies (Nichols et al., 1967). The California group has emphasized experimental studies and studies on mild trachoma in American Indians (Hanna et al., 1965; Hanna, 1968). In the American Indian population, trachoma has become milder, apparently under the combined effects of control measures and environmental improvement; a collaborative study has confirmed that only FA techniques demonstrated chlamydiae in this population (Schachter et al., 1971). Thus, it appears that the extreme sensitivity of the FA techniques may be useful in studies of severe trachoma and be required in studies of mild forms. In recent studies of severe endemic trachoma in Tunisia, we compared matched Giemsa- and FA-stained conjunctival scrapings (Dawson et al., 1947a,b, 1975). The FA is slightly more sensitive than Giemsa in this situation (Yoneda et al., 1975). Following treatment the prevalence of agent-positive smears fell dramatically with both techniques, so they appear to be detecting the same phenomenon, replicating chlamydial agent.

FA techniques have also been shown to be a most sensitive cytologic tool for studying chlamydial oculogenital infections (Schachter et al., 1967, 1970). FA added little to the diagnosis of inclusion blennorrhea (where all tests are likely to be positive), and was slightly more sensitive than Giemsa in diagnosing adult inclusion conjunctivitis or cervical infections, but was much more sensitive in detecting chlamydial infections of the male urethra. It appears, then, that FA methods have an advantage in infections with small amounts of agent. In these studies on oculogenital infections, FA staining of smears was compared to egg isolation in the period before tissue culture isolation techniques became routine. Although there have been no large-scale comparative studies, it seems certain that the tissue culture method for isolation is the preferred method to detect chlamydial genital tract infections (Gordon et al., 1969).

The FA technique has several shortcomings. Even though it appears to be the most sensitive and specific cytologic procedure, it is very time-consuming, requiring rigorous interpretation and criteria, and the staining fades rapidly so smears cannot be re-examined at a later date.

Fluorescent Antibody Technique   Either direct or indirect methods are acceptable. The indirect method may be better suited for laboratories initiating such studies, because staining reagents are commercially available, and theoretically there may be some advantages in the sensitivity of the test.

Slides are air dried, fixed with cold ($-20°$ C) acetone, and stored at $-20°$ C to $-70°$ C before staining. The slides are overlaid with rabbit antiserum for 1 hour in a moist chamber; this antiserum ideally would include antibodies to the serotypes prevalent in the area. The alternate, and possibly more practical, method would be use of a broadly reactive serum. At the WHO Collaborating Centre for Reference and Research on Trachoma and Other Chlamydial Infections, we use hyperimmune rabbit serum against an LGV strain (LGV 434B–Type L-2); high-titered human convalescent LGV serum might be equivalent, but it is hard to obtain. The slides are then washed twice with phosphate-buffered saline (PBS), pH 7.2 to 7.4, 5 minutes each time, and then stained for 1 hour with commercially prepared fluorescein-labeled goat antirabbit globulin. After having been washed with PBS for 15 minutes, the slides are mounted in 90% glycerol in PBS and examined by dark field fluorescent or interference microscopy with appropriate filters.

The reagents for the tests are most easily standardized against monolayers of HeLa or other susceptible cells infected with an LGV isolate (Fig. 17, Plate 12). The cells are incubated at $35°$ C after being infected with an inoculum that produces inclusions in 30% to 90% of the cells. Maximal staining of inclusions is observed 40 to 42 hours postinfection, before the inclusions become too large and the antigen concentration decreases. For a positive reaction, the inclusions must stain brightly. The titers of both the rabbit and fluorescein-conjugated antirabbit serum are determined with these infected monolayers. The antisera used with clinical material are four times more concentrated than the dilution endpoint for bright staining of inclusions in the infected monolayers. For example, a serum with an endpoint at 1:80 would be used at 1:20 as a reagent. Standard tests (blockings, staining of normal cells) are performed to prove the specificity of the reaction. In addition, the sera should be tested to assure that they stain inclusions of all known TRIC immunotypes. The LGV antisera mentioned above meet this criteria, although there is some variation in the brightness of different immunotypes' inclusions. Small quantities of this serum are available from the WHO Collaborating Centre to enable laboratories to initiate studies on *Chlamydia*.

The criteria for detecting chlamydial inclusions in a clinical specimen are based on the presence of a brightly fluorescing mass in the cytoplasm of an epithelial cell, preferably adjacent to the nucleus. Areas of the smears with heaped up cells are difficult to read and must be excluded since all cells are not morphologically identifiable. General brightness or free fluorescing masses should be ignored.

Iodine Stain

Rice (1936) found that chlamydial inclusions contained a glycogen-like material that could be stained with iodine, but the method has been applied only sporadically. It offers the advantages of simplicity and speed. It is easily the fastest staining procedure, and entire slides can be screened in a matter of minutes. Inclusions may also be recognized in the thick areas of the slide, unsuitable for examination by other techniques. The iodine-stained slides can be maintained for permanent record or can be counterstained by the Giemsa method and suitable cells reexamined for confirmation.

The Trachoma Research Unit at the Lister Institute has exploited this technique extensively in their studies on severe endemic trachoma in The Gambia (Gilkes, Smith, and Sowa, 1958; Sowa, Collier, and Sowa 1971; Collier, 1973). Obviously in a heavily infected environment, the ease of reading slides can compensate for relatively poor sensitivity, for this is the least sensitive of the cytologic techniques. This is particularly true in testing inclusion conjunctivitis (Schachter et al., 1967) (Table 2). The technique is not applicable

Table 2
**Comparison of Different Laboratory Procedures
for Demonstrating Chlamydial Oculogenital Infections**

Procedure	Percent Positive*
Iodine stain	32
Giemsa stain	60
Immunofluorescence	86
Isolation (yolk sac)	62
Isolation (tissue culture)	90
Complement fixation (>1:16)	57
Microimmunofluorescence (>1:8)	100

* All patients had proven infection.

to scrapings from the genital tract, since normal specimens may have glycogen-containing cells.

The iodine stain probably has greatest application today in the staining of monolayers employed in chlamydial isolation attempts (Figs. 15, 17, Plates 11, 12). Here speed is the requisite feature, and since many specimens can be screened, the occasional missed positive is acceptable. This technique does not stain inclusions of *C. psittaci*, and the possibility that these organisms may be involved in the disease must be ignored if this stain is to be used.

Iodine-Staining Technique Scrapings are air-dried, fixed in absolute methanol, and stained with Lugol iodine or 5% iodine in 10% potassium iodide for 3 to 5 minutes. Slides are examined as wet mounts. The matrix of inclusions may appear as a reddish-brown mass recognizable under low magnification (Fig. 16, Plate 12). The slides may be decolorized with methanol and restained with Giemsa's stain.

Macchiavello's and Giminez Stains

Any of the above-mentioned techniques can be used to stain inclusions in impression smears. The Macchiavello and Giminez stains are not used in routine diagnosis but are usually applied to impression smears.

Cultured Agents The Macchiavello and Giminez staining methods are generally used to detect elementary bodies in yolk sac smears. These methods are quite similar in principle, but the Giminez is probably simpler for inexperienced workers. The Macchiavello stain gives similar results but may require greater attention to detail. Although the Giemsa method is occasionally used for detecting elementary bodies in yolk sac smears, it is not the method of choice; it requires considerable experience because the elementary bodies do not stain in marked contrast to the yolk sac material. The FA, Giemsa, and iodine stains can be used to demonstrate TRIC agent inclusions in cell culture with the same relationships of sensitivity, specificity, and speed of reading discussed above. The methods are listed below.

Modified Macchiavello's Stain
Stock solutions:
Basic fuchsin — 0.25 gm in 100 ml double-distilled water
Citric acid* — 0.5 gm in 200 ml double-distilled water
Methylene blue — 1.0 gm in 100 ml double-distilled water

After drying in air, the smear or impression preparation is fixed by heat. The basic fuchsin solution, first passed through filter paper in a small funnel, is dropped onto the film and left for 5 minutes before being quickly drained off. The slide is first washed in tap water and then dipped for a few seconds in the citric acid solution, best held in a Coplin jar. The slide is then washed thoroughly with tap water and stained with 1% methylene blue for 20 to 30 seconds; it is washed again in tap water, and dried.

The citric acid solution must be fresh. Exposure to citric acid for more than a few seconds will decolorize the chlamydiae, and they will all stain blue. In a properly prepared slide most elementary bodies will stain red against a blue background.

Giminez's Modification of Macchiavello's Technique
Stock solutions:
1. 10% (w/v) basic fuchsin in 95% ethanol   100 ml
   4% (w/v) aqueous phenol   250 ml
   distilled water   650 ml
2. 0.1 M sodium phosphate buffer solution
   at pH 7.45 (mix 3.5 ml of 0.2 M NaH_2PO_4, 15.5 ml of
   0.2 M Na_2HPO_4, and 19 ml of distilled water)
3. 0.8% aqueous malachite green oxalate

To prepare a working solution of carbol fuchsin, mix 4 ml of stock solution with 10 ml of buffer (pH 7.45); filter immediately and filter again before each staining. The working solution remains satisfactory for about 40 hours.

A very thin smear, air-dried (heat fixation is not necessary for cytologic reasons, but should be employed for safety), is covered with the filtered carbol basic fuchsin working solution and held for 1 to 2

---

* It is important to use a fresh solution daily.

minutes; after thorough washing in tap water, it is covered with the malachite green solution for 6 to 9 seconds and again washed in tap water. The slides are finally dried with absorbent paper. Elementary bodies stain red; the background will be greenish.

SEROLOGIC DIAGNOSIS

There are no wholly satisfactory serologic methods for diagnosing human chlamydial infections and no single test that is generally applicable. A test that is useful for diagnosing one of the diseases may be totally useless in the diagnosis of some of the other infections. At best, the current status of chlamydial diagnostic serology leaves much to be desired. Problems stem from inadequate antibody response for certain tests, inability to obtain appropriately paired sera because of long incubation periods or inapparent infections, and high background reactor rates in high-risk populations.

For practical purposes, only two serologic methods can be recommended. These are the complement fixation (CF) test (Meyer, Eddie, and Schachter, 1969), and Wang's microimmunofluorescent (micro-IF) technique (Wang and Grayston, 1970). The complement fixation test is most useful in the diagnosis of psittacosis and LGV (systemic infections), considerably less helpful in diagnosing TRIC agent oculogenital infections, and virtually useless in the diagnosis of trachoma, a wholly superficial infection. The CF test was first used by Bedson in the early 1930s for diagnosing psittacosis infections. The recently developed micro-IF test has not been used in the routine diagnosis of psittacosis, although it may be adapted to this use in the future (Jones and Treharne, 1974), but it is most useful in the diagnosis of chlamydial oculogenital infections and trachoma. Neither of these tests is as useful in diagnosing *C. trachomatis* infections as serologic tests may be for routine diagnosis of other microbial infections. Both tests are more useful in serologic surveys than in the diagnosis of individual infections.

A variety of other serologic techniques have been utilized for research projects. Some of these tests have not been tried in the routine diagnosis of human infections, while others have been found ineffective. For example, the microagglutination tests once used in diagnosing avian chlamydial infections were found successful only with sera from certain avian species. While agglutination tests are standard in some laboratories, they have not been applicable to human sera in our tests. The radioisotope immune precipitation test has been applied in specialized serologic surveys and appears to be considerably more sensitive than the complement fixation test, although it is of similar specificity (Gerloff and Watson, 1967; Reeve et al., 1974). The long-range usefulness of this test has not been determined, but it will probably be limited because it is expensive and group-reactive.

Chlamydiae produce a hemagglutinin (for certain avian and murine erythrocytes), and both direct and indirect hemagglutination techniques have been described (Barron and Riera, 1969; Lewis, Thacker, and Engleman, 1972). The immunodiffusion tests that have been described appear to be relatively group-specific (although enhanced specificity has been demonstrated in some tests), and the sensitivity of this technique currently offers no advantages (Collins and Barron, 1970).

Sera from some avian species do not fix guinea pig complement. Several modifications of the CF test, most notably the indirect CF test (Karrer, Meyer, and Eddie, 1950; Meyer and Schachter, 1969), have been developed to allow use of the test with avian sera. With regard to diseases discussed in this book, this technique is useful for determining possible sources of human psittacosis infections.

The CF test is a group-specific test. It measures antibodies to an antigenic determinant common to all chlamydiae. The active moiety is apparently an eight-carbon sugar, 2-keto-3-deoxyoctanoic acid (Dhir et al., 1972). In contrast, the micro-IF test measures specific antibodies that are not detected by the CF test. Wang and Grayston initially introduced the micro-IF in 1970 for the serotyping of *Chlamydia trachomatis,* but further studies from the same and other laboratories found it also to be a highly sensitive and specific indicator of antichlamydial antibodies (Hanna et al., 1972; Jones, 1974; Philip et al., 1974; Reeve et al., 1974; Wang and Grayston, 1974; Grayston and Wang, 1975).

Bedson first used the CF test for the diagnosis of psittacosis (Bedson and Western, 1930), and it was applied to the diagnosis of lymphogranuloma venereum when the antigenic relationship between the two organisms was recognized. The early psittacosis antigens, derived from mouse lung or spleen heavily infected with chlamydiae, suffered from considerable variability in potency and stability. Although some egg work was done with psittacosis strains, the LGV antigen was the first to be used extensively as a yolk sac preparation (Lygranum®) (Rake and Jones, 1942; Rake et al., 1941; Shaffer and Rake, 1947). A major contribution was made when Nigg and associates found that boiled and phenolized antigens were stable, potent preparations (Nigg, Hilleman, and Bowser, 1946). This CF antigen is extremely stable, and preparations kept in the refrigerator and treated aseptically maintain titers for many years. The CF technique described below has been used constantly in the Hooper Foundation, with little modification since the 1940s, in over 200,000 tests.

The CF tests and micro-IF tests when applied to individual sera are generally carried through an appropriate dilution range to allow determination of endpoints against the antigens. In survey work it may be possible to simplify testing by screening sera at the specific dilutions that are considered to be indicative of significant titers, in order to determine prevalence of antichlamydial antibodies. The micro-IF test may involve many antigens — up to 15 serotypes may be used (Kuo, et al., 1974; Wang, Grayston, and Gale, 1973; Treharne, Darougar, and Jones, 1973; Grayston and Wang, 1975), but many studies could focus on antigenic types prevalent in the specific geographic area and associated with the disease conditions under consideration. This simplification of the test is particularly applicable in studies on childhood trachoma. Even in other studies it may be possible, in fact, to use only one or two types in the micro-IF test. For instance, our studies on genital tract infections in San Francisco revealed that at least 75% of reactive sera had detectable antibodies to either type E or LGV-2; similar results have been obtained in Washington, D.C. (Philip et al., 1974). Wang and Grayston (1974) have found type-specific patterns in 79% of their sera from isolate-positive patients. Even in this study it is apparent that approximately 75% of these patients' sera react with type E or LGV-2, although much higher titers were observed with homologous serotypes.

Clinical Indications

Cytologic or chlamydial isolation methods are the alternatives to serodiagnosis. These alternatives require a degree of special training or technology, and present some complications. In the case of psittacosis, the organism may be recovered from sputum or blood, but this presents a risk to laboratory workers. The LGV agent may be isolated from pus aspirated from a bubo. The TRIC agent infections can be diagnosed by demonstration of inclusions in epithelial cells scraped from the affected site (conjunctiva, urethra, or cervix); they may also be diagnosed by agent isolation, preferably by using a tissue culture technique or, less effectively, in the embryonated hen's egg. The three routinely used techniques for tissue culture isolation of chlamydiae are clearly the methods of choice for diagnosing active TRIC agent infections (Jones, 1974; Kuo, et al., 1972; Wentworth and Alexander, 1974).

The complement fixation test should be used routinely whenever LGV is considered in the differential diagnosis, such as in the case of young men being examined for inguinal lymphadenopathy, with or without systemic complications. In untreated cases, if a laboratory is available, efforts should be made to isolate chlamydiae from aspirates of fluctuant nodes. The bubonic form of LGV is less often seen in women. Women usually present with what are considered to be the later sequelae of LGV (vaginal-rectal syndrome involving rectal strictures or proctitis).

For LGV the disadvantages of the CF test are not its lack of specificity (for there are no known, defined cross-reactions), but the ubiquitous nature of some of the chlamydial parasites and the group specificity of the test. There will be high rates of low-titer reactors in VD clinic populations. Thus, the positive serologic result may support a diagnosis of LGV but cannot prove it. Serologic proof of the diagnosis would be based on demonstration of rising titers (a greater than fourfold difference in paired acute and convalescent sera), but in most cases the patient has had the chlamydial infection for too long a period before the test is performed. Even in acute lymphadenopathy in the male, there is usually a three- to four-week period from infection to presentation. Since it may be necessary to rely on a single titer, higher CF titers are more suggestive of LGV (1:64 or greater, even though any titer above the 1:8 or 1:16 range is considered significant). The titers in men take on greater meaning than those in women, because the common chlamydial infections causing nongonococcal urethritis in the male tend not to produce either as high a rate or as high a titer as do the genital tract infections in women (cervicitis). It is uncommon to find a man with simple chlamydial urethritis having a CF titer above the 1:16 level (Table 3). Any patient tested for LGV should also have a serologic test for syphilis. Some patients will have both, and VDRL-reactive sera may react with both LGV and normal yolk sac antigens.

The clinician may choose to utilize the delayed hypersensitivity (Frei) test, which is only applied in diagnosing LGV, but is actually group reactive and positive at varying rates among patients with

Table 3
Distribution of Chlamydial CF Titers
in Patients with Proven Infections

Disease	No. Tested	No. with CF Titer				
		<1:16	1:16	1:32	1:64	≥1:128
Lymphogranuloma venereum	15	0	1	2	0	12
Psittacosis	30	0	2	5	5	18
Adult inclusion conjunctivitis	93	46	28	11	6	2
Cervicitis, females	55	30	9	6	4	6
Urethritis, males	60	51	8	1	0	0

psittacosis or the TRIC agent infections. However, Frei test antigens currently available are not particularly potent, and routine use of this test is not recommended. In our experience the CF test is virtually always positive in LGV patients who have positive Frei tests, and is positive in some LGV patients (from whom the agent was recovered) who have negative skin tests (Schachter et al., 1969). CF antibody levels tend to be persistent, but rapid declines in CF titers have been noted both spontaneously and after effective chemotherapy. One can not interpret falling titers in convalescence as support of the diagnosis.

The complement fixation test should be performed whenever a diagnosis of psittacosis is considered. The presence of a pneumonitis, a persistent influenzal disease, or any acute or chronic febrile disease following exposure to birds would be clinical indication that psittacosis should be considered in the differential diagnosis. Here the CF test is much more satisfactory for diagnosis, since acute and convalescent sera can be obtained and often demonstrate rising titers. In fact, in our experience, the great majority of psittacosis cases may be diagnosed in this manner. The diagnosis may have to be based upon a single high titer if the patient has a persistent or relapsing disease, but such a titer would clearly support the clinical impression. The problems of cross-reactions and previous exposure to other chlamydiae are clearly the same as discussed earlier. High rates of seroreactors may be found in individuals with occupational or other long-term contact with birds. In general, psittacosis infections produce high CF antibody levels (1:64 or greater). If a patient has had early and persistent treatment with tetracycline, the antibody levels may be suppressed. There have been a number of human infections (proven by agent isolation) where no serologic response was obtained because of early therapy (Meyer and Eddie, 1956).

The CF test has not been useful in the diagnosis of trachoma (Schachter et al., 1973). Nor is it particularly useful in the diagnosis of oculogenital infections since, at best, only 50% of individuals with eye and genital tract infections will have significant (greater than 1:16) CF titers (Schachter et al., 1970). In the uncomplicated genital tract infections such as urethritis or cervicitis, the CF reactor rates are even less. The CF test is almost useless in the diagnosis of urethritis, since only 15% of men with proven urethritis caused by chlamydiae have shown significant CF levels. However, approximately 40% of the women with chlamydial cervicitis have significant CF levels (Schachter et al., 1970). CF titers in the background populations (i.e., sexually active men and women) will show a similar distribution in reactor rates. Women will have a higher background rate of CF reactors than men.

The micro-IF test measures specific antibodies to antigenic determinants present in the cell walls of the elementary body particles.

It is much more sensitive than the CF test (Philip et al., 1974). For example, in one series of 55 isolate-positive patients, we found 29 with significant CF reactions while all 55 were positive in the micro-IF. The respective geometric mean titers were 1:12 and 1:164. The micro-IF test can be applied to patients with LGV or TRIC agent ocular or oculogenital infections. The presence of a reaction in a single serum specimen simply reflects previous exposure. Changing titers may be seen in patients who are examined relatively early in the course of an infection, but patients are seldom seen at this time. One advantage of the micro-IF is that information on the specific serotype responsible for the infection may be obtained. The micro-IF offers the added advantage of determining the immunoglobulin class of the reactive antibodies; the presence of IgM antibodies may lend further support to diagnosis of early infections. Unfortunately, many of these infections tend to be chronic and the best estimate is that the IgM antibody response may last for approximately one month following infection (Wang and Grayston, 1974). In one study only 33% of patients with active infections had IgM antibodies (Philip et al., 1974).

Another advantage of the micro-IF is that it may be used to test secretions for antibody activity. Thus the demonstration of antichlamydial antibody in tears may support a diagnosis of trachoma (McComb and Nichols, 1969; Hanna et al., 1973). Undoubtedly this test will be applied in the future to genital tract secretions.

The major disadvantage of this test is that its results reflect the high prevalence of chlamydial infection in certain groups (Schachter et al., 1975b,c). In other words, in appropriate populations there may be very high reactor rates from previous exposure to the chlamydiae. These micro-IF antibodies may persist for life, although in some patients they disappear spontaneously (Wang and Grayston, 1974), possibly reflecting brief antigenic exposure. Patients attending VD clinics in Seattle had reactor rates in excess of 60% compared to control rates of 25% (Grayston and Wang, 1975). The reactor rates we have found in different populations are shown in Table 4. The significant level in the micro-IF test has been chosen at 1:8.

Test Procedures

The complement fixation test may be performed in either the tube system or the micro system. We strongly prefer the standardization of reagents in the tube system, regardless of which system is being used for test. We find the micro titer systems most useful in screening

Table 4
Antichlamydial Antibodies in Selected Populations
Tested at the Hooper Foundation

Group	CF ≥1:16 (%)	Micro-IF ≥1:8 (%)
Screening studies		
Normal adults, all ages	2–3	25–45
Pediatric sera	<1	10
Trachoma-endemic population	5–15	>80
Males, venereal disease study,		
young adults without disease	5–10	20–25
Males, symptomatic attending VD clinic	10	60
Females, venereal disease study,		
young adults	15–20	50–70
Prostitutes	30–60	Up to 85
Proven chlamydial infections		
(isolation)		
Lymphogranuloma venereum	100	100
Psittacosis	100	ND*
Adult inclusion conjunctivitis	50	100
Male, urethritis	15	90
Female, cervical infection	45	99

*Not determined.

large numbers of sera but prefer to retest all positives in the tube system. We occasionally find that sera giving titers in the 1:4 to 1:8 range in the micro system are positive at 1:16 (which we consider the significant level) in the tube system. The micro system uses standard plates and volumes one-tenth of those used in the tube test. The complement fixation test is performed on serum specimens heated at 56° C for 30 minutes (preferably acute and convalescent paired sera tested together). In each test a positive control serum of high titer is included together with a known negative serum.

The reagents for the CF test are standardized by the Kolmer technique and include special buffered saline, group antigen, antigen (normal yolk sac) control, the positive serum, the negative serum, guinea pig complement,* rabbit antisheep hemolysin, and sheep red cells. The hemolytic system is titrated and the complement unitage is determined. The test may be performed by either the water bath technique or the overnight (icebox) technique, the former being preferable. Doubling dilutions of the serum (from 1:2) are made in a 0.25 ml volume of saline. The serum is also tested for reactivity

---

*The guinea pig complement should be carefully tested for chlamydial antibodies since many herds are enzootically infected with a chlamydial agent, guinea pig inclusion conjunctivitis.

to normal yolk sac antigen and for anticomplementary activity. The antigen is added at 4 units (0.25 ml), and 2 exact units of complement (0.5 ml) are added. Standard reagent controls are always included. The normal yolk sac control is used at the same dilution as the group antigen. The tubes are shaken well and incubated in a water bath at 37° C for 2 hours, after which 0.5 ml of sensitized sheep red cells are added and the tubes shaken and placed in the water bath for another hour. The tubes are read for hemolysis on a 1+ to 4+ scale, roughly equivalent to 25% to 100% inhibition of red cell lysis. The endpoint of the serum is considered the highest dilution producing less than 50% (2+) hemolysis after a complete inhibition of hemolysis has been observed. It is general practice in our laboratory to shake the tubes to resuspend the settled cells, and then to refrigerate the tubes overnight and recheck the results the following morning.

The micro-IF test is performed against chlamydial organisms grown in yolk sac (Wang and Grayston, 1974). The individual yolk sacs are selected for elementary body richness and are pretitrated to give an even distribution of particles. It is generally found that a 1% to 3% yolk sac suspension (PBS, pH 7.0) is satisfactory. The antigens are stored as frozen aliquots and, after thawing, are well mixed in a Vortex mixer before use. Antigen dots are placed on a slide in a specific pattern using separate pen points for each antigen (Fig. 18). Up to nine clusters of dots which include all the antigenic types to be tested can be conveniently placed on each slide. The antigen dots are air dried and fixed on slides with acetone (15 minutes at room temperature). Slides may be stored frozen. When thawed, water may condense on the slides but they can be conveniently dried with a portable hair dryer set for blower only (i.e., no heat).

For the test, serial dilutions of serum (or tears or exudate) are placed on the individual clusters. The clusters of dots are sufficiently separated to avoid the running of serum from cluster to cluster. After the serum dilutions have been added, the slides are incubated for one-half to one hour in a moist chamber at 37° C. They are then placed in a buffered saline wash for five minutes, followed by a second five-minute wash. The slides are then dried and stained with fluorescein conjugated antihuman globulin. These conjugates are pretitrated in a known positive system to determine appropriate working dilutions. This reagent may be prepared against any class of globulin being considered (IgA or secretory piece for secretions, IgG, or IgM). Counter stains such as bovine serum albumin conjugated with rhodamine may be included.

The slides are then washed twice again, dried, and examined by standard fluorescent microscopy. Use of a monocular tube is recommended to allow greater precision in determining fluorescence for

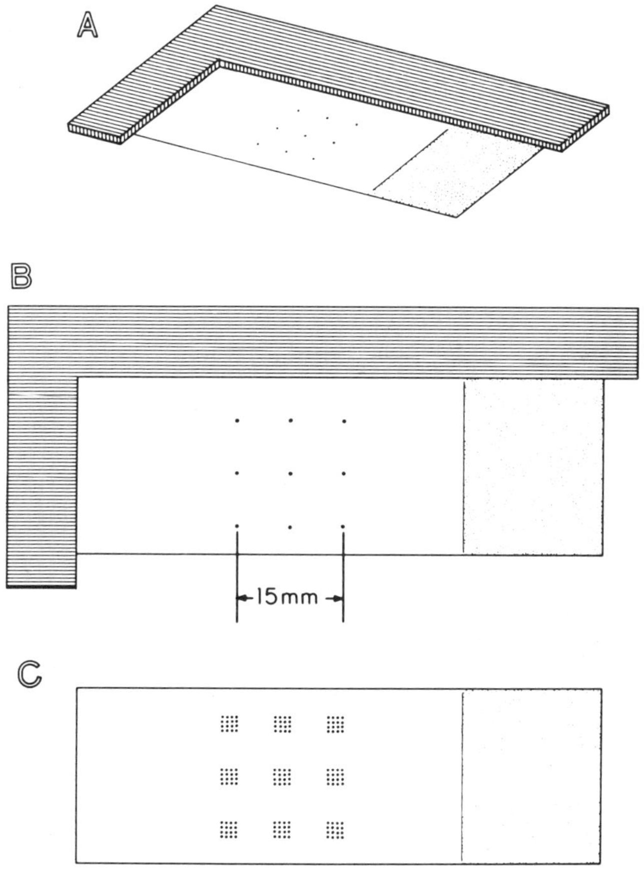

Fig. 18. Use of a template for placement of clusters of antigen dots. (Courtesy of Dr. S.-P. Wang)

individual elementary body particles. The endpoints are read as the dilution giving bright fluorescence clearly associated with the well-distributed elementary bodies throughout the antigen dot. Identification of the type-specific response is based upon dilution differences reflected in the endpoints for different prototype antigens (Jones, 1974; Wang and Grayston, 1974).

For each run of either CF or micro-IF, known positive and negative sera should always be included. These sera should always duplicate their titers as previously observed within the experimental (1 dilution) error of the system.

Reagents The commercially available antigens have occasionally presented sizeable problems. In the CF test, an antigen with the highest possible titer should be used for greatest dilution of the crude preparations and for reasons of economy. Several commercial preparations are available but none can be recommended. We have often seen commercial preparations with titers in the 1:8 or 1:16 range result in unsatisfactory working dilutions of 1:2 to 1:4.

In the CF system, a major problem has been obtaining complement free of antibodies to chlamydiae. Guinea pig inclusion conjunctivitis (Murray, 1964) is a very common chlamydial infection in guinea pig colonies. The antigens can appear to be anticomplementary when they are simply reacting with the antibody present in the complement. This can often be shown when the complement does not react with the normal yolk sac control. One should always attempt to purchase complement certified to be nonreactive with chlamydial antigens. Unfortunately, the certification is not always accurate (because the antigens used by the companies have not been potent). As a matter of routine we buy complement in large lots. One vial is reconstituted, heat inactivated, and titrated for antichlamydial antibodies (we have tested many lots with antibody titers of 1:16 or 1:32). When the complement titration is carried out, a parallel assay is performed in the presence of antigen. We prefer the high-titered complement to less potent preparations that may be available at slightly lower prices.

In the micro-IF test the major reagent problem has been the lack of reliability of immunoglobulin preparations against human IgM. Some of the commercial preparations have been completely nonreactive when tested in systems that have been shown to react when other reagents are used (Juchau et al., 1972).

The CF hemolytic system reagents may be readily obtained commercially. Hyland Laboratories and Microbiological Associates have proven relatively reliable sources of complement, although the previous warning on antibodies in the complement applies. Sheep cells can usually be obtained locally but must be checked for fragility.

There is, however, no commercially available source of antigen which is highly potent. Therefore, the antigens must be prepared in the laboratory. There are several methods available that produce suitable antigens. The deoxycholate-extracted group antigen (Ross and Jenkin, 1962) or the ether-extracted (Volkert and Christensen, 1955) (and acetone-precipitated, if preferred) group antigens are perfectly satisfactory.

Virtually any chlamydial strain can be used to prepare a group antigen, as it appears to be the major antigenic component for all strains. Comparative tests have shown that some strains or isolates are to be preferred over others; for instance, the psittacosis antigens have been superior to the LGV antigens even with LGV serum

(Bucca, 1958). The 6 BC strain* that has been used at the Hooper Foundation for many years is available from the American Type Culture Collection or the WHO Collaborating Centre for Reference and Research on Trachoma and Other Chlamydial Infections, at the Hooper Foundation.

The technique of preparation involves inoculation of a 7-day-old embryonated hen's egg via the yolk sac with a standardized inoculum (0.25 ml containing approximately 10^5 egg LD_{50}), which kills most of the embryos in approximately 96 hours. Embryos dying before 72 hours are discarded. When approximately 50% of the embryos are dead, all the eggs are refrigerated for 3 to 24 hours. The yolk sacs are harvested and examined microscopically (using Giminez or Macchiavello's stain) for elementary bodies. If rich in particles, they are pooled and weighed. Yolk sacs are then ground thoroughly with sterile sand (or homogenized), and a 20% suspension in nutrient broth (pH 7.0) is prepared. Sterility tests are performed and the material is held in the refrigerator for six weeks. During this period the antigen preparation is occasionally shaken. The suspension is then centrifuged lightly (200 X for 30 minutes) to remove coarse tissue debris and then steamed at 100° C for 30 minutes. After cooling, phenol is added to a final concentration of 0.5%. This antigen is aliquoted and stored in the refrigerator for use. It should titer at least 1:256, and, if stored properly and protected from contamination by using aseptic technique, the antigens will be stable for years. Small quantities of antigen are available from the WHO Collaborating Centre for Reference and Research on Trachoma and Other Chlamydial Infections for reference purposes. The normal yolk sac control is prepared in a similar manner from uninfected embryos.

The routine immunofluorescent reagents used in the micro-IF test are available from Antibodies, Inc., the Hyland Laboratories, and Microbiological Associates, among others. The yolk sac antigens, however, are not available commercially and must be prepared in the laboratory. For a complete battery of tests, antigen types A, B, Ba, C, D, E, F, G, H, I, J, and K, and LGV antigens L-1, L-2, and L-3 must be included. For routine screening of human sera a simplified antigen pattern involving fewer antigen dots is useful. Closely related antigens may be pooled, for example D and E, L-1 and L-2, G and F, C and J (Wang et al., 1975). The antigens are generally prepared from infected yolk sac suspensions. Tissue culture preparations may

---

* This is a fully virulent psittacosis strain, and appropriate precautions must be taken.

204

be used, although they tend not to be as rich in particles. The yolk sacs are inoculated with suspensions of chlamydiae titrated to kill the embryos in approximately 7 days. In some instances more time may be required. When 50% of the eggs are dead, the rest are chilled, the yolk sacs are harvested, and individual yolk sacs are examined microscopically; those rich in elementary bodies are selected for use. They are homogenized to approximately 5% with sterile PBS and the final antigen dilution selected on the basis of morphologic screening in a fluorescent system. The working dilution (usually 1% to 3%) may be frozen in aliquots at $-60°$ C and stored until needed for making slides. When frozen, the antigen suspensions and the slides are stable, but thawed suspensions should be used within 1 to 2 weeks.

Interpretation of Results

The percentage of "normal" patients with antibody against the chlamydiae (normal background) reflects the diseases prevalent in the community and will vary depending upon the geographic area where the tests are performed and the specific population group being tested.* In the CF test, for example, at a 1:16 level the general population in the San Francisco area tests 2% to 3% positivity. However, if one were testing veterinarians, one would find between 10% and 20% with significant CF levels depending on the type of practice. Among sexually active young adults, the background is approximately 5% for men and 15% to 20% for women. CF titers of 1:64 or higher are rarely seen in the normal population and are uncommon in sexually active males, although they do occur more often in sexually active females. CF titers of this level are more common in psittacosis or lymphogranuloma venereum. Among patients with Reiter's syndrome, 10% have CF titers over 1:64 and another 15% have titers over 1:16 (Chapter 8).

There has not been similar broad experience with the micro-IF test, but the published results together with unpublished data from the Hooper Foundation indicate no problem with the group-specific cross-reactions. For example, we have tested psittacosis convalescent sera with CF titers of 1:512 and found them completely nonreactive in the micro-IF test. But there is a substantial prevalence of seroreactors with this test. For example, among sexually active young adults, we find 25% of men and 60% to 70% of women with detectable micro-IF titers. Thus, as a diagnostic test, a single positive

---

* Table 4 presents the results obtained at the Hooper Foundation using these two tests in parallel, in different population studies.

titer could again only be used to determine previous exposure. In epidemiologic studies, type-specific reactions could be of considerable interest in detecting predominant serotypes, transmission chains, patterns of clustering, etc. IgM antibodies in the micro-IF test may give greater support for a diagnosis of active or recently acquired infection, but experience indicates that only 28% to 33% of patients with active infections have these antibodies and some patients who have IgM antibodies detected by micro-IF do not have demonstrable chlamydial infection (Philip et al., 1974; Reeve et al., 1974). In the pediatric population we have found approximately 10% of children with micro-IF titers. The stimulus for this antibody response is not known, but some may be a consequence of asymptomatic neonatal infections.

Patients with LGV tend to have high CF titers and very high and broadly reactive micro-IF antibody responses (Philip et al., 1974; Wang and Grayston, 1974). We often find that LGV patients have CF titers of 1:128 or 1:256 and micro-IF titers of 1:4,000 or higher. The highest micro-IF titers we have observed have been in sera obtained from prostitutes; these titers have been as high as 1:16,000 to 1:32,000 and have not correlated with CF titers as well as the LGV sera. Specific antichlamydial IgA or IgG in tears may indicate active chlamydial infection of the conjunctiva (McComb and Nichols, 1969). Similar studies have not yet been reported with genital tract secretions.

In either CF or micro-IF it is clear that a fourfold or greater rise in titer will support the diagnosis of chlamydial infection in the clinical syndrome being considered. Unfortunately this is usually not observed, and often the clinician must simply use a single titer which must be interpreted in terms of the patient's disease and the background prevalence of antibody titers.

ISOLATION OF CHLAMYDIAE

For practical purposes there are only three experimental systems that need be considered for the isolation of chlamydiae. All known chlamydiae grow in the yolk sac (YS) of the embryonated hen's egg. With centrifugation of the inoculum it appears that all chlamydiae (with some variability) will grow in tissue culture; psittacosis and LGV agents are capable of serial growth in tissue culture without centrifugation. The psittacosis agents will grow in mice after intracerebral (IC), intraperitoneal (IP), and intranasal (IN) inoculation. LGV agents may be recovered by infecting mice IC and IN, although the IN route is rarely used. Mice are of no use in recovering TRIC agents.

206

The specimens to be tested include ocular and genital tract epithelial cell scrapings for TRIC agents, bubo pus, and genital tract specimens for LGV agents, and blood, sputum, and biopsied tissues for psittacosis.

For maximal results it is imperative that adequate specimens be collected. With genital tract specimens the specimens must be obtained (either by swabbing or scraping) from the transitional zone of the cervix or the endourethra (4 to 6 cm from the meatus). Culture of discharges or of urine is inadequate.

General guidelines for the handling of specimens are listed below. The diluents and antibiotics used to control bacterial contamination will differ with the isolation system being used, resulting in some minor variations. Samples from birds and mammals are also listed — for cases when they may be tested in efforts to determine sources of human infections. Fresh samples are preferred, but frozen material ($-60°$ C) is acceptable.

Processing of Specimens

Blood   If there is a clot, grind it and add beef heart broth or tissue culture medium to make a 10% suspension.

Sputum or Throat Washings   Sputum is cultured for bacteria on blood agar plates. To prepare the emulsion, suspend sputum, depending on its consistency, in 2 to 10 times its volume of sterile antibiotic-containing broth (pH 7.2 to 7.4) or tissue culture medium; emulsify thoroughly by shaking with glass beads in a sterile, tightly stoppered container. Refrigerate the material for 18 to 24 hours at about $0°$ to $4°$ C to extract the chlamydiae, or inoculate into the isolation system after 1 to 2 hours treatment with antibiotics. It may be advisable to centrifuge extracts for 20 to 30 minutes at 300 rpm to remove coarse material.

Pleural Fluid or Vomitus   Determine the extent of bacterial contamination of pleural fluid by culturing on blood agar plates. Treat with antibiotic solution, then refrigerate the specimen until used for inoculation. Vomitus is also cultured on blood plates to determine the type of contaminant and treated with antimicrobial drugs. When much vomitus is available, the coarse material is sedimented by centrifugation; the supernatant fluid is treated in the manner used for fecal specimens (see below).

Bubo Pus   Grind the viscous material. Suspend in nutrient broth or tissue culture medium to at least 20% of weight. Even when pus is not viscous, dilution is advisable. If the bubo is not fluctuant, sterile saline may be injected and aspirated for isolation attempts. Test for bacterial contaminants, treat with antibiotics, and inoculate the material into mice intracerebrally, into eggs by the yolk sac route, or into cell cultures.

Fecal Samples   The droppings from caged birds or fecal pellets pressed out from the cloaca of live or dead birds are suspended in antibiotic hormone broth, or in a solution of 10% horse serum in buffered water; the proportion in either diluent is 1:3 by volume. The suspension is shaken thoroughly and extracted overnight at about 0° to 4° C.   After centrifugation at 300 X g for 10 minutes, the supernatant fluid is removed. Streptomycin sulfate is added in a concentration of 2 mg/ml of supernatant fluid and the mixture is held for 1 hour at room temperature.

Equally efficient is the following procedure: Fecal pellets are emulsified in the antibiotic broth in the proportion of 1:3 by volume; the solution is centrifuged and 0.5 ml of the supernatant fluid is injected intraperitoneally into 3 to 5 mice.

A third method has been recommended by Storz et al. (1965). Fecal samples are collected from the rectum of sheep, cattle, or other mammals using a fresh wooden tongue depressor for each animal. Immediately after collection, the samples are taken to the laboratory, ground, and brought to a 10% suspension in Earle's balanced salt solution containing 0.5 mg of streptomycin per ml. The samples are centrifuged for 30 minutes at 1,800 X g. Supernatant fluid is gently withdrawn, mixed with an equal amount of fresh diluent, and centrifuged again. This procedure is repeated once more. About 3 ml of supernatant fluid is then withdrawn, and 0.5 ml each of 1:40 and of 1:400 dilutions is inoculated into the yolk sacs of 7-day-old chicken embryos. Appropriate bacteriologic controls are also prepared.

Tissues   Frozen tissue is thawed in a refrigerator at about 4° C for 18 to 24 hours. The specimen is weighed, minced with sterile scissors, and ground to a paste. Grinding may be done with such equipment as (a) a Ten Broeck tissue grinder; (b) a 150 × 20 mm Pyrex test tube in which a narrower, but longer and stronger test tube (200 × 10 mm) with a roughened outer surface acts as a pestle (the risk of contamination is less with this device than with a mortar); (c) a sterile mortar and sterile carborundum (size 60); (d) a scissors for mincing and a special metal container for grinding that can be hermetically closed and operated on a blender base. This method is particularly useful for breaking up large pieces of organ, but there is greater potential for aerosol formation.

After the tissue has been ground thoroughly, the volume of diluent required to make a 10% to 20% emulsion is added to the tube, and the suspension is thoroughly mixed. Plain nutrient broth (pH 7.2 to 7.4) is employed as diluent or, if material is contaminated, hormone broth containing antibiotics is used. If testing is not urgent, holding the suspensions in the refrigerator for 18 to 24 hours is advisable, since it permits additional sedimentation and diffusion of the chlamydiae into the diluent.

Before being refrigerated, a sample of the treated or untreated emulsion is cultured on blood plates and on eosin-methylene blue plates to detect possible bacterial contamination. Should it be grossly contaminated, the bacteria must be partially or completely removed before inoculation.

Mouse Inoculation

The mice to be used should be proven susceptible to chlamydiae as there are some genetic variations in this regard. Mice should be obtained from a colony shown to be free of latent chlamydial infection. There have been at least seven reports of subclinical chlamydial infections in mouse colonies. These agents have been identified as *C. psittaci* (DeBurgh, Jackson, and Williams, 1945; Gerloff and Watson, 1970; Ata, Stephenson, and Storz, 1971) as well as *C. trachomatis* (Nigg and Eaton, 1944), and some have been viscerotropic while others were pneumotropic. These infections were revealed by persistent blind passage of "normal" mouse tissue.

Intraperitoneal Injection   Most psittacine, turkey, and egret isolates will be revealed by inoculation by this route; those from pigeons, chickens, or ducks may produce significantly enlarged spleens and ascitic fluid but do not regularly cause death.

Administer 0.5 ml of the prepared 10% or 20% sterile emulsion. Virulent material from parrots, parakeets, man, and some turkeys, injected by this route in this amount, causes death of the mouse in 3 to 30 days, usually within 3 to 10 days. Some animals recover. Specific death of the animal within 2 or 3 days of infection indicates the presence of high concentrations of a virulent toxic isolate, such as certain turkey or egret isolates.

If mice die within 2 or 3 days, little that is abnormal can be seen with the naked eye; spleen and liver may look normal in size and architecture. Some animals may show signs of vascular damage.

Quite characteristic, and often the only sign, is a bloated duodenum covered with a thin viscous exudate. In some animals, the surface of the liver and intestines may be moist and covered with a thin, sticky exudate that contains abundant endothelial cells packed with chlamydial particles.

When death occurs within 5 to 15 days, the spleen is enlarged, and early necrotic lesions of the liver can be seen. Microscopically, hemorrhages and necrosis are common in the liver; the phagocytic cells of liver and spleen may be packed with chlamydiae. The abdominal cavity may be filled with stringy, turbid, fibrinous exudate.

If animals survive to the 21st day, they should be sacrificed and further blind passage of emulsions of their spleen and liver made. In our experience, if chlamydiae are not found by the third passage, they cannot be isolated no matter how many more passages are made. Mice that recover and are sacrificed three weeks after infection have few gross lesions. In general the intestines are slightly distended and pale. Exudate may be present in the abdominal cavity. The spleen is conspicuously enlarged, the liver friable and mottled, the kidneys grayish. Elementary bodies are sparse in tissue smears, but animal passage has shown that they may exist as long as 300 days after initial infection. Most survivors have an infection immunity.

This technique offers the advantages of simplicity, reliability, and the use of large inocula. If it is desired, the animals may receive multiple (at daily intervals) inoculations from the original specimen. In addition the mice may "filter" out bacteria that have not been controlled by antibiotics or centrifugation and dilution.

Intracranial Injection   Human tissue specimens, sterile exudates from the pericardial or air sacs of birds, or peritoneal fluid and suspensions prepared from infected mice may be safely injected by this route, which may furnish excellent specimens for rapid histologic diagnosis. Inoculate 0.03 ml of a 10% emulsion. Somnolence and paralysis often develop within 24 to 48 hours, and death follows within 3 to 5 days.

This route has the advantage of not involving the respiratory tract, precluding the possibility of activating latent mouse pneumonitis. Smears made from the dura teem with chlamydiae. This technique is a relatively fast and sensitive method for isolating psittacosis and ornithosis agents (somewhat less effective with LGV). This route of inoculation suffers a disadvantage in terms of small volume of inoculum and in the susceptibility of the mice to bacteria that may contaminate the specimen.

Intranasal Instillation   Instill 0.03 to 0.05 ml of a 10% tissue suspension, with the mouse under light anesthesia (ether is suitable). If the material inoculated is virulent or with established isolates, signs of infection — hunched posture, apathy, and increasingly labored respiration — develop rapidly, and death follows within 2 to 20 days. Bacterial contamination must be ruled out. In typical successful isolation attempts, death may take place between the 8th and 16th day if the agent is present in high titer. However, with less virulent material all symptoms may gradually disappear; in such cases, blind passage should be performed 21 days postinoculation. Blind passage is usually required. Segments or entire lobes of the lung may be extensively consolidated. Discrete foci of pneumonia are manifested as limiting infective dilutions are approached. These areas are gray, almost translucent, 1 to 3 mm in diameter, and lie in apparently normal lung.

Fewer elementary bodies are seen in smears from lungs infected for more than 10 days, and there may be difficulty finding them in old lesions; repassage may furnish excellent material for microscopy.

This route of inoculation is of some use with psittacosis agents, less so for LGV.

The Yolk Sac Method

The yolk sac (YS) method has long been used in psittacosis work, and was shown by Wall (1946) to be the method of choice in isolating LGV agents. It was used by T'ang et al. (1957) in the first isolation of the trachoma agent. Until tissue culture procedures were developed, the YS technique was the only practical way to culture TRIC agents.

The YS technique is not particularly sensitive for the isolation of TRIC agents because it may require many elementary bodies to produce one egg LD_{50}. With more virulent psittacosis strains, a single particle may be lethal. This system is much more sensitive for the recovery of *C. psittaci* strains, in general. The technique is cumbersome, making it difficult to screen large numbers of specimens, and can be quite time-consuming. It may take anywhere from one to six weeks to obtain a definitive result.

The eggs to be used must be derived from a flock fed an antibiotic-free diet. They should be free from mycoplasma.

Yolk Sac Isolation Technique　Clinical specimens are collected in an appropriate antibiotic broth. A suitable one contains streptomycin, neomycin, and nystatin (2.5 mg/ml, 0.5 mg/ml, and 100 units/ml, respectively). Other antibiotics may also be used (vancomycin, ristocetin, gentamicin, and amphotericin). The specimen is held for 1 hour at room temperature before inoculation of 0.25 ml into the yolk sac using a 1½-inch 22-gauge needle. Prior to inoculation, the fertile eggs are incubated at 38.5° to 39° C in a moist atmosphere. When 7 days old, embryonated hens' eggs are candled for viability and the location of air sacs and embryos marked with a pencil. The shell over the air sacs is painted with tincture of iodine and a hole gently punched. The specimen is inoculated at a slight angle away from the embryo; we recommend that three or four eggs be used for each specimen. The eggs are labeled with a pencil or marking pen. After inoculation the shell is again swabbed with iodine and the hole sealed (with glue or tape). The eggs are then incubated in a moist environment at 35° C and candled daily for 13 days. Eggs that die in the first 3 days after inoculation are discarded.

The yolk sacs of eggs dying thereafter are harvested. This procedure entails painting the shell with iodine, cracking and removing the shell over the air sac, dissecting the shell and chorioallantoic membranes away, and removing the YS with forceps. Excess yolk material may be stripped away. It is important that all instruments are sterile, and that fresh instruments are used for each specimen. Impression smears are made and stained (Giminez or the modified Macchiavello method). Sterility tests are performed on YS with thioglycolate broth. If the embryos are still viable 13 days postinoculation, the eggs are chilled for several hours and yolk sacs harvested, ground in nutrient broth, centrifuged lightly, and passed to another group of four 7-day-old embryonated hens' eggs (1 ml 50% YS/egg). After two blind passages, attempts are terminated as negative.

The generally acceptable criteria for positive isolation are the finding of elementary bodies in the impression smears, serially transmissible egg mortality, the presence of group antigen in the YS, and the absence of contaminating bacteria (Schachter, 1970).

The clinical specimens should not be held at ambient temperature for more than 2 to 3 hours. They may be refrigerated for up to 18 hours (with significant loss of infectivity) and should be frozen at $-70°$ C (or in liquid nitrogen) for longer storage.

The specimens may be collected with a scraper or a swab. If swabs are used, they should be of a pretested type that will not inactivate TRIC agents.

Psittacosis isolation attempts may be positive within 5 to 10 days of the first passage. Some isolates require more adaptation but, once adapted, will often reach titers of 10^8 or 10^9 egg LD_{50}/gm. In titrations, these strains will kill eggs within 8 to 9 days at limiting dilutions and surviving embryos are rarely infected.

Positive LGV isolation attempts usually become apparent in the latter part of the first passage or early in the second passage. The adaptation process is slower, and usually more than five passages are required before the peak titers ($>10^7$ LD_{50}/gm) are obtained. Surviving embryos in these early passages are often infected. Until peak titers are reached, the isolated LGV agents may not possess all the properties usually attributed to LGV strains. For example, LGV and TRIC agents are generally stated to differ on the grounds that LGV agents will kill mice by the IC route, while TRIC agents will not. This is not true in early passage LGV isolates (Schachter and Meyer, 1969b). These LGV isolates do not kill mice because it apparently requires in excess of 10^5 LD_{50} to kill a mouse, and these levels are not obtained in early passage in eggs.

With TRIC strains there is considerable variation, but the positive isolation attempt usually results in egg lethality in the second week of the second passage. Rarely will specific lethality occur in the first passage, although occasionally elementary bodies are seen at blind passage. Egg infectivity titers greatly exceed egg lethality titers, with $ID_{50}:LD_{50}$ ratios as high as 10^4 or 10^5. These TRIC agent isolates often require much adaptation and display great variability in their behavior in ovo. After 4 or 5 passages the isolates often stabilize at 10^6 to 10^7 LD_{50}/gm; they kill the eggs more slowly than psittacosis or LGV agents, with specific lethality commencing on the 6th to 7th day, and continuing to the 12th or 13th day. Some isolates never develop a regular pattern of egg lethality. We once carried an isolate through 30 passages, each requiring an inoculum of 1 ml of a 50% YS suspension to maintain the agent. Regular lethality was never observed, and use of higher dilutions resulted in loss of agent. It will be of interest to see whether differences in biological behavior (for example, in ovo) can be attributed to the different serotypes currently being recognized.

In summary, the YS technique will continue to be used by many laboratories. It still results in yields of agent that cannot be matched in tissue culture systems. It will continue to be used for isolation of chlamydiae, particularly in laboratories that are not using tissue culture regularly or that have problems in obtaining tissue culture reagents.

Tissue Culture Methods for Isolation

Psittacosis and LGV agents have been successfully propagated in cell culture systems for several decades. The trachoma agent was not isolated till 1957, and the initial attempts to establish strains in cell culture failed. Some egg-propagated trachoma isolates were successfully adapted by difficult techniques (Mitsui et al., 1964); Gordon found that centrifugation of inoculum into irradiated McCoy cells allowed the growth of trachoma agents (Gordon and Quan, 1965b). This technique was soon applied to isolation of the agent from clinical specimens, and it has been adapted for the isolation of psittacosis agents (Lewis and Thacker, 1973).

The early cell culture isolation technique used sonication of specimens and two passages (Gordon et al., 1969). When a yolk sac technique and the cell culture technique were performed in parallel, the tissue culture method was found to be approximately four times more sensitive than the yolk sac method. This has not been the experience of all investigators. In some studies the two techniques have yielded essentially equivalent results (Ford and McCandlish, 1971). With removal of the requirements for sonication of the specimen, the tissue culture technique has been considerably simplified and has reached a degree of sensitivity where approximately 80% of conjunctival specimens presumed to be positive yield isolates (Darougar et al., 1972). In our hands, the two techniques appear to have essentially the same sensitivity with ocular specimens from inclusion conjunctivitis and cervical specimens. We find the advantages of the tissue culture method are its speed, simplicity, and ability to handle large volumes of specimens. In addition, the cell culture systems are less affected by bacterial contamination. With the cervical specimens and the eye specimens, there appears to be, in many instances, more agent than is collected in specimens from the male urethra. With the specimens from the male urethra, it appears that the tissue culture method is more sensitive.

Isolates can be passed readily in cell culture unless the original inoculated coverslip contains less than 10 inclusions. If the agent is first passed several times in tissue culture, yielding increasing inclusion counts with each passage, and then inoculated into eggs, it is usually readily established in the yolk sac. Occasionally, however, attempts to adapt these strains in the eggs do fail, and in many instances the transition from cell culture to egg system is equivalent to inoculating a clinical specimen into the egg. The timing of agent recovery in YS is similar to that observed in the primary isolation attempts to establish these strains. Presumably this is due to requirement for adaptation of growth in the yolk sac. However, Croy, Kuo, and Wang (1975) have shown marked differences in susceptibility of cell lines to infection with different chlamydial serotypes. Perhaps different types grow better in cell culture than in eggs. Some of our results support this speculation. In some studies, the chlamydiae recovered from patients with trachoma did not have the same distribution of serotypes prevalent in the community, as determined by serologic survey (Hanna, personal communication).

Although the irradiated cell technique was introduced by

Gordon, it has been largely the work of the group at The Institute of Ophthalmology in London that has led to the refinement of the technique to the procedures that are generally used today. The changes from the original techniques involved the introduction of routine use of swabbing, rather than scraping, for the collection of the specimens (Darougar and Jones, 1971), and the use of high-temperature (35°– 38° C) and higher forces of centrifugation (2,700 X g) (Darougar, Kinnison, and Jones, 1971). It is apparent that there is no difference in the collection methods, and swabbing is easier from the viewpoint of patient comfort and maintenance of patient-physician relationship. These workers have also introduced the use of liquid nitrogen refrigeration for storage of specimens. They have found that the collection of the specimens in their standard sucrose phosphate antibiotic solution followed by freezing in liquid nitrogen (Gordon et al., 1969) is a convenient method for transporting field specimens. The medium for liquid nitrogen refrigeration is supplemented with 3% fetal bovine serum to protect the organism from damage during freezing and thawing. The group currently uses a simplified one-passage technique, reading one coverslip and passing positive material to establish isolates, or staining and examining the second coverslip if the first has no inclusions. The evolution of these procedures has been reviewed (Darougar et al., 1972).

Darougar, Cubitt, and Jones (1974) found that increasing the temperature of centrifugation to 33° C resulted in a fourfold increase in the number of inclusions compared to that obtained after centrifugation at 18° C. They had essentially equivalent results by using bench centrifuges (with wind shields) at 2,500 X g. These workers felt that increasing the gravitational force could significantly increase the rate of positivity with the specimens collected from patients with chronic or low-grade chlamydial infections; therefore, they have recommended the use of 15,000 X g to obtain higher recovery rates in mild or chronic chlamydial infections where the titer of recoverable agent is probably minimal.

Hobson et al. (1974) have used conventional monolayers of McCoy cells rather than heavily irradiated cells, and have recovered chlamydiae from a similar proportion (20%) of cervical swabs as reported from other laboratories. The obvious advantage of using unirradiated cells is that the procedure is simplified and can be used by laboratories lacking radiation facilities. We have utilized this technique and must point out that, while inclusions can be formed in the unirradiated cells, the visualization and counting of the inclusions is much more difficult in normal than in irradiated cells.

Blyth and Taverne (1974) also emphasized that there is nothing unique about the susceptibility of the irradiated McCoy cell to chlamydial infection. As a matter of fact, they found that both BHK-21 and HeLa cells were as sensitive as the irradiated McCoy cells in titrating TRIC isolates, and BHK-21 and McCoy cells were equal in isolating TRIC agents. In some studies they found more inclusions in the BHK-21 cells. A crucial aspect of this study was the maintenance of these cells in a nonreplicating form, which may well have allowed them to spread and become larger. These workers (and our laboratory studies are in total agreement) discovered that inclusions could be found at similar levels in irradiated and nonirradiated McCoy cells, but that they were much larger and easier to visualize in the bizarre products of irradiation. The irradiation appears to induce giant cell formation, thus creating a large cytoplasmic space in which inclusions can develop. This is probably the real advantage of the irradiated cell line.

Wentworth and Alexander (1974) simplified the isolation system by introducing the use of 5-iodo 2-deoxyuridine (IUDR) treatment of cells as a substitute for irradiation. They found that cells pretreated for three days with IUDR (25 μg/ml) were equally as effective in recovering and propagating chlamydial strains. The obvious advantage of this system is that it allows tissue culture isolation techniques to be performed in areas where irradiation facilities are not available. This technique may well become the system of choice.

Cytochalasin B, another antimetabolite, has also been used to treat cells as a substitute for radiation, and has been shown to render McCoy cells as sensitive to a chlamydial infection as irradiation (Sompolinsky and Richmond, 1974).

Kuo et al. (1972) have used DEAE-treated HeLa cells for the isolation of chlamydiae from cervical scrapings. They found their system to be as sensitive as the irradiated McCoy cells. Croy, Kuo, and Wang (1975) found the HeLa-229 cell line to be the most sensitive of the 11 they tested, and that it supported growth of some chlamydial serotypes better than the IUDR-treated McCoy cells.

Because most chlamydial isolation attempts are performed using coverslips in glass or plastic vials, efforts have been made to increase the volume of specimens which can be handled by using microtiter plates with cells on 5-mm coverslips. Since each plate contains 96 wells, 384 tests could be run in a single centrifugation (McComb and Puzniak, 1974). The problem with this procedure is that the plastic plates tend to crack or rupture at forces over 2,000 X g, and the current routine for isolation uses approximately 3,000 X g. It is unnecessary to utilize this particular method for increasing the volumes of specimens (although this method is attractive because it is cheaper in terms of media). An alternate method uses a six-place horizontal head with the cups machined to take a second bottom (by use of an aluminum plate placed into the machined groove above the level of one set of vials), making it possible to double the number of vials used in each cup. Thus, we can currently run in excess of 150 tubes in each centrifugation run without risk of damage to the specimens.

There is no clearly superior cytologic staining method for screening tissue culture isolation attempts. The options are largely limited to iodine, Giemsa, and fluorescent antibody techniques. It appears that there may be some difference depending on cell type. For example, the HeLa cells do not lend themselves to routine use of the iodine-staining procedure because they occasionally have light iodine-staining material in the cytoplasmic background. The iodine stain is somewhat limited by being positive for a relatively short time within the developmental cycle of the inclusion. Since different isolates may have slightly different growth rates, any set incubation time is a compromise. On the other hand, the iodine stain offers an obvious advantage in giving good contrast with the background, and lends itself to rapid scanning. Iodine will not stain *C. psittaci* inclusions.

The Giemsa stain is probably slightly more sensitive than the iodine, but requires more time to read. The use of Giemsa stain followed by dark field microscopy avoids this problem; when the elementary bodies within the inclusion are viewed by dark field illumination they are very bright yellow and contrast sharply with the background cells (Fig. 15). Unfortunately, there appears to be some variability in this procedure, and not all preparations of stain and coverslips work well in a dark field system. The reason for this variation is not known. The FA staining procedure obviously presents problems in reagents (Fig. 17). While it appears to be a quick method, it probably offers no advantages in terms of sensitivity. Kuo et al. (1972) compared Giemsa and direct FA staining methods to demonstrate inclusions in a HeLa cell isolation system and found that results were essentially the same although it took only 5 to 10 minutes to read the FA slides, whereas it took 20 to 30 minutes to read a Giemsa coverslip.

Tissue Culture Technique

Many cell lines are suitable. The McCoy cells are most commonly used. Confluent monolayers of the cells are grown in the standard growth medium (10% fetal calf serum in Eagle's minimal essential medium supplemented with glutamine and 30 μM/ml glucose). The cells are irradiated (5,000 r), and 1 to 7 days later the cells are seeded onto coverslips. Round coverslips (12 mm) placed in short, 15-mm diameter, disposable flat-bottom vials are especially suitable. Each tube receives approximately 125,000 cells, and they may be used 1 to 7 days after planting. If large numbers of specimens are tested routinely, it is preferable to prepare fresh cells twice each week. The number of cells transferred should be sufficient to obtain light, confluent monolayers.

The clinical specimen is collected by scraping or using suitable swabs,* and is placed into standard growth medium containing streptomycin (200 μg/ml) or gentamicin (10 μg/ml), vancomycin (100 μg/ml), and fungizone (4 μg/ml). Other antibiotics are also suitable. Although sonication of specimens may be preferred, a simple and satisfactory method for dispersing the specimen is to have 2 or 3 glass beads in each collection tube; these tubes are then shaken mechanically for 30 to 60 seconds before inoculation. The inoculum (0.25–0.5 ml) is placed into 2 to 4 vials containing the cell monolayers on coverslips. The vials are then centrifuged at 2,700 to 3,000 X g at 33° to 35° C for one hour. Depending on the clinical source, the inoculum is either replaced with 1 ml growth medium, or medium is added to reach that volume. The tubes are then incubated at 37° C (5% CO_2 atmosphere may be required if loose caps are used) for 65 hours. At that time one coverslip is stained with iodine (after methanol fixation) and examined microscopically for inclusions. At least 90% of positive isolation attempts are positive in the first passage. If an attempt to establish isolates is to be made (or if blind passage is being done), the remaining tubes are shaken vigorously and passed at day 3 or 4 to fresh tubes by the same method. Alternatively the other coverslips may be stained and examined for inclusions. If there is any urgency in establishing the diagnosis, one coverslip may be examined at 40 to 48 hours incubation. The inclusions are not seen as easily as after 65 hours — but can usually be identified.

As a replacement for irradiation, the cells may be treated with IUDR. The light monolayers are treated for 3 days with media containing 25 μg/ml IUDR. The medium containing the antimetabolite is then removed; the cells are washed and treated as before.

According to Kuo et al. (1972), rewashing the cells with DEAE-dextran (25 μg/ml) enhances infectivity. It also may increase the size of the inclusions.

---

* It is important that the laboratory be coordinated with the clinical investigator. Uniformity of technique and standardization of reagents (including swabs) are vital in obtaining optimal results. We have found some cotton swabs toxic for chlamydiae, and dacron swabs interfere with iodine staining procedures. We routinely use alginate swabs of sizes designed for the anatomic sites to be sampled. These swabs do not interfere with microscopy as we use the iodine stain.

218

We have used irradiation and IUDR treatment of McCoy or L-929 cells and have found essential equivalence among the four possible variations.

The tissue culture technique has been in routine use at the Hooper Foundation since 1970. It has been used to isolate chlamydiae from patients with all the diseases covered in this book and from birds and lower mammals. The basic methodology is the same, but some variations must be made to accommodate the different specimens and the properties of the different chlamydiae.

With trachoma, inclusion conjunctivitis, and the genital tract infections the technique is exactly as described above. In LGV, the aspirated bubo pus is diluted (10^{-1} and 10^{-2}) and treated as above. Second passages are always made because detritus from the inoculum may make it difficult to read the slides. In an alternate procedure which we have used for LGV and use routinely for *C. psittaci* isolation attempts, the inoculated monolayers are incubated for 10 days, with routine examination at 5 days and 10 days or whenever a cytopathic effect is noted. The cells are stained by Giemsa's method and examined for inclusions (Fig. 19, Plate 12). This technique has

Table 5

Application of Diagnostic Tests for Chlamydial Infections

	Psitta-cosis	LGV	Tracho-ma	Inclusion Conjunctivitis		Urethritis	Cervi-citis
				Adult	Newborn		
Diagnostic Test							
A Cytology							
Iodine	−	−	±	±	+	−	−
FA	−	−	++	++	++	+	+
Giemsa	−	−	++	+	++	±	+
B Serology							
CF	++	+	−	±	−	−	±
Micro-IF	?	+	+	+	+	+	+
C Isolation							
Yolk sac	++	++	+	+	++	+	+
Mice	++	+	−	−	−	−	−
Tissue Culture	++	++	++	++	++	++	++

Note: This table emphasizes diagnostic tests. Some tests, particularly the micro-IF, are extremely useful in epidemiologic surveys — less so for diagnosis.

  $+$ = often successful.

$++$ = a most useful technique.

  $\pm$ = rarely successful, usually not worth performing.

  $-$ = not useful.

yielded positive results in psittacosis (including avian specimens), ornithosis, human infections with feline pneumonitis agents, and chlamydial infections in cats and other mammals. In most instances the agent was isolated in other systems (eggs or mice), and in some instances the material was known to be positive on cytologic grounds. Although it was more sensitive, the major advantage of the tissue culture system was simply that it allowed use of one method for all these specimens. In some instances it was no faster than with mice (psittacosis) or eggs (psittacosis and feline pneumonitis). However, some of the isolates were not lethal to mice and more of the eggs were lost to bacterial contamination.

Thus it appears that at this time the tissue culture isolation techniques are to be considered the methods of choice (Table 5). This is particularly true of the ocular and genital tract TRIC agent infections. If the equipment and technical expertise are available, these are the methods that should be developed in laboratories beginning studies on chlamydial infections.

BIBLIOGRAPHY

Abrams, A.J.: 1968. Lymphogranuloma venereum. *JAMA* 205:199-202.

Agarwal, L.P., R.P. Saxena, and B.M.S. Gupta: 1955. Antibiotic and chemotherapeutic agents in treatment of trachoma. *Am. J. Ophthalmol.* 40:553-556.

Alepa, F.P.: 1968. LGV stimulation of lymphocytes in Reiter's syndrome. *Arth. Rheum.* 11:462-463, abstract.

Alergant, C.D.: 1957. Lymphogranuloma inguinale in the male in Liverpool, England, 1947 to 1954. *Br. J. Vener. Dis.* 33:47-51.

Alexander, E.R., J. Chandler, T.A. Pheifer, S.-P. Wang, M. English, and K.K. Holmes: 1977. Prospective study of perinatal *Chlamydia trachomatis* infection, pp. 148-152. In: *Nongonococcal Urethritis and Related Infections.* K.K. Holmes and D. Hobson (eds.). Washington, D.C.: American Society for Microbiology.

Alexander, E.R., S.-P. Wang, and J.T. Grayston: 1967. Further classification of TRIC agents from ocular trachoma and other sources by the mouse toxicity prevention test. *Am. J. Ophthalmol.* 63:1469-1478.

Alexander, J.J.: 1968. Separation of protein synthesis in meningopneumonitis agent from that in L cells by differential susceptibility to cycloheximide. *J. Bacteriol.* 95:327-332.

Alexander, J.J.: 1969. Effect of infection with the meningopneumonitis agent on deoxyribonucleic acid and protein synthesis by its L-cell host. *J. Bacteriol.* 97:653-657.

Allen, J.H.: 1944. Inclusion blennorrhea: Part I. Manifestations in the newborn. *Am. J. Ophthalmol.* 27:833-846.

Allison, A.C. and H.R. Perkins: 1960. Presence of cell walls like those of bacteria in *Rickettsiae. Nature* 188:796-798.

Amor, B.: 1969. Apport de la virologie dans la connaissance des rhumatismes inflammatoires. *Gaz. Med. Fr.* 76:4985-4996.

Amor, B., F. Coste, and F. Delbarre: 1965. Sur l'origine virale possible du syndrome oculo-uréthro-synovial. *Presse Med.* 73:1825-1830.

Amor, B., F. Coste, and F. Delbarre. 1967. Mise en évidence, par culture, d'agents du genre *Bedsonia* dans le liquide articulaire en cas de Rhumatisme de Fiessinger-Leroy-Reiter (F.L.R.). *C. R. Acad. Sci.* 264 (Ser. D):1365-1367.

Amor, B., A. Kahan, F. Lecoq, and F. Delbarre: 1972. Le test de transformation lymphoblastique par les antigèns bedsoniens (TTL Bedsonien). *Rev. Rhum.* 39:671-676.

222

Anderson, D.R., H.E. Hopps, M.F. Barile, and B.C. Bernheim: 1965. Comparison of the ultrastructure of several rickettsiae, ornithosis virus, and Mycoplasma in tissue culture. *J. Bacteriol.* 90:1387–1404.

Anderson, J.P.: 1973. Ornithosis in Somerset. Experience in the South Somerset clinical area 1964–71. *Postgrad. Med. J.* 49:533–534.

Anderson, J.P. and F.A.J. Bridgwater: 1968. Ornithosis in a chest clinic practice. *Br. J. Dis. Chest* 62:155–166.

Annamunthodo, H.: 1962. Intestinal lymphogranuloma, pp. 71–123. In: *Lymphogranuloma Venereum. Epidemiological, Clinical, Surgical and Therapeutic Aspects Based on a Study in the Caribbean.* M.M. Sigel (ed.). Coral Gables, Fla.: The University of Miami Press.

Armstrong, C.: 1930. Psittacosis. Epidemiological considerations with reference to the 1929–30 outbreak in the United States. *Public Health Rep.* 45:2013–2033.

Armstrong, C., W.B. Daniels, F.G. MacMurray, and H.C. Turner: 1956. Complement fixation in a cat scratch disease employing Lygranum C.F. as antigen. *JAMA* 161:149–150.

Arnstein, P., B. Eddie, and K.F. Meyer: 1968. Control of psittacosis by group chemotherapy of infected parrots. *Am. J. Vet. Res.* 29:2213–2227.

Assaad, F.A., T. Sundaresan, and F. Maxwell-Lyons: 1971. The household pattern of trachoma in Taiwan. *Bull. W.H.O.* 44:605–615.

Assaad, F.A., T.K. Sundaresan, C.Y. Yang, and L.J. Yeh: 1971. Clinical evaluation of the Taiwan trachoma control programme. *Bull. W.H.O.* 45:491–509.

Ata, F.A., E.H. Stephenson, and J. Storz: 1971. Inapparent respiratory infection of inbred Swiss mice sulfadiazine-resistant, iodine-negative chlamydiae. *Infect. Immun.* 4:506–507.

Aust, O.: 1929. Beitrage zur Trachomforschung. *Graefe's Arch. Ophtalmol.* 123:93–139.

Bader, J.P. and H.R. Morgan: 1961. Latent viral infection of cells in tissue culture. VII. Role of water-soluble vitamins in psittacosis virus propagation in L cells. *J. Exp. Med.* 113:271–281.

Badger, L.F.: 1930. Psittacosis outbreak in a department store. *Public Health Rep.* 45:1403–1409.

Badger, L.F.: 1934. Psittacosis outbreak in a department store in Pittsburgh. *Public Health Rep.* 49:583–584.

Banks, J., B. Eddie, J. Schachter, and K.F. Meyer: 1970a. Plaque formation by *Chlamydia* in L cells. *Infect. Immun.* 1:259–262.

Banks, J., B. Eddie, M. Sung, N. Sugg, J. Schachter, and K.F. Meyer: 1970b. Plaque reduction technique for demonstrating neutralizing antibodies for *Chlamydia. Infect. Immun.* 2:443–447.

Barron, A.L. and M.C. Riera: 1969. Studies on hemagglutination by *Chlamydia. Proc. Soc. Exp. Biol. Med.* 131:1087–1090.

Barron, A.L., Z. Zakay-Rones, and H. Bernkopf: 1965. Hemagglutination of chicken erythrocytes by the agent of psittacosis. *Proc. Soc. Exp. Biol. Med.* 119:377–381.

Barros, E.: 1930. La psitacosis en la República Argentina. *Rev. Assoc. Med. Argent.* XLIII:1–48.

Barros, E.: 1940. La psitacosis durante el decenio 1929–1939. *La Prensa Med. Argent.* 27:9–121.

Barwell, C.F.: 1952. Some observations on the antigenic structure of psittacosis and lymphogranuloma venereum viruses. II. Treatment of virus suspensions by various reagents and the specific activity of acid extracts. *Br. J. Exp. Pathol.* 33:268–279.

Barwell, C.F.: 1955. Laboratory infection of man with virus of zoötic abortion of ewes. *Lancet* 2:1369–1371.

Becker, Y.: 1974. The agent of trachoma. Recent studies on the biology, biochemistry and immunology of a prokaryotic obligate parasite of eukaryocytes, pp. 1–99. In: *Monographs in Virology.* Vol. 7. J.L. Melnick (ed.). Basel: S Karger.

Becker, Y. and Y. Asher: 1972. Synthesis of trachoma agent proteins in emetine-treated cells. *J. Bacteriol.* 109:966–970.

Becker, Y., Y. Asher, N. Himmel, and Z. Zakay-Rones: 1969. Rifampicin inhibition of trachoma agent in vivo. *Nature* 224:33–34.

Becker, Y., E. Hochberg, and Z. Zakay-Rones: 1969. Interaction of trachoma elementary bodies with host cells. *Isr. J. Med. Sci.* 5:121–124.

Bedson, S.P.: 1935. The use of the complement-fixation reaction in the diagnosis of human psittacosis. *Lancet* 2:1277–1280.

Bedson, S.P.: 1936. Observations bearing on the antigenic composition of the psittacosis virus. *Br. J. Exp. Pathol.* 17:109–121.

Bedson, S.P.: 1959. The psittacosis-lymphogranuloma group of infective agents. The Harben Lectures. *J. R. Inst. Public Health Hyg.* 22:67–143.

Bedson, S.P. and J.O.W. Bland: 1932. A morphological study of psittacosis virus, with description of a developmental cycle. *Br. J. Exp. Pathol.* 13:461–466.

Bedson, S.P. and J.O.W. Bland: 1934. The developmental forms of the psittacosis virus. *Br. J. Exp. Pathol.* 15:243–247.

Bedson, S.P. and G.T. Western: 1930. Aetiology — experimental observations, pp. 59–95. In: *A Disease of Parrots Communicable to Man (Psittacosis). Rep. Public Health Med. Subj.* No. 61; E.L. Sturdee and W.M. Scott (eds.). London.

Bedson, S.P., G.T. Western, and S. Levy Simpson: 1930a. Observations on the aetiology of psittacosis. *Lancet* 1:235–236.

Bedson, S.P., G.T. Western, and S. Levy Simpson: 1930b. Further observations on the aetiology of psittacosis. *Lancet* 1:345–346.

Bedson, S.P., C.F. Barwell, E.J. King, and L.W.J. Bishop: 1949. The laboratory diagnosis of lymphogranuloma venereum. *J. Clin. Pathol.* 2:241–249.

Beem, M.O. and E.M. Saxon: 1977a. Respiratory tract colonization and a distinctive pneumonia syndrome in infants infected with *Chlamydia trachomatis. N. Engl. J. Med.* 293:306–310.

Beem, M.O. and E.M. Saxon: 1977b. Letter to the editor. *N. Engl. J. Med.* 296:1124.

Bell, S.D., J.C. Synder, and E.S. Murray: 1959. Immunization of mice against toxic doses of homologous elementary bodies of trachoma. *Science* 130:626–627.

Benedict, A.A. and E. O'Brien: 1956. Antigenic studies on the psittacosis-lymphogranuloma venereum group of viruses. II. Characterization of complement-fixing antigens extracted with sodium lauryl sulfate. *J. Immunol.* 76:293–300.

Benedict. A.A., R.L. Tips, and D. Eddy: 1955. Antigenic studies on the psittacosis-lymphogranuloma venereum group of viruses. I. Acid-soluble complement-fixing and skin test antigens. *Tex. Rep. Biol. Med.* 13:206–212.

Berman, S., E. Freundlich, K. Glaser, A. Abrahamov, E. Ephrati-Elizur, and H. Bernkopf: 1955. Ornithosis in infancy. *Pediatrics* 15:752–760.

Bietti, G.B.: 1963. Progrès de la chimiothérapie et de l'anti-biothérapie du trachome; épreuves d'éfficacité, nouveaux produits, traitement intermittent. *Bull. W.H.O.* 28:395–415.

Bietti, G.B., M.J. Freyche, and R. Vozza: 1962. La diffusion actuelle du trachome dans le monde. *Rev. Int. Trach.* 39:113–310.

Bietti, G.B., C. Pannarale, and C. Milano: 1967. Further contributions to the intermittent therapy of trachoma with new long-acting sulfonamides. *Am. J. Ophthalmol.* 63:1569–1577.

Bietti, G.B. and G.H. Werner: 1967. *Trachoma Prevention and Treatment.* Springfield, Ill.: Charles C Thomas, pp. 5–227.

Binford, C.H. and G.H. Hauser: 1944. An epidemic of a severe pneumonitis in the Bayou Region of Louisiana. III. Pathological observations. Report of autopsy on two cases with a brief comparative note on psittacosis and Q fever. *Public Health Rep.* 59:1363–1373.

Blagojevic, M., D. Savic, and O. Litricin: 1973. Les moyens et les possibilités pratiques d'aboutir au controle complet du trachome. *Rev. Int. Trach.* 50:7–174.

Blyth, W.A. and J. Taverne: 1974. Cultivation of TRIC agents: a comparison between the use of BHK-21 and irradiated McCoy cells. *J. Hyg.* (Camb.) 72:121–128.

Bowie, W.R., E.R. Alexander, J.F. Floyd, J. Holmes, Y. Miller, and K.K. Holmes: 1976. Differential response of chlamydial and ureaplasma-associated urethritis to sulphafurazole (sulfisoxazole) and aminocyclitols. *Lancet* 2:1276–1278.

Bowie, W.R., S.-P. Wang, E.R. Alexander, J. Floyd, P.S. Forsyth, H.M. Pollock, J.S.L. Lin, T.M. Buchanan, and K.K. Holmes: 1977. Etiology of nongonococcal urethritis: evidence for *Chlamydia trachomatis* and *Ureaplasma urealyticum*. *J. Clin. Invest.* 59:735–742.

Braley, A.E.: 1939. Relation between the virus of trachoma and the virus of inclusion blennorrhea. *Arch. Ophthalmol* 22:393–398.

Brewerton, C.A., H. Caffrey, A. Nicholls, D. Walters, and D.C.O. James: 1974. HL-A and arthropathies associated with ulcerative colitis and psoriasis. *Lancet* 1:956–958.

Brewerton, D.A., M. Caffrey, A. Nicholls, D. Walters, J.K. Oates, and D.C.O. James: 1973. Reiter's disease and HL-A 27. *Lancet* 2:996–998.

Briones, O.C., L. Hanna, E. Jawetz, C.R. Dawson, and H.B. Ostler: 1974. Type-specific antibodies in human *Chlamydia trachomatis* infections of the eye. *J. Immunol.* 113:1262–1270.

Brodie, B.C.: 1836. *Pathological and Surgical Observations on the Diseases of the Joints, with Alterations and Additions.* London: Longman, Rees, Orme, Brown, Green, and Longman.

Bucca, M.A.: 1958. Comparison of CF and HI tests on psittacosis-LGV serums. *Public Health Rep.* 73:461–464.

Buckley, S.M., E. Whitney, and F. Rapp: 1955. Identification by fluorescent antibody of the developmental forms of psittacosis virus in tissue cultures. *Proc. Soc. Exp. Biol.* 90:226–230.

Burnet, F.M.: 1935. Enzootic psittacosis amongst wild Australian parrots. *J. Hyg.* (Camb.) 35:412–420.

Burnet, F.M.: 1936. Laboratory investigation of suspected psittacosis. *Med. J. Aust.* 1:363–364.

Buschke, A. and W. Curth: 1931. Über die extragenitale Lokalisation des Lymphogranuloma Inguinale. (Nicolas-Favresche Krankheit). *Klin. Wochenschr.* 10:1709–1711.

Caldwell, G.G., N.J. Lindsey, H. Wulff, D.D. Donrelly, and F.N. Bohl: 1974. Epidemic of adenovirus type 7 acute conjunctivitis in swimmers. *Am. J. Epidemiol.* 94:230–234.

Caminopetros, J.: 1935. Recherches épidémiologiques et expérimentales sur la maladie de Nicholas et Favre. Longue persistance du virus de cette maladie dans l'organisme humain. *Bull. Soc. Pathol. Exot.* 28:408–414.

Cardwell, E.S., Jr. and E.R. Pund: 1940. Malignancies related to venereal disease. *J. Med. Assoc. Ga.* 29:60–62.

Chandler, J.W., E.R. Alexander, T.A. Pheiffer, S.-P. Wang, K.K. Holmes, and M. English: 1977. Ophthalmia neonatorum associated with maternal chlamydial infections. *Tr. Am. Acad. Ophthalmol. Otolaryn.* 83:302–308.

Chanock, R., L. Chambon, W. Chang, F. Goncalves Ferreira, P. Gharpure, L. Grant, J. Hatem, I. Iman, S. Kalra, K. Lim, J. Madalengoitia, L. Spence, P. Teng, and W. Ferreira: 1967. WHO respiratory disease survey in children. *Bull. W.H.O.* 37:363–369.

Chiang, W.T., E.R. Alexander, P.Y. Wei, and J.W. Fresh: 1968. Genital infection with TRIC agents in Taiwan. *Am. J. Obstet. Gynecol.* 100:422–431.

Cockburn, T.A.: 1953. An epidemic of conjunctivitis in Colorado: Associated with pharyngitis, muscle pain, and pyrexia. *Am. J. Ophthalmol.* 36:1534–1539.

Cole, H.N.: 1933. Lymphogranuloma inguinale, the fourth venereal disease; its relation to stricture of the rectum. *JAMA* 101:1069–1076.

Coles, A.C.: 1930. Micro-organisms in psittacosis. *Lancet* 1:1011–1012.

Coll, R. and I. Horner: 1967. Cardiac involvement in psittacosis. *Br. Med. J.* 4:35–36.

Collier, L.H.: 1973. Life at the Border. A review of the work of the MRC Trachoma Unit. *Ann. Rep. Lister Inst. Prev. Med.* 1–26.

Collier, L.H. and W.A. Blyth: 1966a. Immunogenicity of experimental trachoma vaccines in baboons. I. Experimental methods and preliminary tests with vaccines prepared in chick embryos and in HeLa cells. *J. Hyg.* (Camb.), 64:513–528.

Collier, L.H. and W.A. Blyth: 1966b. Immunogenicity of experimental trachoma vaccines in baboons. II. Experiments with adjuvants, and tests of cross-protection. *J. Hyg.* (Camb.), 64:529–544.

Collier, L.H. and W.A. Blyth: 1967. Immunogenicity of experimental trachoma vaccines in baboons. III. Experiments with inactivated vaccines. *J. Hyg.* (Camb.), 65:97–107.

Collins, A.R. and A.L. Barron: 1970. Demonstration of group and species-specific antigens of chlamydial agents by gel diffusion. *J. Infect. Dis.* 121:1–8.

Colón, J.I.: 1962. The role of folic acid in the metabolism of members of the psittacosis group of microorganisms. *Ann. N.Y. Acad. Sci.* 98:234–249.

Coutts, W.E.: 1936. Contribution to knowledge of lymphogranulomatosis venerea as a general disease. *J. Trop. Med. Hyg.* 39:13–19.

Credé, K.S.F.: 1884. *Die Verhütung der Augenentzündung der Neugeborenen (Ophthalmoblennorrhea neonatorum) der häufigsten und wichtigsten Ursache der Blindheit.* Berlin: A Hirschwald, 63 pp.

Credé, K.S.F.: 1963. The prophylactic treatment of ophthalmia neonatorum. *Surv. Ophthalmol.* 8:367-368.

Crocker, T.T., S.R. Pelc, B.L. Nielsen, J.M. Eastwood, and J. Banks: 1965. Population dynamics and deoxyribonucleic acid synthesis in HeLa cells infected with an ornithosis agent. *J. Infect. Dis.* 115:105-122.

Croy, T.R., C.-C. Kuo, and S.-P. Wang: 1975. Comparative susceptibility of eleven mammalian cell lines in infection with trachoma organisms. *J. Clin. Microbiol.* 1:434-439.

Daniels, W.B. and F.G. MacMurray: 1952. Cat scratch disease; nonbacterial regional lymphadenitis: a report of 60 cases. *Ann. Intern. Med.* 37:697-713.

Darougar, S., S. Cubitt, and B.R. Jones: 1974. Effect of high-speed centrifugation on the sensitivity of irradiated McCoy cell culture for the isolation of *Chlamydia. Br. J. Vener. Dis.* 50:308-312.

Darougar, S. and B.R. Jones: 1971. Conjunctival swabbing for the isolation of TRIC agent *(Chlamydia). Br. J. Ophthalmol.* 55:585-590.

Darougar, S., B.R. Jones, J.R. Kinnison, J.D. Vaughn-Jackson, and E.M.C. Dunlop: 1972. Chlamydial infection: Advances in the diagnostic isolation of *Chlamydia,* including TRIC agent, from the eye, genital tract, and rectum. *Br. J. Vener. Dis.* 48:416-420.

Darougar, S., J.R. Kinnison, and B.R. Jones: 1971. Simplified irradiated McCoy cell culture for isolation of chlamydiae, pp. 63-70. In: *Trachoma and Related Disorders Caused by Chlamydial Agents.* R.L. Nichols (ed.). Amsterdam: Excerpta Medica.

Davis, D.E. and J.P. Delaplane: 1958. The lesions of ornithosis in turkeys, pp. 89-110. In: *Progress in Psittacosis Research and Control.* F.R. Beaudette (ed.) New Brunswick, N.J.: Rutgers University Press.

Dawson, C.R., T. Daghfous, M. Messadi, I. Hoshiwara, and J. Schachter: 1976. Severe endemic trachoma in Tunisia. *Br. J. Ophthalmol.* 60:245-252.

Dawson, C.R., T. Daghfous, M. Messadi, I. Hoshiwara, D.W. Vastine, C. Yoneda, and J. Schachter: 1974a. Severe endemic trachoma in Tunisia. II. A controlled therapy trial of topically applied chlortetracycline and erythromycin. *Arch. Ophthalmol.* 92:198-203.

Dawson, C.R., T. Daghfous, M. Messadi, I. Hoshiwara, D.W. Vastine, C. Yoneda, and J. Schachter: 1974b. Microbiologic findings in a controlled trial of rifampicin and tetracycline for the treatment of severe endemic trachoma in Tunisia. *Rev. Int. Trach.* 4:59-64.

Dawson, C.R. and R. Darrell: 1963. Infections due to adenovirus type 8 in the United States. I. An outbreak of epidemic keratoconjunctivitis originating in a physician's office. *N. Engl. J. Med.* 268:1031-1034.

Dawson, C.R., R. Darrell, L. Hanna, and E. Jawetz: 1963. Infections due to adenovirus type 8 in the United States. II. Community-wide infection with adenovirus type 8 *N. Engl. J. Med.* 268:1034–1037.

Dawson, C.R., R.M. Elashoff, L. Hanna, I. Hoshiwara, and H.B. Ostler: 1971. The evaluation of a controlled trachoma therapy trial with oral tetracycline, pp. 545–558. In: *Trachoma and Related Disorders Caused by Chlamydial Agents.* R.L. Nichols (ed.). Amsterdam: Excerpta Medica.

Dawson, C.R. and L. Hanna: 1971. A resumé of experience in controlled trials with topical and systemic tetracycline and systemic sulfonamide. *Ophthalmol. Dig.* 33:30–36.

Dawson, C.R., L. Hanna, and E. Jawetz: 1967. Controlled treatment trials of trachoma in American Indian children. *Lancet* 2:961–964.

Dawson, C.R., L. Hanna, and B. Togni: 1972. Adenovirus type 8 infections in the United States. IV. Observations on the pathogenesis of lesions in severe eye disease. *Arch. Ophthalmol.* 87:258–268.

Dawson, C.R., L. Hanna, T.R. Wood, V. Coleman, O.C. Briones, and E. Jawetz: 1969. Controlled trials with trisulfapyrimidines in the treatment of chronic trachoma. *J. Infect. Dis.* 119:531–590.

Dawson, C.R., L. Hanna, T.R. Wood, and R. Despain: 1970a. Adenovirus type 8 keratoconjunctivitis in the United States. III. Epidemiologic, clinical and microbiologic features. *Am. J. Ophthalmol.* 69:473–480.

Dawson, C.R., I. Hoshiwara, T. Daghfous, M. Messadi, D.W. Vastine, and J. Schachter: 1975. Topical tetracycline and rifampicin therapy of endemic trachoma in Tunisia. *Am. J. Ophthalmol.* 79:803–811.

Dawson, C.R., E. Jawetz, L. Hanna, L. Rose, T.R. Wood, and P. Thygeson: 1966. Experimental inclusion conjunctivitis in man. II. Partial resistance to infection. *Am. J. Epidemiol.* 84:411–425.

Dawson, C.R., E. Jawetz, L. Hanna, W. Winn, and J.G. Thompson: 1960. A family outbreak of adenovirus 8 infection (epidemic keratoconjunctivitis). *Am. J. Hyg.* 72:279–283.

Dawson, C.R., B.R. Jones, and S. Darougar: 1976. Blinding and nonblinding trachoma. The assessment of intensity of upper tarsal inflammatory disease and disabling lesions. *Bull. W.H.O.* 52:279–283.

Dawson, C.R., C. Mordhorst, and P. Thygeson: 1962. Infection of rhesus and cynomolgus monkeys with egg-grown viruses of trachoma and inclusion conjunctivitis. *Ann. N.Y. Acad. Sci.* 98:167–176.

Dawson, C.R. and J. Schachter: 1967. TRIC agent infections of the eye and genital tract. *Am. J. Ophthalmol.* 63:1288–1298.

Dawson, C.R., J. Schachter, H.B. Ostler, R.M. Gilbert, D.E. Smith, and E.P. Engleman: 1970b. Inclusion conjunctivitis and

Reiter's syndrome in a married couple. *Arch. Ophthalmol.* 83:300–306.

Dawson, C.R., T.R. Wood, L. Rose, L. Hanna, and P. Thygeson: 1967. Experimental inclusion conjunctivitis. III. Keratitis and other complications. *Arch. Ophthalmol.* 78:341–349.

Dawson, M.H. and R.L. Boots: 1939. Arthritis associated with lymphogranuloma venereum. *JAMA* 113:1162–1163.

DeBurgh, P., A.V. Jackson, and S.E. Williams: 1945. Spontaneous infection of laboratory mice with a psittacosis-like organism. *Aust. J. Exp. Biol. Med. Sci.* 23:107–110.

Dekking, F. and A.C. Ruys: 1951. Psittacose et ornithose en Hollande. *Rev. Belge Pathol. Med. Exp.* 21:92–98.

Detels, R., E.R. Alexander, and S.P. Dhir: 1966. Trachoma in Punjabi Indians in British Columbia. A prevalence study with comparisons to India. *Am. J. Epidemiol.* 84:81–91.

Dhir, S.P., L.P. Agarwal, R. Detels, S.-P. Wang, and J.T. Grayston: 1967. Field trial of two bivalent trachoma vaccines in children of Punjab Indian villages. *Am. J. Ophthalmol.* 63:1639–1644.

Dhir, S.P., S. Hakomori, G.E. Kenny, and J.T. Grayston: 1972. Immunochemical studies on chlamydial group antigen (presence of a 2-keto-3-deoxycarbohydrate as immunodominant group). *J. Immunol.* 109:116–122.

Dickerson, M.S.: 1962. Texas outbreaks. Turkey ornithosis in man. *Tex. State J. Med.* 58:916–920.

Doherty, R.L., J.G. Carley, P.E. Lee, K.F. Meyer, and B. Eddie: 1961. The effect of chlortetracycline on Australian parrots naturally infected with psittacosis. *Med. J. Aust.* 11:134–139.

Dömök, I.: 1963. Ornithosis epidemics of the last two years in Hungary. *Arch. Gesamte. Virusforsch.* 13:323–325.

Donaldson, P., D.E. Davis, J.R. Watkins, and S.E. Sulkin: 1958. The isolation and identification of ornithosis infection in turkeys by tissue culture and immunocytochemical staining. *Am. J. Vet. Res.* 19:950–954.

Doury, P., S. Pattin, and J.-L. Durosoir: 1973. Le test de transformation lymphoblastique avec l'antigène Bedsonien dans les Syndromes de Fiessinger-Leroy-Reiter anciens et récents et dans les spondylarthrites ankylosantes. *Rev. Rhum.* 40:643–649.

Drachman, T.S.: 1953: A recent outbreak of psittacosis in upper Westchester County, New York. *Am. J. Public Health* 43:165–172.

Duke-Elder, W.S.: 1965. Inflammations of the conjunctiva and associated inflammations of the cornea. Specific types of keratoconjunctivitis—The TRIC viruses, pp. 254–303. In: *System of Ophthalmology,* Vol. VIII, Diseases of the Outer Eye, Part 1. London: Henry Kimptom.

Dunlop, E.M.C., M.K. Al-Hussaini, A. Freedman, J.A. Garland, I.A. Harper, B.R. Jones, J.W. Race, M.S. du Toit, J.D. Treharne, and J.M. Wright: 1966a. Infections by TRIC agent and other members of the Bedsonia group with a note on Reiter's disease: III. Genital infection and diseases of the eye. *Trans. Ophthalmol. Soc. U.K.* 86:321–334.

Dunlop, E.M.C., I.A. Harper, M.K. Al-Hussaini, J.A. Garland, J.D. Treharne, D.J.M. Wright, and B.R. Jones: 1966b. Relation of TRIC agent to 'non-specific' genital infection. *Br. J. Vener. Dis.* 42:77–87.

Dunlop, E.M.C., B.R. Jones, and M.K. Al-Hussaini: 1964. Genital infection in association with TRIC virus infection of the eye. III. Clinical and other findings. Preliminary report. *Br. J. Vener. Dis.* 40:33–42.

Dunlop, E.M.C., B.R. Jones, S. Darougar, and J.D. Treharne: 1972a. Chlamydia and non-specific urethritis. *Br. Med. J.* 2:575–577.

Dunlop, E.M.C., J.D. Vaughn-Jackson, S. Darougar, and B.R. Jones: 1972b. Chlamydial infection: Incidence in 'non-specific' urethritis. *Br. J. Vener. Dis.* 48:425–428.

Durand, M., J. Nicolas, and M. Favre: 1913. Lympho-granulomatose inguinale subaiguë d'origine génital probable, peut-être vénérienee. *Bull. Mem. Soc. Méd. Hôp.* 35:274–288.

Durfee, P.T., M.M. Pullen, R.W. Currier, and R.L. Parker: 1975. Human psittacosis associated with commercial processing of turkeys. *J. Am. Vet. Med. Assoc.* 167:804–808.

Eaton, M.D., M.D. Beck, and H.E. Pearson: 1941. A virus from cases of atypical pneumonia: Relation to the viruses of meningopneumonitis and psittacosis. *J. Exp. Med.* 73:641–654.

Eddie, B., K.F. Meyer, F.L. Lambrecht, and D.P. Furman: 1962. Isolation of ornithosis bedsoniae from mites collected in turkey quarters and from chicken lice. *J. Infect. Dis.* 110:231–237.

Elkeles, G. and E. Barros: 1931. Die Psittacosis (Papageinkrankheit) mit besonderer Berücksichtigung der Pandemie des Jahres 1929/30. *Ergeb. Hyg. Bakteriol. Immunitaetsforsch. Exp. Ther.* 12:529–639.

Engleman, E.P. and H.M. Weber: 1968. Reiter's syndrome. *Clin. Orthop.* 57:19–29.

Enright, J.B. and W.W. Sadler: 1954. Presence in human sera of complement fixing antibodies to virus of sporadic bovine encephalomyelitis. *Proc. Soc. Exp. Biol. Med.* 85:466–468.

Erskine, D.: 1958. Lymphogranuloma venereum: A review of 61 cases. *Br. J. Vener. Dis.* 34:163–165.

Eschenbach, D.A., T.M. Buchanan, H.M. Pollock, P.S. Forsyth,

E.R. Alexander, J.-S. Lin, S.-P. Wang, B.B. Wentworth, W.M. McCormack, and K.K. Holmes: 1975. Polymicrobial etiology of acute pelvic inflammatory disease. *N. Engl.J. Med.* 293:166–171.

Fagan, R.: 1958. Direct comparison of chick embryo and mouse in the isolation of the psittacosis agent, pp. 111–116. In: *Progress in Psittacosis Research and Control.* F.R. Beaudette (ed.). New Brunswick, N.J.: Rutgers University Press.

Fan, V.S.C. and H.M. Jenkin: 1970. Glycogen metabolism in Chlamydia-infected HeLa cells. *J. Bacteriol.* 104:608–609.

Fehr: 1900. Endemische Bad Konjunktivitis. *Berl. Klin. Wochenschr.* 37:10–11.

Fiessinger, N. and E. Leroy: 1916. Contribution à l'étude d'une épidémie de dysenterie dans la Somme (juillet-octobre 1916). *Bull. Soc. Méd. Hôp. Paris* 40:2030–2069.

Findlay, G.M.: 1933. Experiments on the transmission of the virus of climatic bubo (lymphogranuloma inguinale) to animals. *Trans. R. Soc. Trop. Med. Hyg.* 27:35–66.

Findlay, G.M., R.D. MacKenzie, and F.O. MacCallum: 1938. A morphological study of the virus of lymphogranuloma inguinale (climatic bubo). *Trans. R. Soc. Trop. Med. Hyg.* 32:183–188.

Fitz, R.H., G. Meiklejohn, and M.D. Baum: 1955. Psittacosis in Colorado. *Am. J. Med. Sci.* 229:252–261.

Ford, D.K.: 1968. Non-gonococcal urethritis and Reiter's syndrome. *Can. Med. Assoc. J.* 99:900–910.

Ford, D.K. and L. McCandlish: 1969. Isolation of TRIC agents from the human genital tract. *Br. J. Vener. Dis.* 45:44–46.

Ford, D.K. and L. McCandlish: 1971. Isolation of human genital TRIC agents in nongonococcal urethritis and Reiter's disease. *Br. J. Vener. Dis.* 47:196–197.

Forster, R.K., C.R. Dawson, and J. Schachter: 1970. Late followup of patients with neonatal inclusion conjunctivitis. *Am. J. Ophthalmol.* 69:467–472.

Forster, W.G. and J.R. McGibony: 1944. Trachoma. *Am. J. Ophthalmol.* 27:1107–1117.

Fortner, J.: 1936. Sur la question de l'immunité contre la psittacose. *Bull. Off. Int. d'Hyg. Pub.* 28:683–687.

Fortner, J. and R. Pfaffenberg: 1934. Über das gehäufte Wiederauftreten der Psittakose. *Z. Hyg. Infektionskrankheiten* 116:397–416.

Foster, S.O., D.K. Powers, and P. Thygeson: 1966. Trachoma therapy: A controlled study. *Am. J. Ophthalmol.* 61:451–455.

Foy, H.M., S.-P. Wang, G.E. Kenny, W.L. Johnson, and J.T. Grayston: 1967. Isolation of TRIC agents and Mycoplasma from the cervix of pregnant women: Preliminary results. *Am. J. Ophthalmol.* 63:1053–1056.

Fransén, H.: 1969. Ornithosis in Stockholm. *Scand. J. Infect. Dis.* 1:61–66.

Fraser, C.E.O., D.E. McComb, E.S. Murray, and A.B. Mac-Donald: 1975. Immunity to chlamydial infections of the eye. IV. Immunity in owl monkeys to reinfection with trachoma. *Arch. Ophthalmol.* 93:518–521.

Freedman, A., M.K. Al-Hussaini, E.M.C. Dunlop, M.H.M. Emarah, J.A. Garland, I.A. Harper, B.R. Jones, J.W. Race, M.S. du Toit, J.D. Treharne, D.J.M. Wright: 1966. Infection by TRIC agent and other members of the Bedsonia group; with a note on Reiter's disease. *Trans. Ophthalmol. Soc.* 86:313–320.

Frei, W.: 1925. Eine neue Hautreaktion bei Lymphogranuloma inguinale. *Klin. Wochenschr.* 4:2148–2149.

Freyche, M.J.: 1949–1950. Antibiotics and sulfonamides in the treatment of trachoma. *Bull. W.H.O.* 2:523–544.

Friis, R.R.: 1972. Interaction of L cells and *Chlamydia psittaci:* Entry of the parasite and host responses to its development. *J. Bacteriol.* 110:706–721.

Fritsch, H., O. Hofstätter, K. Lindner: 1910. Experimentelle Studien zur Trachomfrage. *Graefe's Arch. Ophtalmol.* 76:547–558.

Frommel, G.T., F.W. Bruhn, and J.D. Schwartzman: 1977. Isolation of *Chlamydia trachomatis* from infant lung tissue. *N. Engl. J. Med.* 296:1150–1152.

Galasso, G.T. and G.P. Manire: 1961. Effect of antiserum and antibiotics on persistent infection of HeLa cells with meningopneumonitis virus. *J. Immunol.* 86:382–385.

Gale, C., B.S. Pomeroy, and V.L. Sanger: 1959. Characterization in mice of a turkey ornithosis virus of low virulence. *J. Infect. Dis.* 104:295–299.

Gale, J.L., W.T. Chiang, J.M. Gordon, and J.S. Lai: 1970. Human genital infection with *Chlamydia* in Taiwan. *J. Formosan Med. Assoc.* 69:610.

Gale, J.L., S.-P. Wang, and J.T. Grayston: 1971. Chronic trachoma in two Taiwan monkeys ten years after infection, pp. 489–493. In: *Trachoma and Related Disorders Caused by Chlamydial Agents.* R.L. Nichols (ed.). Amsterdam: Excerpta Medica.

Garcia, P.P.: 1940. Impresiones clinico-epidemiológicas sobre el último paroxismo de psitacosis en la capital federal. *La Prensa Med. Argent.* XXVII:3–152.

Garrett, A.J., M.J. Harrison, and G.P. Manire: 1974. A search for the bacterial mucopeptide component, muramic acid, in *Chlamydia. J. Gen. Microbiol.* 80:315–318.

Gaugler, R.W., E.M. Neptune, Jr., G.M. Adams, T.L. Sallee, E. Weiss, and N.N. Wilson: 1969. Lipid synthesis by isolated *Chlamydia psittaci. J. Bacteriol.* 100:823–826.

Gerlach, F.: 1936. Menschen als Psittakosevirusträger nach "stummer" Infektion mit Psittakosevirus. *Z. Hyg. Infektionskr.* 118:709–723.

Gerloff, R.K., D.B. Ritter, and R.O. Watson: 1966. DNA homology between the meningopneumonitis agent and related microorganisms. *J. Infect. Dis.* 116:197–202.

Gerloff, R.K., D.B. Ritter, and R.O. Watson: 1970. Studies on thermal denaturation of DNA from various chlamydiae. *J. Infect. Dis.* 121:65–69.

Gerloff, R.K. and R.O. Watson: 1967. The radioisotope precipitation test for psittacosis group antibodies. *Am. J. Ophthalmol.* 63:1492–1498.

Gerloff, R.K. and R.O. Watson: 1970. A *Chlamydia* from the peritoneal cavity of mice. *Infect. Immun.* 1:64–68.

Gilbert, R.J., J. Schachter, E.P. Engleman, and K.F. Meyer: 1973. Antibiotic therapy in experimental bedsonial arthritis. *Arth. Rheum.* 16:30–33.

Gilkes, M.J., C.H. Smith, and J. Sowa: 1958. Staining of the inclusion bodies of trachoma and inclusion conjunctivitis. *Br. J. Ophthalmol.* XLII:473–477.

Gill, S.D. and R.B. Stewart: 1970a. Glucose requirements of L cells infected with *Chlamydia psittaci. Can. J. Microbiol.* 16:997–1001.

Gill, S.D. and R.B. Stewart: 1970b. Respiration of L cells infected with *Chlamydia psittaci. Can. J. Microbiol.* 16:1033–1039.

Gill, S.D. and R.B. Stewart: 1970c. Effect of metabolic inhibitors on the production of *Chlamydia psittaci* by infected L cells. *Can. J. Microbiol.* 16:1079–1085.

Giroud, P.: 1969. Des agents de la psittacose a ceux du trachome. Agents bedsoniens ou néorickettsiens. *La Presse Med.* 77:475–479.

Gogolak, F.M.: 1954. The mouse erythrocyte hemagglutinin of feline pneumonitis virus. *J. Infect. Dis.* 95:220–225.

Gogolak, F.M. and M.R. Ross: 1955. The properties and chemical nature of the psittacosis virus hemagglutinin. *Virology* 1:474–496.

Goldberg, J. and L. Banov, Jr.: 1956. Complement fixation titres in tertiary lymphogranuloma venereum: a study of results after treatment with broad-spectrum antibiotics. *Br. J. Vener. Dis.* 32:37–39.

Gordon, F.B., V.W. Andrew, and J.C. Wagner: 1957. Development of resistance to penicillin and to chlortetracycline in psittacosis virus. *Virology* 4:156–171.

Gordon, F.B., I.A. Harper, A.L. Quan, J.D. Treharne, R.St.C. Dwyer, and J.A. Garland: 1969. Detection of *Chlamydia (Bedsonia)* in certain infections of man. I. Laboratory procedures: Comparison of yolk sac and cell culture for detection and isolation. *J. Infect. Dis.* 120:451–462.

Gordon, F.B. and A.L. Quan: 1965a. Occurrence of glycogen in inclusions of the psittacosis-lymphogranuloma venereum-trachoma agents. *J. Infect. Dis.* 115:186–196.

Gordon, F.B. and A.L. Quan: 1965b. Isolation of the trachoma agent in cell culture. *Proc. Soc. Exp. Biol. Med.* 118:354–359.

Gordon, F.B., A.L. Quan, T.I. Steinman, and R.N. Philip. 1973. Chlamydial isolates from Reiter's syndrome. *Br. J. Vener. Dis.* 49:376–380.

Gordon, I.: 1958. The diagnosis of human infection, pp. 139–149. In: *Progress in Psittacosis Research and Control.* F.R. Beaudette (ed.). New Brunswick, N.J.: Rutgers University Press.

Gordon, M.H.: 1930a. Virus studies in relation to psittacosis, pp. 96–107. In: *A Disease of Parrots Communicable to Man (Psittacosis). Rep. Public Health Med. Subj.* No. 61; E.L. Sturdee and W.M. Scott (eds.). London.

Gordon, M.H.: 1930b. Virus studies concerning the aetiology of psittacosis. *Lancet* 1:1174–1177.

Goscienski, P.J. and R.R. Sexton: 1972. Follow-up studies in neonatal inclusion conjunctivitis. *Am. J. Dis. Child.* 124:180–182.

Goto, T., H. Shioda, H. Nakamura, H. Naito, S. Matsushima, J. Murano, K. Shimano, and M. Matumoto: 1961. Psittacosis in Japan: Clinical observations of 42 serologically diagnosed human cases. *Jap. J. Exp. Med.* 31:249–258.

Gow, J.A., H.B. Ostler, and J. Schachter: 1974. Inclusion conjunctivitis with hearing loss. *JAMA* 229:519–520.

Graber, R.E. and B.S. Pomeroy: 1958. Ornithosis (psittacosis): An epidemiological study of a Wisconsin human outbreak transmitted from turkeys. *Am. J. Public Health* 48:1469–1483.

Grace, A.W.: 1941. Lymphogranuloma venereum. *Bull. N.Y. Acad. Med.* 17:627–646.

Grace, A.W.: 1943. Anorectal lymphogranuloma venereum. *JAMA* 122:74–78.

Grace, A.W., L. Frank, and R.J. Wyse: 1952. Effect of cortisone upon hypersensitivity due to lymphogranuloma venereum. *Arch. Dermatol. Syphil.* 65:348–350.

Grace, A.W., G. Rake, and M.F. Shaffer: 1940. A new material (Lygranum) for the performance of the Frei test for lymphogranuloma venereum. *Proc. Soc. Exp. Biol. Med.* 45:259–263.

Gradle, H.: 1938. Discussion of Loe, F.: Sulfanilamide treatment of trachoma. *JAMA* 111:1371–1372.

Graham, D.M.: 1965. Growth and neutralization of the trachoma agent in mouse lungs. *Nature* 207:1379–1380.

Gray, S.H., G.A. Hunt, P. Wheeler, and J.O. Blache: 1936. Lymphogranuloma inguinale: Its incidence in St. Louis. *JAMA* 106:919–921.

Grayston, J.T.: 1971. Trachoma vaccine, pp. 311–315. In: Proceedings: *International Conference on the Application of Vaccines Against Viral, Rickettsial, and Bacterial Diseases of Man.* December 14–18, 1970. Scientific Publication 226, Pan American Health Organization, Washington, D.C.

Grayston, J.T., K.S.W. Kim, E.R. Alexander, and S.-P. Wang: 1971. Protective studies in monkeys with trivalent and monovalent trachoma vaccines, pp. 377–385. In.: *Trachoma and Related Disorders Caused by Chlamydial Agents.* R.L. Nichols (ed.). Amsterdam: Excerpta Medica.

Grayston, J.T. and S.-P. Wang: 1975. New knowledge of chlamydiae and the diseases they cause. *J. Infect. Dis.* 132:87–105.

Greaves, A.B.: 1963. The frequency of lymphogranuloma venereum in persons with perirectal abscesses, fistulae in ano, or both: with particular reference to the relationship between perirectal abscesses of lymphogranuloma origin in the male and inversion. *Bull. W.H.O.* 29:797–801.

Greaves, A.B., M.R. Hilleman, S.R. Taggart, A.B. Bankhead, and M. Field: 1957. Chemotherapy in bubonic lymphogranuloma venereum. A clinical and serological evaluation. *Bull. W.H.O.* 16:277–289.

Greaves, A.B. and S.R. Taggart: 1953. Serology, Frei reaction, and epidemiology of lymphogranuloma venereum. *Am. J. Syphil.* 37:273–282.

Greenblatt, R.B.: 1952. Antibiotics in treatment of lymphogranuloma venereum and granuloma inguinale. *Ann. N.Y. Acad. Sci.* 55: 1082–1089.

Greenblatt, R.B., E.R. Pund, E.S. Sanderson, R. Jorpin, and R.B. Dienst: 1964. *Management of Chancroid, Granuloma Inguinale, Lymphogranuloma Venereum in General Practice.* Public Health Service Publication No. 255, revised 1964. Washington, D.C.: U.S. government Printing Office, pp. 1–57.

Grimble, A.S. and K.L. Amarasuriya: 1975. Non-specific urethritis and the tetracyclines. *Br. J. Vener. Dis.* 51:198–205.

Grist, N.R. and C. McLean: 1964. Infections by organisms of psittacosis/lymphogranuloma venereum group in the West of Scotland. *Br. Med. J.* 2:21–25.

Guerra, P.A., A. Buogo, E. Marubini, and M. Ghione: 1967.

Analysis of clinical and laboratory data of an experiment with trachoma vaccine in Ethiopia. *Am. J. Ophthalmol.* 63:1631–1638.

Guiard, F.P.: 1897. Des uréthritis non gonococciques. *Ann. Mal. Org. Genito-Urin.* 15:449–499.

Günther, F.: 1930. Beobachtungen über den Verlauf und die Epidemiologie der Psittacose. *Klin. Wochenschr.* 9:203–205.

Haagen, E. and G. Mauer: 1938. Ueber eine auf den Menschen übertragbare Viruskrankheit bie Sturmvögeln und ihre Beziehung zur Psittakose. *Zentralbl. Bakteriol.* 143:81–88.

Haddad, N.A. and S.K. Ballas: 1968. Seasonal mucopurulent conjunctivitis. *Am. J. Ophthalmol.* 65:225–228.

Haim, A. and C. Mathewson, Jr.: 1937. Incidence of lymphogranuloma inguinale in San Francisco. *JAMA* 108:961–965.

Halberstaedter, L. and S. von Prowazek: 1907a. Über Zelleinschlüsse parasitärer Natur beim Trachom. *Arb. Gesundheitsa.* XXVI:44–47.

Halberstaedter, L. and S. von Prowazek: 1907b. Zur Ätiologie des Trachoms. *Dtsch. Med. Wochenschr.* 33:1285–1287.

Halberstaedter, L. and S. von Prowazek: 1909. Ueber Chlamydozoenbefunde bei Blennorrhoea neonatorum non gonorrhoica. *Klin. Wochenschr.* 46:1839–1840.

Hales, R.H. and H.B. Ostler: 1973. Newcastle disease conjunctivitis with subepithelial infiltrates. *Dr. J. Ophthalmol.* 57:694–697.

Handsfield, H.H., E.R. Alexander, S.-P. Wang, A.H.B. Pedersen, and K.K. Holmes: 1976. Differences in the therapeutic response of chlamydia-positive and chlamydia-negative forms of nongonococcal urethritis. *J. Am. Wener. Dis. Assoc.* 2:5–9.

Handsfield, H.H., K.K. Holmes, and B.B. Wentworth: 1972. Etiology and treatment of non-gonococcal urethritis. Read before the Twelfth Interscience Conference on Antimicrobial Agents and Chemotherapy, Atlantic City, N.J., September 26–29, 1972.

Hanna, L.: 1968. An evaluation of the fluorescent antibody technic in the diagnosis of trachoma and inclusion conjuctivitis. *Rev. Int. Trach.* 45:345–359.

Hanna., L., E. Jawetz, O.C. Briones, H. Keshishyan, I. Hoshiwara, H.B. Ostler, and C.R. Dawson: 1973. Antibodies to TRIC agents in tears and serum of naturally infected humans. *J. Infect. Dis.* 127:95–98.

Hanna, L., E. Jawetz, B. Nabli, I. Hoshiwara, B. Ostler, and C. Dawson: 1972. Titration and typing of serum antibodies in TRIC infections by immunofluorescence. *J. Immunol.* 108:102–107.

Hanna, L., M. Okumoto, P. Thygeson, L. Rose, and C.R. Dawson: 1965. TRIC agents isolated in the United States. X.

Immunofluorescence in the diagnosis of TRIC agent infection in man. *Proc. Soc. Exp. Biol. Med.* 119:722–728.

Hanna, L., J. Schachter, and E. Jawetz: 1974. Chlamydiae (Psittacosis-lymphogranuloma venereum-trachoma group), pp. 795–804. In: *Manual of Clinical Microbiology,* 2nd Ed. E.H. Lennette, E.H. Spaulding, and J.P. Truant (eds.). Washington, D.C.: American Society for Microbiology.

Hansman, D.: 1969. Inclusion conjunctivitis. *Med. J. Aust.* 1:151–153.

Hardy, D., P.G. Surman, W.H. Howarth, and M.C. Path: 1967. A system of representation of cytologic features of external eye infections with special reference to trachoma. *Am. J. Ophthalmol.* 63:1535–1537.

Hardy, G.C.: 1941. Vaginal flora in children. *Am. J. Dis. Child.* 62:939–954.

Harrison, M.J.: 1970. Enhancing effect of DEAE-dextran on inclusion counts of an ovine *Chlamydia (Bedsonia)* in cell culture. *Aust. J. Exp. Biol. Med. Sci.* 48:207–213.

Harrison, M.J.: 1972. Conditions for growth of an ovine *Chlamydia (Bedsonia)* in cell culture. *Aust. J. Exp. Biol. Med. Sci.* 50:447–466.

Hasseltine, H.E.: 1932. Some epidemiological aspects of psittacosis. *Am. J. Public Health* XXII:795–803.

Hegler, C.: 1934. Psittacosis (Papageienkrankheit), pp. 1085–1097. In: *Handbuch der Inneren Medizin.* G. V. Bergmann, R. Staehelin, and V. Salle (eds.). Berlin: Springer Verlag.

Hellerström, S.: 1929. A contribution to the knowledge of lymphogranuloma inguinale. *Acta Derm. Venereol.* Suppl. I:5–224.

Hellerström, S. and E. Wassén: 1930. Meningo-enzephalitische Veränderungen bei Affen nach intracerebraler Impfung mit Lymphogranuloma inguinale, pp. 1147–1151. In: Proceedings: *VII Congres International de Dermatologie et de Syphiligraphie.*

Heymann, B.: 1909. Ueber die "Trachomkörperchen." *Dtsch. Med. Wochenschr.* 35:1692–1694.

Heymann, B.: 1910. Ueber die Fundorte der Powazek'schen Körperchen. *Berl. Klin. Wochenschr.* 47:663–666.

Hickam, J.B.: 1945. Cutaneous and articular manifestations in lymphogranuloma venereum. *Arch. Dermatol. Syphil.* 51:330–336.

Higashi, N. and A. Tamura: 1960. A plaque assay for meningopneumonitis virus in monolayers of strain L cells. *Virology* 12:578–588.

Hilleman, M.R.: 1945. Immunological studies on the psittacosis-lymphogranuloma group of viral agents. *J. Infect. Dis.* 76:96–114.

Hilleman, M.R., D.A. Haig, and R.J. Helmold: 1951. The indirect complement fixation, hemagglutination and conglutinating complement absorption tests for viruses of the psittacosis-lymphogranuloma venereum group. *J. Immunol.* 66:115–130.

Hilton, A.L., S.J. Richmond, J.D. Milne, F. Hindley, and S.K.R. Clarke: 1974. *Chlamydia* A in the female genital tract. *Br. J. Vener. Dis.* 50:1–10.

Hobson, D., F.W.A. Johnson, E. Rees, and I.A. Tait: 1974. Simplified method for diagnosis of genital and ocular infections with Chlamydia. *Lancet* 2:555–556.

Hoge, V.M.: 1934. Psittacosis in the United States. Incidence, scientific aspects, and administrative control measures. *Public Health Rep.* 49:451–462.

Holmes, K.K., H.H. Handsfield, S.-P. Wang, B.B. Wentworth, M. Turck, J.B. Anderson, and E.R. Alexander: 1975. Etiology of nongonococcal urethritis. *N. Engl. J. Med.* 292:1199–1206.

Hopsu-Havu, V.K. and C.E. Sonck: 1973. Infiltrative, ulcerative, and fistular lesions of the penis due to lymphogranuloma venereum. *Br. J. Vener. Dis.* 49:193–202.

Hoshiwara, I.: 1971. Ophthalmological care for American Indians. *Arch. Ophthalmol.* 86:368.

Hoshiwara, I., H.B. Ostler, L. Hanna, F. Cignetti, V.R. Coleman, and E. Jawetz: 1973. Doxycycline treatment of chronic trachoma. *JAMA* 224:220–223.

Hoshiwara, I., D.K. Powers, and G. Krutz: 1971. Comprehensive trachoma control program among the Southwestern American Indians, pp. 1935–1939. In: *Proceedings: XXI International Congress of Ophthalmology,* March 8–14, 1970, Mexico D.F. M.P. Solanes (ed.). International Congress Series No. 222. Amsterdam: Excerpta Medica.

Howe, L.: 1896. Loi pour la prévention de la cécité résultant de l'ophtalmie des nouveaux-née. *Bull. Mem. Soc. Fr. Ophtalmol.* 14:108–116.

Huet, M.: 1958. A propos de Haemophilus aegyptius. *Arch. L'Institut Pasteur de Tunis* 35:55–60.

Huntemüller and Padderstein: 1913. Befunde bei Schwimmbadkonjunktivitis. *Dtsch. Med. Wochenschr.* 39:63–66.

Hunter, J.A.: 1786. *A Treatise on the Venereal Disease.* London.

Hurst, E.W., J.K. Landquist, P. Melvin, J.M. Peters, N. Senior, J.A. Silk, and G.J. Stacey: 1953. The therapy of experimental psittacosis and lymphogranuloma venereum (inguinale). II. The activity of quinoxaline-1: 4-dioxide and substituted and related compounds, with a note on the morphological changes induced in lymphogranuloma virus by these compounds and by antibiotics. *Br. J. Pharmacol. Chemother.* 8:297–305.

Hurst, E.W., J.M. Peters, and P. Melvin: 1950. The therapy of experimental psittacosis and lymphogranuloma venereum (Inguinale). I. The comparative efficacy of penicillin, chloramphenicol, aureomycin, and terramycin. *Br. J. Pharmacol. Chemother.* 5:611–624.

Irons, J.V., M.L. Denley, and T.D. Sullivan: 1955. Psittacosis in turkeys and fowls as a source of human infection, pp. 44–65. In: *Psittacosis. Diagnosis, Epidemiology and Control.* F.R. Beaudette (ed.). New Brunswick, N.J.: Rutgers University Press.

Irons, J.V., T.D. Sullivan, and J. Rowen: 1951. Outbreak of psittacosis (ornithosis) from working with turkeys or chickens. *Am. J. Public Health* 41:931–937.

Jacobs, N.F., Jr. and S.J. Kraus: 1975. Gonococcal and nongonococcal urethritis in men: clinical and laboratory differentiation. *Ann. Intern Med.* 82:7–12.

Jadin, J. and P. Giroud: 1963. Neorickettsial infections in Africa. *Ann. Soc. Belg. Med. Trop.* 43:883–892.

Jannach, J.R.: 1958. Myocarditis in infancy with inclusions characteristic of psittacosis. *Am. J. Dis. Child.* 96:734–740.

Jawetz, E.: 1969. Chemotherapy of chlamydial infections, pp. 253–282. In: *Advances in Pharmacology and Chemotherapy,* Vol. 7. S. Garattini, A. Goldin, F. Hawking, and I.J. Kopin (eds.). New York: New York Academic Press.

Jawetz, E., L. Hanna, C.R. Dawson, R. Wood, and O. Briones: 1967. Subclinical infections with TRIC agents. *Am. J. Ophthalmol.* 63:1413–1424.

Jenkin, H.M.: 1960. Preparation and properties of cell walls of the agent of meningopneumonitis. *J. Bacteriol.* 80:639–647.

Jenkin, H.M.: 1967. Comparative lipid composition of psittacosis and trachoma agents. *Am. J. Ophthalmol.* 63:1087–1098.

Jenkin, H.M. and V.S.C. Fan: 1971. Contrast of glycogenesis of *Chlamydia trachomatis* and *Chlamydia psittaci* strains in HeLa cells. In: *Trachoma and Related Disorders Caused by Chlamydial Agents.* R.L. Nichols (ed.). Amsterdam: Excerpta Medica.

Jenkin, H.M., S. Makino, D. Townsend, M.C. Riera, and A.L. Barron: 1970. Lipid composition of the hemagglutinating active fraction obtained from chick embryos infected with *Chlamydia psittaci:* 6 BC. *Infect. Immun.* 2:316–319.

Jenkin, H.M., M.R. Ross, and J.W. Moulder: 1961. Species-specific antigens from the cell walls of the agents of meningopneumonitis and feline pneumonitis. *J. Immunol.* 86:123–127.

Jones, B.R.: 1964. Ocular syndromes of TRIC virus infection and their possible genital significance. *Br. J. Vener. Dis.* 40:3–18.

240

Jones, B.R.: 1974. Laboratory tests for chlamydial infection: Their role in epidemiological studies of trachoma and its control. *Br. J. Ophthalmol.* 58:438–454.

Jones, B.R.: 1975. Prevention of blindness from trachoma. *Trans. Ophthalmol. Soc. U.K.* 95:16–33.

Jones, B.R. and L.H. Collier: 1962. Inoculation of man with inclusion blennorrhea virus. *Ann. N.Y. Acad. Sci.* 98:212–228.

Jones, B.R., L.H. Collier, and C.H. Smith: 1959. Isolation of virus from inclusion blennorrhoea. *Lancet* 1:902–905.

Jones, B.R. and J.D. Treharne: 1974. Micro-immunofluorescence type-specific serological tests for chlamydial infection applied to psittacosis, ornithosis, lymphogranuloma venereum, trachoma, paratrachoma and 'nonspecific' urethritis. *Proc. R. Soc. Med.* 67:735–736.

Jones. H., G. Rake, and B. Stearns: 1945. Studies on lymphogranuloma venereum. III. The action of the sulfonamides on the agent of lymphogranuloma venereum. *J. Infect. Dis.* 76:55–69.

Jorgensen, M.B. and K.A. Steffensen: 1956. Ornithosis. An analysis of 44 human cases with positive complement fixation tests. *Dan. M. Bull.* 3:20–24.

Juchau, S.V., W.D. Linscott, J. Schachter, and E. Jawetz: 1972. Inhibition of antichlamydial IgM antibody by IgG antibody in immunofluorescence tests. *J. Immunol.* 108:1563–1569.

Jüergensen, T.: 1874. Handbuch der speziellen Pathologie und Therapie. Handbuch der Krankheiten des Respirations-Apparates 2:3. Leipzig: Vogel.

Kalter, S.S.: 1961. Cat scratch disease: results of complement fixation and skin tests. School of Aerospace Medicine. U.S.A.F. Aerospace Medical Center (ATC), Brooks Air Force Base, Texas.

Karrer, H., B. Eddie, and R. Schmid: 1950. Barnyard fowl as a source of human ornithosis. Case report. *Calif. Med.* 73:55–57.

Karrer, H., K.F. Meyer, and B. Eddie: 1950. The complement fixation inhibition test and its application to the diagnosis of ornithosis in chickens and in ducks. I. Principles and technique of the test. *J. Infect. Dis.* 87:13–23.

Kellogg, D.S., Jr.: 1974. *Calymmatobacterium granulomatis,* pp. 323–325. In: *Manual of Clinical Microbiology,* 2d Ed. E.H. Lennette, E.H. Spaulding, and J.P. Truant (eds.). Washington, D.C.: American Society for Microbiology.

Kemmerer, G., H.G. Haussmann, G. Schoop, and E. Kauker: 1956. Zur Klinik und Epidemiologie der durch Tauben übertragenen menschlichen Ornithose. *Dtsch. Med. Wochenschr.* 81:930–933.

Keshishyan, H., L. Hanna, and E. Jawetz: 1973. Emergence of rifampin-resistance in *Chlamydia trachomatis. Nature* 244:173–174.

King, A.J., C. F. Barwell, and R.D. Catterall: 1956. Intradermal tests in the diagnosis of lymphogranuloma venereum. *Br. J. Vener. Dis.* 32:209–216.

Kingsbury, D.T.: 1969. Estimate of the genome size of various microorganisms. *J. Bacteriol.* 98:1400–1401.

Kingsbury, D.T. and E. Weiss: 1968. Lack of deoxyribonucleic acid homology between species of the genus *Chlamydia. J. Bacteriol.* 96:1421–1423.

Kinsella, T.D., W.L. Norton, and M. Ziff: 1968. Complement-fixing antibodies to *Bedsonia* organisms in Reiter's syndrome and ankylosing spondylitis. *Ann. Rheum. Dis.* 27:241–244.

Kono, R., E. Miyamura, S. Tajiri, S. Shiga, A. Sasagawa, P.F. Irani, S.M. Katrak, and N.H. Wadia: 1974. Neurologic complications associated with acute hemorrhagic conjunctivitis virus infection and its serologic confirmation. *J. Infect. Dis.* 129:590–593.

Kordová, N., J.C. Wilt, and M. Sadiq: 1971. Lysosomes in L cells infected with *Chlamydia psittaci* 6 BC strain. *Can. J. Microbiol.* 17:955–959.

Korns, R.F.: 1955. Psittacosis in ducks and persons exposed to ducks, pp. 80–89. In: *Psittacosis. Diagnosis, Epidemiology and Control.* F.R. Beaudette (ed.). New Brunswick, N.J.: Rutgers University Press.

Koteen, H.: 1945. Lymphogranuloma venereum. *Medicine* 24:1–69.

Kramer, M.J. and F.B. Gordon: 1971. Ultrastructural analysis of the effects of penicillin and chlortetracycline on the development of a genital tract *Chlamydia. Infect. Immun.* 3:333–341.

Kroner, T.: 1884. Zur Ätiologie der Ophthalmoblennorrhoea neonatorum. *Zentralbl. Gynaekol.* 8:643–645.

Krumwiede, C., M. McGrath, and C. Oldenbusch: 1930. The etiology of the disease psittacosis. *Science* 71:262–263.

Kukowka, A., H. Stephan, and W. Krebs: 1960. Entenform als Ausgangspunkt von Ornithoseerkrankungen bei Menschen. *Dtsch. Gesundheitsw.* 15:2477–2484.

Kuo, C.-C., S.-P. Wang, and J.T. Grayston: 1973. Effect of polycations, polyanions and neuraminidase on the infectivity of trachoma-inclusion conjunctivitis and lymphogranuloma venereum organisms in HeLa cells: Sialic acid residues as possible receptors for trachoma-inclusion conjunctivitis. *Infect. Immun.* 8:74–79.

Kuo, C.-C., S.-P. Wang, and J.T. Grayston: 1975. Comparative infectivity of trachoma organisms in HeLa 229 cells and egg cultures. *Infect. Immun.* 12:1078–1082.

Kuo, C.-C., S.-P. Wang, J.T. Grayston, and E.R. Alexander: 1974. TRIC Type K, a new immunological type of *Chlamydia* trachomatis. *J. Immunol.* 113:591–596.

Kuo, C.-C., S.-P. Wang, B.B. Wentworth, and J.T. Grayston: 1972. Primary isolation of TRIC organisms in HeLa 229 cells treated with DEAE-Dextran. *J. Infect. Dis.* 125:665–668.

Lassus, A., K.K. Mustakallio, and O. Wager: 1970. Auto-immune serum factors and IgA elevation in lymphogranuloma venereum. *Ann. Clin. Res.* 2:51–56.

Law, W.A.: 1943. Treatment of lymphogranuloma inguinale with anthiomaline. *Lancet* 1:300–304.

Lepinay, A., R. Robineaux, J. Orfila, L. Orme-Rosselli, and J.M. Boutry: 1971. Ultrastructure et cytochimie ultrastructurale des membranes de *Chlamydia psittaci. Archiv. Gesamte Virusforsch.* 33:271–280.

Levin, I., S. Romano, M. Steinberg, and R.A. Welsh: 1964. Lymphogranuloma venereum: rectal stricture and carcinoma. *Dis. Colon Rectum* 7:129–134.

Levinthal, W.: 1930. Die Aetiologie der Psittakosis. *Klin. Wochenschr.* 9:654–659.

Levison, D.A., W. Guthrie, C. Ward, D.M. Green, and P.G.C. Robertson: 1971. Infective endocarditis as part of psittacosis. *Lancet* 2:844–847.

Lewis, V.J. and W.L. Thacker: 1973. Susceptibility of McCoy cells to infection by *Chlamydia psittaci. Can. J. Microbiol.* 19:617–621.

Lewis, V.J., W.L. Thacker, and A.F. Cacciapuoti: 1973. Detection of *Chlamydia psittaci* by immunofluorescence. *Appl. Microbiol.* 24:8–12.

Lewis, V.J., W.L. Thacker, and H.M. Engleman: 1972. Indirect hemagglutination test for chlamydial antibodies. *Appl. Microbiol.* 24:22–25.

Liccione, W.T.: 1936. Venereal stricture of the rectum: Adenocarcinoma as a late complication of lymphogranuloma venereum. *Am. J. Surg.* 31:551–555.

Lillie, R.D.: 1930. Psittacosis: Rickettsia-like inclusions in man in experimental animals. *Public Health Rep.* 45:773–778.

Lillie, R.D.: 1933. I. The pathology of psittacosis in man. *Nat. Inst. Health Bull.* 161:1–66. Washington, D.C.: United States Government Printing Office.

Lin, H.-S.: 1968. Inhibition of thymidine kinase activity and deoxyribonucleic acid synthesis in L cells infected with the meningopneumonitis agent. *J. Bacteriol.* 96:2054–2065.

Lin, H.-S., and J.W. Moulder: 1966. Patterns of response to sulfadiazine, D-cycloserine and D-alanine in members of the psittacosis group. *J. Infect. Dis.* 116:372–376.

Lindner, K.: 1909. Uebertragungsversuche von gonokokkenfreien Blennorrhoea neonatorum auf Affen. *Wien. Klin. Wochenschr.* 22:1555.

Lindner, K.: 1910. Zur Ätiologie der gonokokkenfreien Urethritis. *Wien. Klin. Wochenschr.* 23:283–284.

Lindner, K.: 1911. Gonoblennorrhöe, Einschlussblennorrhoe, und Trachoma. *Graefe's Arch. Ophtalmol.* 78:380.

Luger, N.M. and E.B. Cheatham, Jr.: 1950. The incidence of lymphogranuloma venereum as determined by the quantitative complement fixation test. *Am. J. Syphil.* 34:351–355.

Lwoff, A.: 1957. The concept of virus. *J. Gen. Microbiol.* 17:239–253.

McChesney, J.A., A. Zedd, H. King, C.M. Russell, and J.O. Hendley: 1973. Acute urethritis in male college students. *JAMA* 226:37–39.

McClintock, A.T.: 1925. *Pleomorphism in Bacterial Protoplasm. A Study in Psittacosis.* Archives of the Andrew Todd McClintock Memorial Foundation. Vol. 1, 240 pp. Wilkes-Barre, Pa. (Private printing.)

McComb, D.E. and R.L. Nichols: 1969. Antibodies to trachoma in eye secretions of Saudi Arab children. *Am. J. Epidemiol.* 90:278–284.

McComb, D.E., J.H. Peters, C.E.O. Fraser, E.S. Murray, A.B. MacDonald, and R.L. Nichols: 1971. Resistance to trachoma infection in owl monkeys correlated with antibody status at the outset in an experiment to test the response to topical trachoma antigens, pp. 396–406. In: *Trachoma and Related Disorders Caused by Chlamydial Agents.* R.L. Nichols (ed.). Amsterdam: Excerpta Medica.

McComb, D.E. and C.I. Puzniak: 1974. Micro cell culture method for isolation of *Chlamydia trachomatis. Appl. Microbiol.* 28:727–729.

McGavran, M.H., C.W. Beard, R.F. Berendt, and R.M. Nakamura: 1962. The pathogenesis of psittacosis. Serial studies on rhesus monkeys exposed to a small particle aerosol of the Borg strain. *Am. J. Pathol.* 40:653–670.

McGuire, C. and R. Durant: 1957. The role of flies in the transmission of eye disease in Egypt. *Am. J. Trop. Med. Hyg.* 6:569–575.

MacCallan, A.F.: 1936. *Trachoma.* London: Butterworth and Company.

MacCallum, F.O. and G.M. Findlay: 1938. Chemotherapeutic experiments on the virus of lymphogranuloma inguinale in the mouse. *Lancet* 2:136–138.

Macchiavello, A.: 1944. El virus del trachoma y su cultivo en el saco vitelino del huevo de gallina. *Rev. Ecuat. Hig. Med. Trop.* 2:211.

Makino, S., H.M. Jenkin, H.M. Yu, and D. Townsend: 1970.

Lipid composition of *Chlamydia psittaci* grown in monkey kidney cells in defined medium. *J. Bacteriol.* 103:62–70.

Manire, G.P. and G.T. Galasso: 1959. Persistent infection of the HeLa cells with meningopneumonitis virus. *J. Immunol.* 83:529–533.

Manire, G.P. and K.F. Meyer: 1950. The toxins of the psittacosis-lymphogranuloma group of agents. III. Differentiation of strains by the toxin neutralization test. *J. Infect. Dis.* 86:241–250.

Manire, G.P. and A. Tamura: 1967. Preparation and chemical composition of the cell walls of mature infectious dense forms of meningopneumonitis organisms. *J. Bacteriol.* 94:1178–1183.

Manning, J.D., and J.D. Reid: 1958. The significance of positive complement fixation tests against psittacosis antigen in cat scratch disease. *Am. J. Clin. Pathol.* 29:430–432.

Margileth, A.M.: 1968. Cat scratch disease: nonbacterial regional lymphadenitis. The study of 145 patients and a review of the literature. *Pediatrics* 42:803–818.

Matsumoto, A. and G.P. Manire: 1970a. Electron microscopic observations on the fine structure of cell walls of *Chlamydia psittaci. J. Bacteriol.* 104:1332–1337.

Matsumoto, A. and G.. Manire: 1970b. Electron microscopic observations on the effects of penicillin on the morphology of *Chlamydia psittaci. J. Bacteriol.* 101:278–285.

Maxwell-Lyons, F.: 1947. Mass treatment with sulphonamides. *Bull. Ophthalmol. Soc. Egypt* 40:51–58.

Maxwell-Lyons, F.: 1953. The twofold problems of acute conjunctivitis and trachoma in Egypt. A survey of the epidemiology and of recent experiments on their prophylaxis. *Rev. Int. Trach.* 30:341–351.

Maxwell-Lyons, F. and C.R. Amies: 1949. The epidemiology and prevention of the acute ophthalmias of Egypt. *Bull. Ophthalmol. Soc. Egypt* 42:116–139.

Mårdh, P.-A., T. Ripa, L. Svensson, and L. Weström: 1977. *Chlamydia trachomatis* infection in patients with acute salpingitis. *N. Engl. J. Med.* 296:1377–1379.

Meiklejohn, G., J.C. Wagner, and G.W. Beveridge: 1946. Studies on the chemotherapy of viruses in the psittacosis-lymphogranuloma group. I. Effect of penicillin and sulfadiazine on ten strains in chick embryos. *J. Immunol.* 54:1–8.

Meyer, K.F.: 1935. Psittacosis. *Proceedings: Twelfth International Veterinary Congress* III:182–205.

Meyer, K.F.: 1941a. Phagocytosis and immunity in psittacosis. *Schweiz. Med. Wochenschr.* 71:436–438.

Meyer, K.F.: 1941b. Pigeons and barnyard fowls as possible sources of human psittacosis or ornithosis. *Schweiz. Med. Wochenschr.* 71:1377–1379.

Meyer, K.F.: 1942. The ecology of psittacosis and ornithosis. *Medicine* 21:175–206.

Meyer, K.F.: 1955. Problems in the control of psittacosis and ornithosis. *Proceedings: 92nd Annual Meeting, Am. Vet. Med. Assoc.* pp. 412–419.

Meyer, K.F.: 1958. Ornithosis: A public health problem. *Proceedings: 62nd Annual United States Livestock Sanitary Assoc.* Nov. 230–243.

Meyer, K.F.: 1959. Some general remarks and new observations on psittacosis and ornithosis. *Bull. W.H.O.* 20:101–119.

Meyer, K.F.: 1965. Ornithosis, pp. 675–770. In: *Diseases of Poultry,* 5th Ed. H.E. Biester and L.H. Schwarte (eds.). Ames, Iowa: The Iowa State University Press.

Meyer, K.F.: 1967. The host spectrum of psittacosis-lymphogranuloma venereum (PL) agents. *Am. J. Ophthalmol.* 63:1225–1246.

Meyer, K.F. and B. Eddie: 1933a. Latent psittacosis infections in mice. *Proc. Soc. Exp. Biol. Med.* 30:483–484.

Meyer, K.F. and B. Eddie: 1933b. Latent psittacosis infections in shell parakeets. *Proc. Soc. Exp. Biol. Med.* 30:484–488.

Meyer, K.F. and B. Eddie: 1933c. Latente Psittakoseinfektion bei Sittichen. *Z. Infektionskr.* 44:237–242.

Meyer, K.F. and B. Eddie: 1939. The value of the complement fixation test in the diagnosis of psittacosis. *J. Infect. Dis.* 65:225–233.

Meyer, K.F. and B. Eddie: 1942. Spontaneous ornithosis (psittacosis) in chickens the cause of a human infection. *Proc. Soc. Exp. Biol. Med.* 49:522–525.

Meyer, K.F. and B. Eddie: 1951. Human carrier of the psittacosis virus. *J. Infect. Dis.* 88:109–125.

Meyer, K.F. and B. Eddie: 1952. Human pneumonitis viruses and their classification. *Arch. Gesamte Virusforsch.* IV:579–590.

Meyer, K.F. and B. Eddie: 1953. Characteristics of a psittacosis viral agent isolated from a turkey. *Proc. Soc. Exp. Biol. Med.* 83:99–101.

Meyer, K.F. and B. Eddie: 1956. The influence of tetracycline compounds on the development of antibodies in psittacosis. *Am. Rev. Tuberc. Pulm. Dis.* 74:566–571.

Meyer, K.F. and B. Eddie: 1962. Immunity against some Bedsonia in man resulting from infection and in animals from infection or vaccination. *Ann. N.Y. Acad. Sci.* 98:288–313.

Meyer, K.F. and B. Eddie: 1964. Psittacosis-lymphogranuloma venereum group (Bedsonia infections), pp. 603–639. In: *Diagnostic Procedures for Viral and Rickettsial Diseases,* 3rd Ed. E.H. Lennette and N.J. Schmidt (eds.). New York: Am. Public Health Assoc., Inc.

Meyer, K.F., B. Eddie, J.H. Richardson, N.L. Shipkowitz, and R.J. Muir: 1958. Chemotherapy in the control of psittacosis in parakeets, pp. 163–196. In: *Progress in Psittacosis Research and control.* F.R. Beaudette (ed.). New Brunswick, N.J.: Rutgers University Press.

Meyer, K.F., B. Eddie, and J. Schachter: 1969. Psittacosis-lymphogranuloma venereum agents, pp. 869–903. In: *Diagnostic Procedures for Viral and rickettsial Infections,* 4th Ed. E.H. Lennette and N.J. Schmidt (eds.). New York: Am. Public Health Assoc., Inc.

Meyer, K.F., B. Eddie, and H. Yanamura: 1939. Complement fixation test with tissue-culture-antigens as aid in recognizing latent avian psittacosis (ornithosis). *Proc. Soc. Exp. Biol. Med.* 41:173–176.

Meyerhoff, M.: 1911. Sur la conjonctivité gonococcique epidemique d'Egypte et ses rapports avec le trachome. *Arch. Ophtalmol.* 21:1–34.

Mills, R.B. and R.E. Kalina: 1972. Reiter's keratitis. *Arch. Ophthalmol.* 87:447–449.

Mitsui, Y., T. Kitamuro, K. Endo, and K. Matsumura: 1964. Trachoma and inclusion conjunctivitis agents: adaptation to HeLa cell cultures. *Science* 145:715–716.

Mitsui, Y., T. Kitamuro, and M. Fujimoto: 1967. Adaptation of TRIC agents to tissue culture and characteristics of tissue culture adapted variants. *Am. J. Ophthalmol.* 65:1191–1205.

Mitsui, Y. and C. Tanaka: 1951. Terramycin, Aureomycin and chloramphenicol in the treatment of trachoma. *Antibiot. Chemother.* 1:146–157.

Mitsui, Y., C. Tanaka, K. Yamashita, and J. Hanabusa: 1954. Erythromycin (Erythrocin®) in ophthalmology with special reference to trachoma. *Kumamoto Med. J.* 7:1–6.

Mollaret, P., J. Reilly, R. Bastin, and P. Tournier: 1951. La découverte du virus de la Lymphoréticulose bénigne d'inoculation: 1. Caractérisation sérologique et immunologique. *Presse Med.* 59:681–682.

Morange, A.: 1895. De La psittacose, ou infection spéciale déterminée par des perruches. Thése. Paris: Académie de Paris.

Morax, V.: 1903. Sur l'étiologie des ophtalmies du nouveau-né et la déclaration obligatoire. *Ann. Ocul.* 129:346–363.

Morax, V.: 1933. *Les Conjonctivites Folliculaires.* Paris: Masson et Cie.

Mordhorst, C.H.: 1967. Studies on oculogenital TRIC agents isolated in Denmark. *Am. J. Ophthalmol.* 63:1282–1288.

Mordhorst, C.H. and C.R. Dawson: 1971. Sequelae of neonatal inclusion conjunctivitis and associated disease in parents. *Am. J. Ophthalmol.* 71:861–867.

Morgan, H.R.: 1952a. Factors related to the growth of psittacosis virus (Strain 6BC). I. Pteroylglutamic acid, vitamin B_{12}, and citrovorum factor. *J. Exp. Med.* 95:269–276.

Morgan, H.R.: 1952b. Factors related to the growth of psittacosis virus (Strain 6BC). II. Purines, pyrimidines, and other components related to nucleic aicd. *J. Exp. Med.* 95:277–283.

Morgan, H.R.: 1956. Latent viral infection of cells in tissue culture. I. Studies on latent infection of chick embryo tissues with psittacosis virus. *J. Exp. Med.* 103:37–47.

Morgan, H.R. and J.P. Bader: 1954. Factors related to the growth of psittacosis virus (Strain 6BC). IV. Certain amino acids, vitamins, and other substances. *J. Exp. Med.* 99:451–460.

Morgan, H.R. and J.P. Bader: 1957. Latent viral infection of cells in tissue culture. IV. Latent infection of L cells with psittacosis virus. *J. Exp. Med.* 106:39–44.

Morris, R., A.L. Metzger, R. Bluestone, and P.I. Terasaki: 1974. HL-A.W27—A clue to the diagnosis and pathogenesis of Reiter's syndrome. *N. Engl. J. Med.* 209:554–556.

Morrison, S.J. and H.M. Jenkin: 1972. Growth of *Chlamydia psittaci* strain meningopneumonitis in mouse L cells cultivated in a defined medium in spinner cultures. *In Vitro* 8:94–100.

Morton, R.S.: 1972. Reiter's disease. *Practitioner* 209:631–638.

Moulder, J.W.: 1962a. *The Biochemistry of Intracellular Parasitism.* Chicago and London: The University of Chicago Press.

Moulder, J.W.: 1962b. Some basic properties of the psittacosis-lymphogranuloma venereum group of agents. Structure and chemical composition of isolated particles. *Ann. N.Y. Acad. Sci.* 98:92–99.

Moulder, J.W.: 1964. *The Psittacosis Group as Bacteria.* (CIBA lectures in Microbial Biochemistry, 1963) New York: John Wiley and Sons, Inc.

Moulder, J.W.: 1966. The relation of the psittacosis group (chlamydiae) to bacteria and viruses. *Ann. Rev. Microbiol.* 20:107–130.

Moulder, J.W.: 1969. A model for studying the biology of parasitism. *Chlamydia psittaci* and mouse fibroblasts (L cells). *Bioscience* 19:875–882.

Moulder, J.W., B.R.S. McCormack, F.M. Gogolak, M.M. Zebovitz, and M.K. Itatani: 1955. Production and properties of·a penicillin-resistant strain of feline pneumonitis virus. *J. Infect. Dis.* 96:57–74.

Moulder, J.W., J. Ruda, J.I. Colon, and R.M. Greenland: 1958. The effect of passage with chloramphenicol upon the behavior of penicillin-resistant feline pneumonitis virus during subsequent passage with penicillin. *J. Infect. Dis.* 102:186–201.

Mufson, M.A., V. Chang, V. Gill, S.C. Romansky, and R.M. Chanock: 1967. The role of viruses, mycoplasmas and bacteria in acute pneumonia in civilian adults. *Am. J. Epidemiol.* 86:526–544.

Mukhija, R.D., U. Gupta, R.A. Bhujwala, V.M. Mahajan, L.K. Bhutani, and K.C. Kandhari: 1973. A study of urethritis in males with particular reference to mycoplasma and TRIC-agent. *Indian J. Med. Res.* 61:1766–1770.

Murray, E.S.: 1964. Guinea pig inclusion conjunctivitis virus. I. Isolation and identification as a member of the psittacosis-lymphogranuloma-trachoma group. *J. Infect Dis.* 114:1–12.

Murray, E.S., C.E.O. Fraser, J.H. Peters, D.E. McComb, and R.L. Nichols: 1971. The owl monkey as an experimental primate model for conjunctival trachoma infection, pp. 386–396. In: *Trachoma and Related Disorders Caused by Chlamydial Agents.* R.L. Nichols (ed.). Amsterdam: Excerpta Medica.

Nabli, B. and M.L. Tarizzo: 1967. The effect of antiseptics and other substances on TRIC agents. *Am. J. Ophthalmol.* 63:1541–1550.

Naib, Z.M.: 1970. Cytology of TRIC agent infection of the eye of newborn infants and their mothers' genital tracts. *Acta Cytol.* 14:390–395.

Nataf, R., T. Daghfous, and M.L. Tarizzo: 1965. Etude comparative de l'action de l'erythromycine et de la chlortetracycline (aureomycine) dans le traitment du trachome. *Rev. Int. Trach.* 42:76–85.

Nataf, R., P. Lepine, and G. Bonamour: 1960. *Oeil et Virus.* Paris: Masson et Cie.

Nichols, R.L., S.D. Bell, N.A. Haddad, and A.A. Bobb: 1969. Studies on trachoma. VI. Microbiological observations in a field trial in Saudi Arabia of bivalent trachoma vaccine at three dosage levels. *Am. J. Trop. Med. Hyg.* 18:723–730.

Nichols, R.L., S.D. Bell, Jr., E.S. Murray, N.A. Haddad, and A.A. Bobb: 1966. Studies on trachoma. V. Clinical observations in a field trial of bivalent trachoma vaccine at three dosage levels in Saudi Arabia. *Am. J. Trop. Med. Hyg.* 15:639–642.

Nichols, R.L., A.A. Bobb, N.A. Haddad, D.E. McComb: 1967. Immunofluorescent studies of the microbiologic epidemiology of trachoma in Saudi Arabia. *Am. J. Ophthalmol.* 63:1372–1408.

Nichols, R.L., K. von Fritzinger, and D.E. McComb: 1971. Epidemiological data derived from immunotyping of 338 trachoma strains isolated from children in Saudi Arabia, pp. 337–357. In: *Trachoma and Related Disorders Caused by Chlamydial Agents.* R.L. Nichols (ed.). Amsterdam: Excerpta Medica.

Nichols, R.L., D.E. McComb, N.A. Haddad, and E.S. Murray: 1963. Studies on trachoma. II. Comparison of fluorescent antibody, Giemsa, and egg isolation methods for detection of trachoma virus in human conjunctival scrapings. *Am. J. Trop. Med. Hyg.* 12:223–229.

Nigg, C. and M.D. Eaton: 1944. Isolation from normal mice of a pneumotropic virus which forms elementary bodies. *J. Exp. Med.* 79:497–510.

Nigg, C., M.R. Hilleman, and B.M. Bowser: 1946. Studies on lymphogranuloma venereum complement fixing antigens. I. Enhancement by phenol or boiling. *J. Immunol.* 53:259–268.

Nocard, E.: 1893. Conseil d'hygiène du Départment de la Seine. Cited in Cox, H.R.: Psittacosis, ornithosis, and related viruses. *Ann. N.Y. Acad. Sci.* 48:393–414, 1947.

Noer, H.R.: 1966. 'Experimental' epidemic of Reiter's syndrome. *JAMA* 198:693–698.

Noguchi, H.: 1928. The etiology of trachoma. *J. Exp. Med.* 48:1–53.

Officer, J.E. and A. Brown: 1960. Growth of psittacosis virus in tissue culture. *J. Infect. Dis.* 107:283–299.

Officer, J.E. and A. Brown: 1961. Serial changes in virus and cells in cultures chronically infected with psittacosis virus. *Virology* 14:88–99.

Olson, B.J. and C.L. Larson: 1944. An epidemic of a severe pneumonitis in the Bayou Region of Louisiana. IV. A preliminary note on etiology. *Public Health Rep.* 59:1373–1374.

Olson, B.J. and W.L. Treuting: 1944. An epidemic of a severe pneumonitis in the Bayou Region of Louisiana. I. Epidemiological study. *Public Health Rep.* 59:1299–1311.

Oriel, J.D., A. Powis, P. Reeve, A. Miller, and C.S. Nicol: 1974. Chlamydial infections of the cervix. *Br. J. Vener. Dis.* 50:11–16.

Oriel, J.D., P. Reeve, P. Powis, A. Miller, and C.S. Nicol: 1972. Chlamydial infection: Isolation of *Chlamydia* from patients with nonspecific genital infection. *Br. J. Vener. Dis.* 48:429–436.

Oriel, J.D., P. Reeve, B.J. Thomas, and C.S. Nicol: 1975. Infection with *Chlamydia* Group A in men with urethritis due to *Neisseria gonorrhoeae. J. Infect. Dis.* 131:376–382.

Ortel, S.: 1964. Die Ornithose-Situation in der DDR auf Grund epidemiologischer und serologischer. *Arch. Exp. Veterinaermed.* 18:89–96.

Ostler, H.B., C.R. Dawson, J. Schachter, and E.P. Engleman: 1971. Reiter's syndrome. *Am. J. Ophthalmol.* 71:986–991.

Ostler, H.B., L. Hanna, I. Hoshiwara, E. Jawetz, and C.R. Dawson: 1971. A comparison of tetracycline and doxycycline in chronic trachoma of American Indians, pp. 540–544. In: *Trachoma and Related Disorders Caused by Chlamydial Agents.* R.L. Nichols (ed.). Amsterdam: Excerpta Medica.

Ostler, H.B., J. Schachter, and C.R. Dawson: 1969. Acute

250

follicular conjunctivitis of epizootic origin. *Arch. Ophthalmol.* 82:587–591.

Ostler, H.B., J. Schachter, and C.R. Dawson: 1970. Ocular infection of rabbits with a bedsonia isolated from a patient with Reiter's syndrome. *Invest. Ophthalmol.* 9:256–262.

Page, L.A.: 1959a. Measurement of pathogenicity of turkey ornithosis agents for mice. *Avian Dis.* 3:23–27.

Page, L.A.: 1959b. Thermal inactivation studies on a turkey ornithosis virus. *Avian Dis.* 3:67–79.

Page, L.A.: 1966a. Revision of the family *Chlamydiaceae* Rake (Rickettsiales): Unification of the psittacosis-lymphogranuloma venereum-trachoma group of organisms in the genus *Chlamydia* Jones, Rake and Stearns, 1945. *Int. J. Sys. Bacteriol.* 16:223–252.

Page, L.A.: 1966b. Interspecies transfer of psittacosis-LGV-trachoma agents: Pathogenicity of two avian and two mammalian strains for eight species of birds and mammals. *Am. J. Vet. Res.* 27:397–407.

Page, L.A.: 1967. Comparison of 'pathotypes' among chlamydial (psittacosis) strains recovered from diseased birds and mammals. *Bull. Wildl. Dis. Assoc.* 3:166–175.

Page, L.A.: 1968. Proposal for the recognition of two species in the genus *Chlamydia* Jones, Rake, and Stearns, 1945. *Int. J. Sys. Bacteriol.* 18:51–66.

Page, L.A.: 1971. Influence of temperature on the multiplication of chlamydiae in chicken embryos, pp. 40–51. In: *Trachoma and Related Disorders Caused by Chlamydial Agents.* R.L. Nichols (ed.). Amsterdam: Excerpta Medica.

Page, L.A.: 1972. Chlamydiosis (ornithosis), pp. 414–447. In: *Diseases of Poultry,* 6th Ed. M.S. Hofstad (ed.). Ames, Iowa: The Iowa State University Press.

Page, L.A.: 1973. Comments on immunity to bovine chlamydial abortion. *J. Am. Vet Med. Assoc.* 163:891–893.

Page, L.A.: 1974. Order II. Chlamydiales Storz and Page 1971, Part 18. The Rickettsias, pp. 914–928. In: *Bergey's Manual of Determinative Bacteriology,* 8th Ed. R.E. Buchanan and N.E. Gibbons (eds.). Baltimore: The Williams and Wilkins Co.

Page, L.A., W.T. Derieux, and R.C. Cutlip: 1975. An epornitic of fatal chlamydiosis (ornithosis) in South Carolina turkeys, *J. Am. Vet. Med. Assoc.* 166:175–178.

Page, L.A. and K. Erickson: 1969. Serologic evidence of natural and experimental transfers of *Chlamydia psittaci* between wild and domestic animals. *Proceedings: Annual Conference, Bull. Wildl. Dis. Assoc.* 5:284–290.

Page, L.A. and P.C. Smith: 1974. Placentitis and abortion in cattle inoculated with chlamydiae isolated from aborted human placental tissue. *Proc. Soc. Exp. Biol. Med.* 146:269–275.

Paronen, I.: 1948. Reiter's disease: A study of 344 cases observed in Finland. *Acta Med. Scand.* Suppl. 212, 112pp.

Pearson, J.W., J.T. Duff, N.F. Gearinger, and M.L. Robbins: 1965. Growth characteristics of three agents of the psittacosis group in human diploid cell cultures. *J. Infect. Dis.* 115:49–58.

Pelc, S.R. and T.T. Crocker: 1961. Differences in utilization of labelled precursors for the synthesis of deoxyribonucleic acid in cell nuclei and psittacosis virus. (Proceedings of the Biochemical Society) *Biochem. J.* 78:20p.

Pfaffenberg, R.: 1936. Die Psittacosis (Papageienkrankheit) in den Jahren 1931–1935. Epidemiologie, Forschungsergebnisse, Bekämpfung. *Ergeb. Hyg. Bakteriol. Immunitaetsforsch. Exp. Ther.* 18:251–331.

Philip, R.N., E.A. Casper, F.B. Gordon, and A.L. Quan: 1974. Fluorescent antibody responses to chlamydial infection in patients with lymphogranuloma venereum and urethritis. *J. Immunol.* 112:2126–2134.

Phillips, P.E. and C.L. Christian: 1970. Myxovirus antibody increases in human connective tissue disease. *Science* 168:982–984.

Pierce, K.R., L.H. Carroll, and R.W. Moore: 1964. Experimental transmission of ornithosis from sheep to turkeys. *Am. J. Vet. Res.* 25:977–980.

Pinkerton, H. and R.L. Swank: 1940. Recovery of a virus morphologically identical with psittacosis from thiamin-deficient pigeons. *Proc. Soc. Exp. Biol. Med.* 45:704–706.

Piraino, F.F.: 1965. The occurrence of psittacosis virus complement fixing (CF), noncomplement fixing (NCF) and neutralizing (N) antibodies in domestic pigeons. *J. Immunol.* 95:1107–1110.

Piraino, F.F. and C. Abel: 1964. Plaque assay for psittacosis virus in monolayers of chick embryo fibroblasts. *J. Bacteriol.* 87:1503–1511.

Pollard, M. and N. Sharon: 1963. Induction of prolonged latency in psittacosis-infected cells by aminopterin. *Proc. Soc. Exp. Biol. Med.* 112:51–54.

Pollard, M. and T.M. Witka: 1947. The antigenic relationship of lymphogranuloma venereum and psittacosis by skin test in humans. *Tex. Rep. Biol. Med.* 5:288–293.

Prentice, M.J., D. Taylor-Robinson, and G.W. Csonka: 1976. Nonspecific urethritis: a placebo-controlled trial of minocycline in conjunction with laboratory investigations. *Br. J. Vener. Dis.* 52:269–275.

Prowazek, S. von: 1907. Chlamydozoa. I. Zusammenfassende

Übersicht *Arch. Protistenk.* 10:336–364.

Public Health Reports: 1944. An epidemic of a severe pneumonitis in the Bayou Region of Louisiana. Reprint No. 2580, 59:1299–1311, 59:1331–1350, 59:1363–1374.

Pund, E.R. and G.R. Lacy, Jr.: 1951. Lymphogranuloma venereum (inguinale), a precipitating cause of carcinoma. Statistical analysis of one hundred and thirty-five cases of carcinoma of penis, vulva and anorectum. *Am. Surg.* 17:711–718.

Rainey, R.: 1954. The association of lymphogranuloma inguinale and cancer. *Surgery* 35:221–235.

Rake, G., M.D. Eaton, and M.F. Shaffer: 1941. Similarities and possible relationships among viruses of psittacosis, meningo-pneumonitis, and lymphogranuloma venereum. *Proc. Soc. Exp. Biol. Med.* 48:528–531.

Rake, G. and H.P. Jones: 1942. Studies on lymphogranuloma venereum. I. Development of the agent in the yolk sac of the chicken embryo. *J. Exp. Med.* 75:323–338.

Rake, G., C.M. McKee, and M.F. Shaffer: 1940. Agent of lympho-granuloma venereum in the yolk-sac of the developing chick embryo. *Proc. Soc. Exp. Biol. Med.* 43:332–334.

Rake, G., M.F. Shaffer, A.W. Grace, C.M. McKee, and H.P. Jones: 1941. New aids in the diagnosis of lymphogranuloma venereum. *Am. J. Syphil.* 25:687–698.

Rake, G., M.F. Shaffer, and P. Thygeson: 1942. Relationship of agents of trachoma and inclusion conjunctivitis to those of lympho-granuloma-psittacosis group. *Proc. Soc. Exp. Biol. Med.* 49:545–547.

Rees, E., I.A. Tait, D. Hobson, and R.W.A. Johnson: 1977. Chlamydia in relation to cervical infection and pelvic inflammatory disease, pp. 67–76. In: *Nongonococcal Urethritis and Related Infections.* K.K. Holmes and D. Hobson (eds.). Washington, D.C.: American Society for Microbiology.

Reeve, P., R.K. Gerloff, E. Casper, R.N. Philip, J.D. Oriel, and P.A. Powis: 1974. Serological studies on the role of *Chlamydia* in the aetiology of non-specific urethritis. *Br. J. Vener. Dis.* 50:136–139.

Reeve, P. and J. Taverne: 1962. Some properties of the complement fixing antigens of the agents of trachoma and inclusion blennorrhoea and the relationship of the antigens to the developmental cycle. *J. Gen. Microbiol.* 27:501–508.

Reinhards, J., A. Weber, and F. Maxwell-Lyons: 1959. Collective antibiotic treatment of trachoma. *Bull. W.H.O.* 21:665–702.

Reinhards, J., A. Weber, B. Nizetic, K. Kupka, and F. Maxwell-Lyons: 1968. Studies in the epidemiology and control of seasonal conjunctivitis and trachoma in Southern Morocco. *Bull. W.H.O.* 39:497–545.

Reinicke, V. and E. Sondergaard: 1969. A familial epidemic of ornithosis. *Scand. J. Infect. Dis.* 1:113–118.

Reiter, H.: 1916: Ueber eine bisher unerkannte Spirochäteninfektion *(Spirochaetosis arthritica). Dtsch. Med. Wochenschr.* 42:1535–1536.

Rice, C.E.: 1936. Carbohydrate matrix of epithelial-cell inclusion in trachoma. *Am. J. Ophthalmol.* 19:1–8.

Richards, P., W.G. Forster, and P. Thygeson: 1939. Treatment of trachoma with sulfonilamide. *Arch. Ophthalmol.* 21:577–580.

Richmond, S.J., A.L. Hilton, and S.K.R. Clarke: 1972. Chlamydial infection: Role of *Chlamydia* Subgroup A in non-gonococcal and post-gonococcal urethritis. *Br. J. Vener. Dis.* 48:437–444.

Ritter, J.: 1880. Beitrage zur Frage des Pneumotyphus. *Dtsch. Arch. Klin. Med.* XXV:53–96.

Rivers, T.M. and G.P. Berry: 1932. Laboratory method of diagnosis of psittacosis in man. *Proc. Soc. Exp. Biol. Med.* 29:942–944.

Rivers, T.M. and F.F. Schwentker: 1934. Vaccination of monkeys and laboratory workers against psittacosis. *J. Exp. Med.* 60:211–238.

Roberts, W., N.R. Grist, and P. Giroud: 1967. Human abortion associated with infection by ovine abortion agent. *Br. Med. J.* 4:37.

Rose, L. and J. Schachter: 1964. Genitourinary aspects of inclusion conjunctivitis. *Invest. Ophthalmol.* 3:680.

Ross, M.R. and H.M. Jenkin: 1962. Cell wall antigens from members of the psittacosis group of organisms. *Ann. N.Y. Acad. Sci.* 98:329–336.

Rota, T.R. and R.L. Nichols: 1971. Infection of cell cultures by trachoma agent: Enhancement by DEAE-dextran. *J. Infect. Dis.* 124:419–421.

Rota, T.R. and R.L. Nichols: 1973. *Chlamydia trachomatis* in cell culture. I. Comparison of efficiencies of infection in several chemically defined media, at various pH and temperature values, and after exposure to diethylaminoethyl-dextran. *Appl. Microbiol.* 26:560–565.

Rowe, S., E. Aicardi, C. Dawson, and J. Schachter: 1977. Purulent conjunctivitis in neonates: significance of *C. trachomatis. Annual Meeting of the Ambulatory Pediatrics Association,* April 25–26, 1977. San Francisco, California, p. 84.

Rubin, H.: 1954. A disease in captive egrets caused by a virus of the psittacosis-lymphogranuloma venereum group. *J. Infect. Dis.* 94:1–8.

Rubin, H., R.E. Kissling, R.W. Chamberlain, and M.E. Eidson: 1951. Isolated of a psittacosis-like agent from the blood of snowy egrets. *Proc. Soc. Exp. Biol. Med.* 78:696–698.

Saad, E.A., O.F. DeGouveia, L.B. Dias, and R. Da Silva: 1961.

Alterazioni delle proteine seriche e dell'istologia epatica della fase tardiva del linfogranuloma venereo. *Arch. Ital. Sci. Med. Trop. Parasitol.* 42:499–514.

Sabin, A.B. and C.D. Aring: 1942. Meningoencephalitis in man caused by the virus of lymphogranuloma venereum. *JAMA* 120:1376–1381.

Sairanen, E., I. Paronen, and H. Mähönen: 1969. Reiter's syndrome: A follow-up study. *Acta Med. Scand.* 185:57–63.

Schachter, J.: 1967a. A bedsonia isolated from a patient with clinical lymphogranuloma venereum. *Am. J. Ophthalmol.* 63:1049–1053.

Schachter, J.: 1967b. Isolation of bedsoniae from human arthritis and abortion tissues. *Am. J. Ophthalmol.* 63:1082–1086.

Schachter, J.: 1970. Recommended criteria for the identification of trachoma and inclusion conjunctivitis agents. *J. Infect. Dis.* 22:105–107.

Schachter, J.: 1971. Complement fixing antibodies to Bedsonia in Reiter's syndrome, TRIC agent infection, and control groups. *Am. J. Ophthalmol.* 71:857–860.

Schachter, J.: 1977. The expanding clinical spectrum of infections with *Chlamydia trachomatis. Sex. Trans. Dis.* 4:116–118.

Schachter, J., P. Arnstein, C.R. Dawson, L. Hanna, P. Thygeson, and K.F. Meyer: 1968. Human follicular conjunctivitis caused by infection with a psittacosis agent. *Proc. Soc. Exp. Biol. Med.* 127:292–295.

Schachter, J. and G. Atwood: 1975. Chlamydial pharyngitis? *J. Am. Vener. Dis. Assoc.* 2:12.

Schachter, J., J. Banks, N. Sugg, M. Sung, J. Storz, and K.F. Meyer: 1974. Serotyping of *Chlamydia.* I. Isolates of ovine origin. *Infect. Immun.* 9:92–94.

Schachter, J., J. Banks, N. Sugg, M. Sung, J. Storz, and K.F. Meyer: 1975a. Serotyping of *Chlamydia:* Isolates of bovine origin. *Infect. Immun.* 11:904–907.

Schachter, J., M.G. Barnes, J.P. Jones, Jr., E.P. Engleman, and K.F. Meyer: 1966. Isolation of bedsoniae from the joints of patients with Reiter's syndrome. *Proc. Soc. Exp. Biol. Med.* 122:283–285.

Schachter, J., C.R. Dawson, S. Balas, and P. Jones: 1970. Evaluation of laboratory methods for detecting acute TRIC agent infection. *Am. J. Ophthalmol.* 70:375–380.

Schachter, J., L. Hanna, E.C. Hill, S. Massad, C.W. Sheppard, J.E. Conte, Jr., S.N. Cohen, and K.F. Meyer: 1975b. Are chlamydial infections the most prevalent venereal disease? *JAMA* 231:1252–1255.

Schachter, J., L. Hanna, M.L. Tarizzo, and C.R. Dawson: 1971. Relative efficacy of different methods of laboratory diagnosis in chronic trachoma in the United States, pp. 469–475. In: *Trachoma and Related Disorders Caused by Chlamydial Agents.* R.L. Nichols (ed.). Amsterdam: Excerpta Medica.

Schachter, J., E.C. Hill, E.B. King, V.R. Coleman, P. Jones, and K.F. Meyer: 1975c. Chlamydial infection in women with cervical dysplasia. *Am. J. Obstet. Gynecol.* 123:753–757.

Schachter, J., L. Lum, C.A. Gooding, and B. Ostler: 1975d. Pneumonitis following inclusion blennorrhea. *J. Pediatr.* 87:779–780.

Schachter, J. and K.F. Meyer: 1969a. Characteristics of some newly isolated lymphogranuloma venereum strains. *Bacteriol. Proc.* M273, abstract.

Schachter, J. and K.F. Meyer: 1969b. Lymphogranuloma venereum. II. Characterization of some recently isolated strains. *J. Bacteriol.* 99:636–638.

Schachter, J., C.H. Mordhorst, B.W. Moore, and M.L. Tarizzo: 1973. Laboratory diagnosis of trachoma: a collaborative study. *Bull. W.H.O.* 48:509–515.

Schachter, J., H.B. Ostler, and K.F. Meyer: 1969. Human infection with the agent of feline pneumonitis. *Lancet* 1:1063–1065.

Schachter, J., L. Rose, C.R. Dawson, and M. Barnes: 1967. Comparison of procedures for laboratory diagnosis of oculogenital infections with inclusion conjunctivitis agents. *Am. J. Epidemiol.* 85:453–458.

Schachter, J., L. Rose, and K.F. Meyer: 1967. The venereal nature of inclusion conjunctivitis. *Am. J. Epidemiol.* 85:445–452.

Schachter, J., D.E. Smith, C.R. Dawson, W.R. Anderson, J.J. Deller, Jr., A.W. Hoke, W.H. Smartt, and K.F. Meyer: 1969. Lymphogranuloma venereum. I. Comparison of Frei test, complement fixation test, and isolation of the agent. *J. Infect. Dis.* 120:372–275.

Schaffner, W., D.J. Drutz, G.M. Duncan, and M.G. Koenig: 1967. The clinical spectrum of endemic psittacosis. *Arch. Intern. Med.* 119:433–443.

Schechter, E.M.: 1966. Synthesis of nucleic acid and protein in L cells infected with the agent of meningopneumonitis. *J. Bacteriol.* 91:2069–2080.

Schiraldi, O. and M. Pesce: 1965. Pleuro-pericardite in soggetti con positivita delle reazioni di deviazione del complemento per l'ornitosi-psittacosi. *IL Policlinico* LXXII:1603–1609.

Schlosstein, L., P.I. Terasaki, R. Bluestone, and C.M. Pearson: 1973. High association of an HL-A antigen, W27, with ankylosing spondylitis. *N. Engl. J. Med.* 288:704–706.

Schmeichler, L.: 1909. Ueber Chlamydozoenbefunde bei nicht-gonorrhoischer Blennorrhöe der Neugeborenen. *Klin. Wochenschr.* 46:2057–2058.

Schmid, H.: 1931. Über eine psittakoseähnliche Epidemie in einen Tierspital. *Z. Klin. Med.* 117:563–593.

Schoenemann, J. von and E. Gasel: 1965. Akute benigne Perikarditis bei Ornithose. *Z. Gesamte. Inn. Med.* 20:121–124.

Schoenholz, W.K.: 1968. Studies of Bedsonia latency: I. Induction of latency in rabbit cornea (Sirc) cell culture and its reversal by changes in culture conditions. *Z. Immunitaetsforsch.* 135:283–293.

Schoenholz, W.K.: 1970. Studies on Bedsonia latency: II. Effect of immune lymphocytes and of rabbit-anti-lymphocyte globulin (RAMLG) on infected macrophages exposed to increased incubation temperature in vitro. *Z. Immunitaetsforsch.* 139:359–371.

Schultz, P.: 1899. Eine hiesige Badeanstalt, der Infektionsort verschiedener Trachomerkrankungen. *Berl. Klin. Wochenschr.* 36:865–866.

Schultz, P.: 1900. Ein Beitrag zum Character, Verlauf und Behandlung der jüngsten Trachomepidemie in Berlin. *Klin. Wochenschr.* 37:11–14.

Seibert, R.H., W.S. Jordan, Jr., and J.H. Dingle: 1956. Clinical variations in the diagnosis of psittacosis. *N. Engl. J. Med.* 254:925–930.

Shaaban, M.M.H., A.A. Shokeir, I.A. Wasfy, and M.K. Al-Hussaini: 1971. Female genital tract infection with TRIC agents in a trachomatous population. *J. Egypt Med. Assoc.* 54:331–337.

Shaffer, M.F., H. Jones, A.W. Grace, D.M. Hamre, and G. Rake: 1944. Use of the yolk sac of the developing chicken embryo in the isolation of the agent of lymphogranuloma venereum. *J. Infect. Dis.* 75:109–112.

Shaffer, M.F. and G. Rake: 1947. Studies on lymphogranuloma venereum: evaluation of the complement fixation test with Lygranum. *J. Lab. Clin. Med.* 32:1060–1086.

Sharp, J.T., M.D. Lidsky, and W.A. Riley: 1968. Clinical studies on gonococcal arthritis and Reiter's syndrome and measurement of gonococcal and Bedsonia antibodies. *Arth. Rheum.* 11:569–578.

Shatkin, A.A., E.R. Agababova, V.R. Martynova, N.I. Sumarokova, S.I. Sidelnikova, N.V. Nikolskaya, and V.Z. Borovik: 1973. Study of the etiological role of *Halprowia*—Microorganisms of PLT group in diseases of joints. Report I. Isolation of *Halprowia arthritidis* from joints in patients with rheumatoid monosinovitis and Reiter's syndrome. *Vopr. Revm.* 2:9–13.

Sheldon, W.H. and A. Heyman: 1947. Lymphogranuloma venereum: A histologic study of the primary lesion, bubonulus, and lymph nodes in cases proved by isolation of the virus. *Am. J. Pathol.* 23:653–665.

Sheldon, W.H., M.J. Wall, J.DeR. Slade, and A. Heyman: 1948.

Lymphogranuloma venereum in a patient with mediastinal lymphadenopathy and pericarditis. *Arch. Intern. Med.* 82:410–416.

Shimizu, Y. and R.A. Bankowski: 1963. The nature of the cross reactions between a bacterium of the genus *Herellea* and the ornithosis virus in complement fixation. *Am. J. Vet. Res.* 24:1283–1290.

Shindarov, L., N. Runevski, and V. Vassileva: 1971. Morphologic and cytochemic studies on the development of *Chlamydia psittaci* in tissue culture of a cold-blooded animal at 20 °C. *Zentralbl. Bakteriol.* 216:9–14.

Shukla, B.R., H.J. Nema, J.S. Mathur, and K. Nath: 1966. Gantrisin and madribon in trachoma. *Br. J. Ophthalmol.* 50:218–221.

Siboulet, A. and P. Galistin: 1962. Arguments in favour of a virus aetiology of nongonococcal urethritis illustrated by three cases of Reiter's disease. *Br. J. Vener. Dis.* 38:209–211.

Sigel, M.M.: 1962. *Lymphogranuloma Venereum. Epidemiological, Clinical, surgical and Therapeutic Aspects Based on a Study in the Caribbean.* Coral Gables, Fla.: The University of Miami Press.

Simmons, P.D. and F. Vosmik: 1974. Cervical cytology in nonspecific genital infection. An aid to diagnosis. *Br. J. Vener. Dis.* 50:313–314.

Simpson, R.G.: 1954. The relation of lymphogranuloma venereum to syphilis and to falsely positive serologic tests for syphilis. *Am. J. Syphil.* 38:422–428.

Siniscal, A.D.: 1957. Epidemiologic aspects of trachoma in the U.S.A. *Bull. W.H.O.* 16:1047–1050.

Smadel, J.E.: 1943. Atypical pneumonia and psittacosis. *J. Clin. Invest.* XXII:57–65.

Smith, D.E., P.G. James, J. Schachter, E.P. Engleman, and K.F. Meyer: 1973. Experimental bedsonial arthritis. *Arth Rheum.* 16:21–29.

Sompolinsky, D., Z. Harari, F. Soloman, E. Caspi, D. Krakowski, and E. Henig: 1973. A contribution to the microbiology of urethritis. *Isr. J. Med. Sci.* 9:438–446.

Sompolinsky, B. and S. Richmond: 1974. Growth of *Chlamydia trachomatis* in McCoy cells treated with Cytochalasin B. *Appl. Microbiol.* 28:912–914.

Sonck, C.E.: 1972. Lymphogranuloma inguinale. Klinische, epidemiologische und immunologische Aspekte. *Hautarzt.* 23:280–286.

Sonck, C.E., J.A. Räsänen, K.K. Mustakallio, and A. Lassus: 1972. Autoimmune serum factors in active and inactive lymphogranuloma venereum. *Br. J. Vener. Dis.* 49:67–68.

Sowa, J., L.H. Collier, and S. Sowa: 1971. A comparison of the iodine and fluorescent antibody methods for staining trachoma inclusions in the conjunctiva. *J. Hyg.* (Camb.) 67:699–717.

Sowa, S., J. Sowa, and L.H. Collier: 1968. Investigations of neonatal conjunctivitis in The Gambia. *Lancet* 2:243–247.

Sowa, S., J. Sowa, L.H. Collier, and W.A. Blyth: 1969. Trachoma vaccine field trials in The Gambia. *J. Hyg.* (Camb.) 67:699–717.

Stanier, R.Y.: 1964. Toward a definition of the bacteria, pp. 445–464. In: *The Bacteria: A Treatise on Structure and Function;* K. Gunsalus and R.Y. Stanier (ed.). Heredity, Vol. 3. New York and London: Academic Press.

Stargardt, K.: 1909. Über Epithelzellveränderungen beim Trachom und andern Konjunctivalerkrankungen. *Graefe's Arch. Ophtalmol.* 69:525–542.

Steele, J.H. and J.H. Scruggs: 1958. The epidemiology of psittacosis, 1951–1956, pp. 32–51. In: *Progress in Psittacosis Research and Control.* F.R. Beaudette (ed.). New Brunswick, N.J.: Rutgers University Press.

Stiller, D.: 1973. Dermacentor occidentalis Marx 1892 (Acarina: Ixodidae) as a potential vector of *Chlamydia.* Ph.D. Dissertation, University of California.

Stokes, G.V.: 1973. Formation and destruction of internal membranes in L cells infected with *Chlamydia psittaci. Infect. Immun.* 7:173–177.

Stokes, G.V.: 1974. Cycloheximide-resistant glycosylation in L cells infected with *Chlamydia psittaci. Infect. Immun.* 9:497–499.

Storz, J.: 1971. *Chlamydia and Chlamydia-Induced Diseases.* Springfield, Ill.: Charles C Thomas.

Storz, J. and L.A. Page: 1971. Taxonomy of the chlamydiae: Reasons for classifying organisms of the genus *Chlamydia,* family Chlamydiaceae, in a separate order, *Chlamydiales* ord. nov. *Int. J. Sys. Bacteriol.* 21:332–334.

Storz, J., J.L. Shupe, M.E. Marriott, and W.R. Thornley: 1965. Polyarthritis of lambs induced experimentally by a psittacosis agent. *J. Infect. Dis.* 115:9–18.

Strauss, J.: 1957. Ornithosis in Czechoslovakia. *Acta Virol.* 1:132–137.

Strauss, J.: 1967. Microbiologic and epidemiologic aspects of duck ornithosis in Czechoslovakia. *Am. J. Ophthalmol.* 63:1246–1259.

Sturdee, E.L. and W.M. Scott: 1930. *A Disease of Parrots Communicable to Man (Psittacosis).* Rep. Public Health Med. Subj., No. 61, Ministry of Health, 132 pp., London.

Sullivan, P. and A. Brewin: 1974. Evidence of skeletal muscle involvement in psittacosis. *West. J. Med.* 121:232–234.

Sutton, G.C., J.A. Demakis, T.O. Anderson, and R.A. Morrissey:

1971. Serologic evidence of a sporadic outbreak in Illinois of infection by Chlamydia (psittacosis-LGV agent) in patients with primary myocardial disease and respiratory disease. *Am. Heart J.* 81:597–607.

Sutton, G.C., J.F. Driscoll, K.M. Gunner, and J.R. Tobin, Jr.: 1964. Exploratory mediastinotomy in primary myocardial disease. *Prog. Cardiovasc. Dis.* 7:83–97.

Sutton, G.C., R.A. Morrissey, J.R. Tobin, Jr., T.O. Anderson: 1967. Pericardial and myocardial disease associated with serological evidence of infection by agents of the psittacosis-lymphogranuloma venereum group (Chlamydiaceae). *Circulation* XXXVI:830–838.

Swanson, J., D.A. Eschenbach, E.R. Alexander, and K.K. Holmes: 1975. Light and electron microscopic study of *Chlamydia trachomatis* infection of the uterine cervix. *J. Infect. Dis.* 131:678–687.

Tamura, A. and M. Iwanaga: 1965. RNA synthesis in cells infected with the meningopneumonitis agent. *J. Mol. Biol.* 11:97–108.

T'ang, F.-F., H.-L. Chang, Y.-T. Huang, and K.-C. Wang: 1957. Trachoma virus in chick embryo. *Natl. Med. J. China* 43:81–86.

Tarizzo, M.L., B. Nabli, and J. Labonne: 1968. Studies on trachoma. II. Evaluation of laboratory diagnostic methods under field conditions. *Bull. W.H.O.* 38:897–905.

Tarizzo, M.L. and R. Nataf: 1970. The treatment of trachoma/Le traitement du trachome. *Rev. Int. Trach.* 47:7–48/49–87.

Taylor, J.W., J.W. Chandler, and M.K. Cooney: 1975. Acute hemorrhagic conjunctivitis associated with adenovirus type 19. *N. Engl. J. Med.* 292:978–979.

Terskikh, I.I., O.M. Popova, A.I. Gromyko, G.K. Zairov, N.A. Chutkov, and A.Yu. Bekleshova: 1969. Nature and peculiarities of the habitat of ornithosis—trachoma causative agents. *Vopr. virusol.* 14:336–342.

Thygeson, P.: 1934. The etiology of inclusion blennorrhea. *Am. J. Ophthalmol.* 17:1019–1035.

Thygeson, P.: 1946. The cytology of conjunctival exudates. *Am. J. Ophthalmol.* 29:1499–1512.

Thygeson, P.: 1949. Acute trachoma. *Arch. Ophthalmol.* 42:655–665.

Thygeson, P.: 1962a. Trachoma virus: Historical background and review of isolates. *Ann. N.Y. Acad. Sci.* 98:6–1

Thygeson, P.: 1962b. The limbus and cornea in experimental and natural human trachoma and inclusion conjunctivitis. *Ann. N.Y. Acad. Sci.* 98:201–209.

Thygeson, P.: 1963. Epidemiologic observations on trachoma in the United States. *Invest. Ophthalmol.* 2:482–489.

Thygeson, P.: 1971. Historical review of oculogenital disease. *Am. J. Ophthalmol.* 71:975–985.

Thygeson, P. and T. Crocker: 1956. Observations on experimental trachoma and inclusion conjunctivitis. *Am. J. Ophthalmol.* 42:76–83.

Thygeson, P. and C.R. Dawson: 1971. Pseudotrachoma caused by molluscum contagiosum virus and various chemical irritants, pp. 1894–1897. In: *Proceedings: XXI International Congress of Ophthalmology,* March 8–14, 1970, Mexico D.F. M.P. Solanes (ed.). International Congress Series No. 222. Amsterdam: Excerpta Medica.

Thygeson, P. and W.F. Mengert: 1936. The virus of inclusion conjunctivitis. Further observations. *Arch Ophthalmol.* 15:377–410.

Thygeson, P. and M. Okumoto: 1967. A new type of chronic follicular conjunctivitis. *Am. J. Ophthalmol.* 63:1277–1282.

Thygeson, P. and F.I. Proctor: 1935. Etiological significance of the elementary body in trachoma. *Am. J. Ophthalmol.* 18:811–813.

Thygeson, P. and P. Richards: 1938. Nature of the filterable agent of trachoma. *Arch. Ophthalmol.* 20:569–584.

Thygeson, P. and W. Stone, Jr.: 1942. Epidemiology of inclusion conjunctivitis. *Arch. Ophthalmol.* 27:91–122.

Timberger, R.J. and D. Armstrong: 1969. Ornithosis without direct bird exposure: response to erythromycin. *Am. Rev. Respir. Dis.* 99:936–939.

Treharne, J.D., S. Darougar, and B.R. Jones: 1973. Characterization of a further microimmunofluorescence serotype of *Chlamydia:* TRIC Type G. *Br. J. Vener. Dis.* 49:295–300.

Treharne, J.D., S.J. Davey, S.J. Gray, and B.R. Jones: 1972. Immunological classification of TRIC agents and of some recently isolated LGV agents by the microimmunofluorescence test. *Br. J. Vener. Dis.* 48:18–25.

Treuting, W.L. and B.J. Olson: 1944. An epidemic of a severe pneumonitis in the Bayou Region of Louisiana. II. Clinical features of the disease. *Public Health Rep.* 59:1331–1350.

Tribby, I.I.E. and J.W. Moulder: 1966. Availability of bases and nucleosides as precursors of nucleic acids in L cells and in the agent of meningopneumonitis. *J. Bacteriol.* 91:2362–2367.

Vaag, A.: 1950. Historien om psittacosen pa Faer/oerne. *Ugeskr. Laeger* 112:804–806.

Valero, A.: 1953. Human ornithosis in Israel. *Harefuah* 45:101–102.

Vastine, D.W., C.R. Dawson, T. Daghfous, M. Messadi, I. Hoshiwara, C. Yoneda, and R. Nataf: 1974. Severe endemic trachoma in Tunisia. I. The effect of topical chemotherapy on conjunctivitis and ocular bacteria. *Br. J. Ophthalmol.* 58:833–842.

Vaughn-Jackson, J.D., E.M.C. Dunlop, S. Darougar, R.St.C. Dwyer, and B.R. Jones: 1972. Chlamydial infection: Results of tests for *Chlamydia* in patients suffering from acute Reiter's disease compared with results of tests of the genital tract and rectum in patients with ocular infection due to TRIC agent. *Br. J. Vener. Dis.* 48:445–451.

Vender, J. and J. W. Moulder: 1967. Initial step in catabolism of glucose by the meningopneumonitis agent. *J. Bacteriol.* 94:867–869.

Vergnani, R.J. and R.S. Smith: 1974. Reiter syndrome in a child. *Arch. Ophthalmol.* 91:165–166.

Verhoeff, F.H.: 1940. Improved method of staining within tissues, Leptotriches of Parinaud's conjunctivitis and gram-positive microorganisms. *JAMA* 115:1546.

Vickery, H.F. and O. Richardson: 1904. Three cases of probable psittacosis, with bacteriological report by Oscar Richardson. *Trans. Assoc. Am. Physicians* 19:364–372.

Volk, J.J. and S.J. Kraus: 1974. Nongonococcal urethritis: A venereal disease as prevalent as epidemic gonorrhea. *Arch. Intern. Med.* 134:511–514.

Volkert, M. and P.M. Christensen: 1955. Two ornithosis complement fixing antigens from infected yolk sacs. *Acta Pathol. Microbiol. Scand.* 37:211–218.

Volkert, M. and M. Matthiesen: 1956. An ornithosis related antigen from a coccoid bacterium. *Acta Pathol. Microbiol. Scand.* 39:117–126.

Vosti, G.J. and H. Roffwarg: 1961. Myocarditis and encephalitis in a case of suspected psittacosis. *Ann. Intern. Med.* 54:764–776.

Wachendörfer, J.G.: 1973: Epidemiology and control of psittacosis. *J. Am. Vet Med. Assoc.* 162:298–303.

Waelsch, L.: 1904. Über nicht-gonorrhoische Urethritis. *Arch. Dermatol.* 70:103–124.

Wall, M.J.: 1946. Isolation of the virus of lymphogranuloma venereum from twenty-eight patients: relative value of the use of chick embryos and mice. *J. Immunol.* 54:59–64.

Wall, M.J.: 1947. Complement fixing antibodies of lymphogranuloma venereum in mice: Their development and response to sulfonamide therapy. *J. Immunol.* 55:353–361.

Wang, S.-P. and J.T. Grayston: 1970. Immunologic relationship between genital TRIC, lymphogranuloma venereum, and related organisms in a new microtiter indirect immunofluorescence test. *Am. J. Ophthalmol.* 70:367–374.

Wang, S.-P. and J.T. Grayston: 1971a. Classification of TRIC and related strains with microimmuno-fluorescence, pp. 305–321. In: *Trachoma and Related Disorders Caused by Chlamydial Agents.* R.L. Nichols (ed.). Amsterdam: Excerpta Medica.

Wang, S.-P. and J.T. Grayston. 1971b. Studies on the identity of the 'fast' egg-killing chlamydia strains, pp. 322–336. In: *Trachoma and Related Disorders Caused by Chlamydial Agents.* R.L. Nichols (ed.). Amsterdam: Excerpta Medica.

Wang, S.-P. and J.T. Grayston: 1974. Human serology in *Chlamydia trachomatis* infection with microimmunofluorescence. *J. Infect. Dis.* 130:388–397.

Wang, S.-P., J.T. Grayston, and E.R. Alexander: 1967. Trachoma vaccine studies in monkeys. *Am. J. Ophthalmol.* 63:1615–1630.

Wang, S.-P., J.T. Grayston, E.R. Alexander, and K.K. Holmes: 1975. A simplified microimmunofluorescence test with trachoma-lymphogranuloma venereum *(Chlamydia trachomatis)* antigens for use as a screening test for antibody. *J. Clin. Microbiol.* 1:250–255.

Wang, S.-P., J.T. Grayston, and J.L. Gale: 1973. Three new immunologic types of trachoma-inclusion conjunctivitis organisms. *J. Immunol.* 110:873–879.

Wang, S.-P., C.-C. Kuo, and J.T. Grayston: 1973. A simplified method for immunological typing of trachoma-inclusion conjunctivitis-lymphogranuloma venereum organisms. *Infect. Immun.* 7:356–360.

Watson, P.G. and D. Gairdner: 1968. TRIC agent as a cause of neonatal eye sepsis. *Br. Med. J.* 3:527–528.

Weiss, E.: 1950. The effect of antibiotics on agents of the psittacosis-lymphogranuloma group: I. The effect of penicillin. *J. Infect. Dis.* 87:249–263.

Weiss, E.: 1967. Transaminase activity and other enzymatic reactions involving pyruvate and glutamate in *Chlamydia* (psittacosis-trachoma group). *J. Bacteriol.* 93:177–184.

Weiss, E.: 1968. Comparative metabolism of rickettsiae and other host dependent bacteria. *Zentralb. Bakteriol.* (orig.) 206:292–298.

Weiss, E. and H.R. Dressler: 1960. Centrifugation of rickettsiae and viruses onto cells and its effect on infection. *Proc. Soc. Exp. Biol. Med.* 103:691–695.

Weiss, E. and H.R. Dressler: 1962. Investigation of the stability of the trachoma agent. *Ann. N.Y. Acad. Sci.* 98:250–260.

Weiss, E., S. Schramek, N.N. Wilson, and L.W. Newman: 1970. Deoxyribonucleic acid heterogeneity between human murine strains of *Chlamydia trachomatis. Infect. Immun.* 2:24–28.

Weiss, E. and N.N. Wilson: 1969. Role of exogenous adenosine triphosphate in catabolic and synthetic activities of *Chlamydia psittaci. J. Bacteriol.* 97:719–724.

Wentworth, B.B. and E.R. Alexander: 1974. Isolation of *Chlamydia trachomatis* by use of 5-iodo-2-deoxyuridine-treated cells. *Appl. Microbiol.* 27:912–916.

Wentworth, B.B., P. Bonin, K.K. Holmes, L. Gutman, P. Wiesner, and E.R. Alexander: 1973. Isolation of viruses, bacteria and other organisms from venereal disease clinic patients: Methodology and problems associated with multiple isolations. *Health Lab. Sci.* 10:75-81.

Weyer, F.: 1964. Weitere Beobachtungen im Rahmen von diagnostischen Tierversuchen bei Ornithose-Psittakose mit Bemerkungen über die Entwicklung der Ornithose-Situation in Deutschland während der letzten Jahre. *Zentralb. Bakteriol.* 193:147-178.

Whitcher, J.P., C.R. Dawson, M. Messadi, T. Daghfous, N. ben Abdullah, F. Triki, and I. Hoshiwara: 1974. Severe endemic trachoma in Tunisia: Changes in ocular bacterial pathogens in children treated by the intermittent antibiotic regimen. *Rev. Int. Trach.* 4:49-54.

Whitcher, J.P., N.J. Schmidt, R. Mabrouk, M. Messadi, T. Daghfous, I. Hoshiwara, and C.R. Dawson: 1976. Acute hemorrhagic conjunctivitis in Tunisia: Report of viral isolations. *Arch. Ophthalmol.* 94:51-55.

Wong, J.L., P.A. Hines, M.D. Brasher, G.T. Rogers, R.F. Smith, and J. Schachter: 1977. The etiology of nongonococcal urethritis in men attending a venereal disease clinic. *Sex. Trans. Dis.* 4:4-8.

World Health Organization Technical Report Series, No. 234. Expert Committee on Trachoma, Third Report 3-48, 1962. Geneva: World Health Organization.

World Health Organization Technical Report Series, No. 330. Fourth WHO Scientific Group on Trachoma Research Report 2-24, 1966. Geneva: World Health Organization.

World Health Organization Statistics Report. Rapport De/Statistiques Sanitaires Mondiales 24:248-329, 1971. Geneva: World Health Organization.

World Health Organization: Guide to the Laboratory Diagnosis of Trachoma. Prepared by the participants in a WHO symposium, 1975. Geneva: World Health Organization.

Williams, R.D. and A.B. Gutman: 1936. Hyperproteinemia with reversal of the albumin:globulin ratio in lymphogranuloma inguinale. *Proc. Soc. Exp. Biol. Med.* 34:91-94.

Wood, W.H., Jr. and H. Felson: 1946. A case of lymphogranuloma venereum associated with atypical pneumonia. *Ann. Intern. Med.* 24:904-908.

Woodroffe, G.M. and J.W. Moulder: 1960. Penicillin-insensitive and non-neutralizable variants of feline pneumonitis virus. *J. Infect. Dis.* 107:195-202.

Woolridge, R.L., K.H. Cheng, I.H. Chang, C.Y. Yang, T.C. Hsu, and J.T. Grayston: 1967. Failure of trachoma treatment with ophthalmic antibiotics and systemic sulfonamides used along or in combination with trachoma vaccine. *Am. J. Ophthalmol.* 63:1577-1583.

Yoneda, C., C.R. Dawson, T. Daghfous, I. Hoshiwara, P. Jones, M. Messadi, and J. Schachter: 1975. Cytology as a guide to the presence of chlamydial inclusions in Giemsa-stained conjunctival smears in severe endemic trachoma. *Br. J. Ophthalmol.* 59:116–124.

Young, V.M.: 1974. Haemophilus, pp. 302–307. In: *Manual of Clinical Microbiology,* 2d Ed. E.H. Lennette, E.H. Spaulding, and J.P. Truant (eds.). Washington, D.C.: American Society for Microbiology.

Yow, E.M., J.C. Brennan, J. Preston, and S. Levy: 1959. the pathology of psittacosis: A report of two cases with hepatitis. *Am. J. Med.* XXVII:739–749.

Zhodzishskii, I.A.: 1966. The etiology of the urethrooculosynovial syndrome. *Urol. Nefrol.* 31:35–40.

Abortion, 153, 154
Achromycin (*see* Tetracyclines)
Adenosine triphosphate (*see* ATP)
Adenovirus, 104–106, 116, 184
   epidemic keratoconjunctivitis,
      104, 105
   follicular conjunctivitis, 104
   keratitis, 105
   pharyngoconjunctival fever,
      104, 105
Allergic diseases, 66, 78
Aminocyclitol, 127
Ankylosing spondylitis, 143, 146
Anorectal syndrome, 50
Antibiotics (*see* Chloramphenicol;
   Erythromycin; Neomycin;
   Penicillins; Rifampicin; Strep-
   tomycin; Sulfonamides;
   Tetracyclines)
Antibody
   complement fixing
      inclusion conjunctivitis, 108
      LGV, 46, 59–61, 193, 196
      measurement of, 199–200
      NGU, 196
      psittacosis, 23, 193, 197
      Reiter's syndrome, 145,
         147–148
      trachoma, 197
      VD populations, 46, 125
   microimmunofluorescent
      genital tract infection, 126
      inclusion conjunctivitis, adult,
         108
      LGV, 61–62
      measurement of, 200–201
      trachoma, 81–82
   neutralizing, 179
   in tears, 87, 198
Antigens, 178, 179–180
Arthritis
   experimental, 149
   LGV, 50
   psoriatic, 146
   Reiter's syndrome, 141, 142
Asymptomatic female in LGV, 46
Atopic disease, 78
ATP, 166

Atypical pneumonia, 16, 17
Axenfeld's conjunctivitis, 67, 76

Baboons (*see* Primates)
Bacteria, 64, 115
   diphtheroids, 73
   Haemophilus, 53, 72, 79, 115,
      Plate 10
   Herrellea, 180
   Moraxella, 72, 76, 79, Plate 10
   Neisseria, 72, 79, 115,
      116, 123, 124, 126–128, 129
      130, 131, 170, Plate 10
   pneumococcus, 72, 79, 115,
      Plate 10
   Staphylococcus aureus, 72, 73,
      76, 79, 115
   Staphylococcus epidermidis, 79
   Streptococcus, 73, 115
Bacterium aerytrycke, 11
Bacterium antitratum, 180
Bacterium granulosis, 64
Bacterium psittacosis, 11
Balanitis, 142
Beal's follicular conjunctivitis, 104
Bedson, Samuel, 2, 11
Bedsonia, 3
Birds, wild, as sources of human
   infection, 32
Blennorrhea, 122, 130
Blepharitis, 76
Blood, isolation of chlamydiae,
   206
Bubo, 48
   pus, 206–207

*Calymmatobacterium granulo-
   matis,* 53
Candida albicans, 128, 130,
   135–136
Carcinomas and LGV, 56–57
Cardiac involvement
   LGV, 51
   psittacosis, 21–23
Cat-scratch disease, 54, 154–156
Catarrh, vernal, 66, 78

Cell culture isolation technique, 81
Cell wall, 179
Central nervous system
    and LGV, 50
    and psittacosis, 19, 22, 28
Cervicitis, 122, 128–131, 134–136
Cervix
    infection, 122, 123, 128–131
    scrapings from, 129
CF test (*see* Complement fixation
    test)
Chancroid, 53
Chemotherapy (*see* Treatment)
Chickens, 12, 14, 15, 31
Chlamydia psittaci
    conjunctival infections, 107
    species defined, 5–6
Chlamydia trachomatis, species
    defined, 5
Chlamydiae
    antigens, cross-reacting, 180
    antigens, specific, 179–180
    bacterial nature, 158–160
    chemical composition, 163–164
    developmental cycle, 160–162
    DNA homology, 170–171
    DNA synthesis, 168–169
    group A, 4, 139
    group B, 4, 139
    growth in cell culture, 172–175
    hemagglutination reaction, 180
    latency in vitro, 175–177
    lipid synthesis, 171
    metabolism, 165–167
    morphologic characteristics, 157
    nutritional requirements, 165
    pathogenicity, 99–100, 138
    penicillins, effect of, 162–163
    polysaccharide synthesis, 171–
        172
    protein synthesis, 167–168
    stability, 177–178
Chlamydial isolation, 205–219 (*see
    also* Isolation of chlamydiae)
Chloramphenicol
    inclusion conjunctivitis,
        neonatal, 114
    LGV, 55–56
    psittacosis, 26
Cicatrization, 66, 69, 103, 113–114
Climatic bubo, 45
Collection medium, 217

Complement fixation (CF) test,
    46, 81, 108
    cat-scratch disease, 155–156
    indirect, 194
    LGV, 46, 59–61, 193, 196
    NGU, 196
    in proven chlamydial infection,
        196
    psittacosis, 23, 193, 197
    reactor rates in VD clinics,
        46, 125
    reagents, 201–203
    Reiter's syndrome, 145, 147–148
    technique, 199–200
    trachoma, 197
Conjunctival scrapings, 79, 105
Conjunctivitis
    acute hemorrhagic, 104, 106–107
    allergic, 66, 78
    angular, 76
    atopic, 78
    Axenfeld's 67, 76
    bacterial, 70, 73, 76, 90
    Beal's, 104
    blepharo-, 76
    catarrh, vernal, 66, 78
    chronic follicular, 76–77
    cicatricial, 75
    cytology, 80–81, 105, 184–186
    epidemic, 106
    follicular (*see* Follicular
        conjunctivitis)
    inclusion (*see* Inclusion
        conjunctivitis)
    membranous, 105, 113
    mucopurulent, 72
    "orphan's," 76
    papillary, 78
    Parinaud's oculoglandular,
        77–78
    phlyctenular, 107
    Reiter's syndrome, 142–143
    swimming pool, 98, 100, 105
    Thygeson's chronic follicular,
        67, 77
    toxic follicular, 76
    viral, 104–107, 115–116
Cornea, 102–103, 143
Corneal ulceration, 66, 72, 95
Corticosteroids, 71, 104, 106, 109,
    143
Credé's method, 111, 119, 121

Cryoglobulins, 52
Cycloserine, 4
Cytologic techniques, 182–193
Cytology, trachoma, 78–81, 184
 (*see also* Laboratory diagnosis)
Cytomegaloviruses, 130

DEAE-dextran, enhancement of
 infectivity, 173–174, 217
DEAE-treated cells, 215
Delayed hypersensitivity (*see*
 Immunity, cellular)
Deoxyribonucleic acid (*see* DNA)
Developmental cycle, 160–162
Diagnosis (*see* Laboratory
 diagnosis)
Diphtheroids, 73
Diplobacillus, 72, 76, 79
DNA, 164
 content, 171
 homology, 170–171
 synthesis, 168–169
Donovan bodies, 53
Drugs (*see* Corticosteroids;
 Erythromycin; Neomycin; Peni-
 cillins; Streptomycin; Sulfona-
 mides; Tetracyclines)
Dry eye syndrome, 66, 70, 89
Ducks, 12, 31

Ectopy, 135
Egg embryo isolation technique,
 81
Egrets, 13
Egypt, 64
Egyptian ophthalmia, 64
Elementary body, 135, 157, 160,
 161, 162
Encephalitis, 22
Eosinophilic leukocytes, 184
Epidemiology
 genital tract infections, 125,
  133, 136
 inclusion conjunctivitis, adult,
  99, 100–101
 inclusion conjunctivitis, neo-
  natal, 113
 LGV, 45–47
 psittacosis, 29–35
 Reiter's syndrome, 143
 trachoma, 64, 70–74, 95
Epididymitis, 138

Erythromycin
 genital tract infections, 134
 inclusion conjunctivitis, adult,
  109
 inclusion conjunctivitis, neonatal, 116
 pneumonia in infants, 118
 psittacosis, 26
 trachoma, 90, 93–94, 95
Esthiomene, 50
Ethiopia, 72, 87
Experimental infection
 inclusion conjunctivitis, 98–100
 in primates, 28–29, 64, 98–100,
  121, 149
 psittacosis, 28–29, 38–39
 Reiter's syndrome, 149
 trachoma, 64, 121
Extragenital LGV, 47

FA (*see* Fluorescent antibody
 stain)
Fallopian tubes, 138
Faroe Islands, 11
Fast-killing strains, 84
Fatality rates, psittacosis, 18, 19
Fecal samples, isolation of
 chlamydiae, 207
Fiessinger-Leroy-Reiter syndrome,
 141
Fistulas, 50
Flies, 74, 90
Fluorescent antibody (FA) stain,
 182–183, 188–189
 methods, 79, 80, 81, 189–190
Follicles, conjunctival, 65, 67
Follicular conjunctivitis, 65, 67,
 98, 102, 138 (*See also* Inclusion conjunctivitis; Trachoma)
 acute, 104
 adenovirus, 104
 chronic, 65, 74
 folliculosis, 75
 herpetic, 106
 inclusion (*see* Inclusion conjunctivitis)
 molluscum, 75
 Newcastle disease virus, 104, 106
Folliculosis, 75
Frei test, 47, 57–59
Fulmars, 11

Gambia, 83, 84
Genital tract infections, 112, 114,
  121–139
    blennorrhea, 122, 131
    cervicitis, 122, 128–131, 134–136
    CF antibodies, 196
    conjunctivitis, 99–101, 112,
      136–137
    epidemiology, 125, 133, 136
    gonorrhea, 129, 134
    historical aspects, 98, 121–124
    micro-IF antibodies, 126, 198
    NGU, 121–128, 134–136, 139
        diagnosis, 128
    PGU, 131–132
  tissue culture isolation methods,
      212–216
    treatment, 132–134
Genito-ano-rectal syndrome in
  LGV, 49–50
Genome, 171
Giemsa stain, 79, 80, 82, 105, 108,
  116, 182, 183–188
    method, 187–188
Giminez stain, 182, 191–192
Glycogen, 172
Gonorrhea, 116, 123–124, 129,
  131–132
Granuloma inguinale, 53
Groove sign, 49
Group A chlamydiae, 4, 139
Group B chlamydiae, 4, 139
Growth cycle, 157, 160–162
Guinea pig inclusion conjuncti-
  vitis, 202

Haemophilus, 53, 72, 79, 115,
  Plate 10
Haemophilus ducreyi, 53
Halberstaedter, L., 4, 64
HeLa cells, 209
Hemagglutination reactions, 180
Hemagglutinin, 171, 194
Hemorrhagic conjunctivitis, 104,
  106, 107
Heparin, 173
Hepatitis, 18
Herbert's pits, 66
Herpes genitalis, 53
Herpesvirus hominis
  cervicitis, 129, 130

  conjunctivitis, 104, 106, 115,
    184
  urethritis, 128, 135
Herrellea, 180
Histocompatibility antigen, 104,
  151
Histopathology, 182
Historical aspects
  genital tract infections, 121–124
  inclusion conjunctivitis, adult,
    98–100
  inclusion conjunctivitis, neo-
    natal, 112
  LGV, 45–47
  psittacosis, 9–12
  Reiter's syndrome, 141
  trachoma, 63–65
HLA B27, 104, 151
Hypersensitivity, 84

IgA in LGV, 52
IgG in ICN, 117
IgM
  in ICN, 117
  in LGV, 61
  in NGU, 126
Immunity
  genital tract infection, 139
  inclusion conjunctivitis, 103
  psittacosis, 26–27
  trachoma, 83
Immunization, trachoma, 83–88
Immunodiffusion, 194
Immunoglobulins
  IgA, 52, 200, 205
  IgG, 117, 200, 205
  IgM, 61, 117, 126, 198, 200, 205
Immunology, 179–180, 193–205
Immunotypes, 72, 99, 179–180
Immunotyping, 179–180
Inclusion blennorrhea, 122, 131
  (*see also* Inclusion conjunc-
  tivitis, neonatal)
Inclusion body, 162–164, 184, 186,
  Plates 9, 10, 11, 12
Inclusion conjunctivitis, adult, 97–
  109, 138, 184
  clinical disease, 99, 102–104
  differential diagnosis, 104–107
  epidemiology, 99, 100–101
  laboratory diagnosis, 107–108

treatment, 108–109
Inclusion conjunctivitis, neonatal, 98, 111–120, 138
  clinical disease, 113–115
  complications, 115
  differential diagnosis, 115–116
  epidemiology, 112, 121
  laboratory diagnosis, 116
  pneumonia in infants, 117–120
  treatment, 116–117
Inclusions, 184, 186
Incubation period
  LGV, 47, 48
  psittacosis, 17
Indirect complement fixation (CF) test, 194
Inflammatory cells, 184
Influenza, 24–25
Initial body, 157, 161–162, Plates 9, 10
Iodine stain, 108, 190–191
  taxonomic significance, 4
Iran, 84, 91
Iritis, 103–104, 109, 143
Irradiated cell technique, 214
Isolation of chlamydiae, 205–219
  genital tract infections, 122, 123, 128
  inclusion conjunctivitis, 107, 108
  LGV, 62, 205
  mice, 208–210
  processing of specimens, 206–208
  psittacosis, 24, 205
  Reiter's syndrome, 145–147
  tissue culture methods, 212–216
  trachoma, 81
  yolk sac method, 210–212
IUDR-treated cell, 215

Keratitis, 66, 73, 102, 105, 106, 109, 114
Keratoconjunctivitis
  atopic, 78
  epidemic, 104, 105
  herpes simplex virus, 106
Keratodermia blennorrhagia, 142
Koch, Robert, 72, 73
Koch-Weeks bacillus, 72, 73, Plate 10

Laboratory diagnosis, 181–219
  cytologic techniques, 182–193
    FA stain, 182–183, 188–190
    Giemsa stain, 79, 80, 82, 105, 108, 116, 182, 183–188
    Giminez stain, 182, 191–192
    iodine stain, 108, 190–191
    Macchiavello stain, 64, 182, 191–192
    specimen collection, 183
  isolation, 205–219
    mouse inoculation, intracranial, 209
    mouse inoculation, intranasal, 209–210
    mouse inoculation, intraperitoneal, 208–209
    specimen processing, 206–208
    tissue culture methods, 212–216
    tissue culture technique, 216–219
    yolk sac method, 210–212
  serologic diagnosis, 193–205
    CF, technique, 199–200
    interpretation, 204–205
    micro-IF, technique, 200–201
Lacrimal secretion, 66, 72, 89
Latency, 135
  in vitro, 175–177
  LGV, 51–52
  psittacosis, 35
Leber cells, 184
Lesion, primary, in LGV, 47–48
LGV (see Lymphogranuloma venereum)
Lindner, Karl, 112, 122
Lipid content, 164
Lipid synthesis, 171
Local antibody, eye, 198
Louisiana outbreak (psittacosis), 12–13
Lower mammals and human infection, 153–156
Lygranum, 58
Lymphadenitis, 48, 154
Lymphadenopathy, 48
Lymphoblastic transformation, 148
Lymphogranuloma inguinale, 45
Lymphogranuloma venereum (LGV), 45–62, 78, 172
  asymptomatic female, 46
  and cancer, 56–57

CF test, 46, 47, 58, 59–61,
  193, 196, 205
chemotherapy, 54–56
clinical manifestations, 47–52
diagnostic methods, 57–62
differential diagnosis, 52–54
epidemiology, 45–47
extragenital, 47, 49, 50–52
Frei test, 47, 57–59
genito-ano-rectal syndrome, 49–
  50
historical aspects, 45–47
incubation period, 47, 48
isolation of agent, 62
latency, 51–52
primary lesion, 47–48
rectal, 47
secondary lesions, 48–49
serologic abnormalities, 52, 59
sex ratio, 48
systemic complications, 50–52
tertiary stage, 49–50
tetracyclines, 55
Lymphoid cells, 184
Lymphopathia venereum, 45
Lysosomes, 162

MacCallan, Arthur, 67
MacCallan classification of tra-
  choma, 67
Macchiavello stain, 64, 182, 191–
  192
Macrophages, 177
Malady of Durand, Nicolas, and
  Favre, 45
Mammalian chlamydiae, 154
McCoy cells, 212–213
Membranous conjunctivitis, 105,
  113
Meningitis, LGV, 50
Meningococcus *(see Neisseria men-
  ingitidis)*
Metabolism, 165–167
  carbohydrate, 171–172
  lipid, 171
  nucleic acid, 168–169
Meyer, Karl F., 3, 11, 35
Microimmunofluorescence (Micro-
  IF) test, 108, 193, 198
  genital tract infections, 126
  inclusion conjunctivitis, adult,
    108

LGV, 61–62
reagents, 203–204
serotypes, 179–180
techniques, 200–201
trachoma, 81–82
Minocycline, 133
Miyagawanella, 3
Molluscum, 75
Monkey inoculation, 84, 86, 87,
  98
Moraxella, 72, 76, 79, Plate 10
Mouse, experimental infection, 38
Mouse, isolation systems in, 208–
  210
Mouse toxicity prevention test, 179
Mucopurulent conjunctivitis, 72
Muramic acid, 162–163
Murine toxin, 179
Musca domestica, 74, 90
Mycoplasma hominis, 130
Mycoplasma pneumoniae, 16

Neisseria gonorrhoeae infection
  in female, 123, 129, 130
  in male, 123, 124, 126, 131–132
  ocular, 72, 73, 79, 114, 115,
    116, Plate 10
Neisseria meningitidis, infection,
  ocular, 72, 79, 115, Plate 10
Neomycin, 210
Neorickettsiae, 6
Neuraminidase, 173, 174
Neutralization, 179
Neutralizing antibody, 179
Newcastle disease virus, 104, 106
NGU *(see* Nongonococcal ure-
  thritis)
Nonbacterial lymphadenitis, 154
Nongonococcal urethritis (NGU)
  chlamydial infections, 122–128
  diagnosis, 128
  etiology, 122–128, 135–136
  history, 122
  postgonococcal, 124–125, 131–
    132, 133
  prevalence, 139
  Reiter's syndrome, 142, 143
  treatment, 132–134
Nonspecific urethritis, 133
Nosocomial infections, 105, 107

Nucleic acids, 168–169, 170–171
Nutritional requirements, 165

Ocelles, 66
Oculoglandular fever, 77
"Oculourethrosynovial syndrome,"
  141
Ointments (*see* Antibiotics)
Ophthalmia neonatorum (*see* In-
  clusion conjunctivitis, neonatal)
Ornithosis, 9, 12
Otitis, 104, 105, 109, 138
Owl monkey, 86

Pandemic of 1929–1930, 2, 10–11
Pannus, 66, 75
Papanicolaou stain, 186
Papillary conjunctivitis, 78
Parakeets, 31, 39
Parinaud's oculoglandular syn-
  drome, 77
Parrots, 31
Pathogenicity
  C. psittaci, 38, 172
  C. trachomatis, 172
Pathology
  LGV, 48–51
  psittacosis, 28–29
  trachoma, 65, 66
Pathotypes, 172
Pelvic inflammatory disease, 138
Penicillins
  effect on chlamydiae, 162–163
  gonorrhea, 131–132
  psittacosis, 26
PGU (*see* Postgonococcal ure-
  thritis)
Phagocytosis, 161
Pharyngoconjunctival fever, 104,
  105
Pigeons, 12, 14, 31
Plasma cells, 184
Pleural fluid, 206
Pneumococcus, 72, 79, 115
Pneumonia,
  atypical, 16–17
  in infants, 117–120
Pneumonitis, 17
  LGV, 51

Postgonococcal urethritis, 124,
  125, 131–132, 134
Poultry, 12, 14, 15, 31
Primates, subhuman
  experimental disease, 28–29, 64,
    98–100, 121, 149
  genital tract infections, 121
  immunization studies, 26, 83,
    84, 87
  inclusion conjunctivitis, 98–100
  psittacosis, 26, 28–29
  Reiter's syndrome, 149
  trachoma, 64, 83, 84, 86, 87
Proctitis, 47, 50, 124
Protein content, 164
Protein synthesis, 167–168
Pseudotrachoma (*see* Follicular
  conjunctivitis, chronic)
Psittacine species, 9, 31
Psittacosis 9–43, 107
  birds, natural history in, 36
  cardiac involvement, 21
  CF test, 23, 193, 197
  clinical picture, 17–23
  complications, 20
  diagnosis in avians, 37–38
  differential diagnosis, 24–25
  epidemiology, 29–35
  experimental host range of
    chlamydiae, 38–39
  fatality rates, 18, 19
  historical aspects, 9–13
  immunity, 26–27
  incubation period, 17
  isolation of agent, 24
  laboratory diagnosis, 23–24
  latency, 35
  Louisiana outbreak, 12–13
  occupational disease, 33–35
  pathology, 28–29
  prevalence, 13–17
  quarantine, 40
  reinfection, 27
  relapse, 20, 26
  transmission of, man-to-man,
    30, 32
  treatment, 25–26
Purulent conjunctivitis, 73, 90
Pus, bubo, 206–207

Q fever, 24
Quarantine centers, psittacosis, 40

272

Radioisotope immune precipitation
test, 193–194
Rectal infection, 124
Rectal LGV, 47, 49–50
Rectal strictures, 50
Reinfection
psittacosis, 27
trachoma, 94
Reiter's syndrome, 104, 141–156
CF test, 145, 147–148
clinical description, 142–143
cytologic studies, 146
diagnosis, 149–150
evidence for chlamydial involvement, 144
experimental studies, 149
historical aspects, 141
isolation attempts, 145–147
postdysenteric form, 143
role of chlamydiae, 150–152
Reticulate particle, 161
Ribonucleic acid (*see* RNA)
Rickettsiae, 6
Rifampicin, 90, 94
RNA, 164

Sacroileitis, 142, 143
Salmonella typhimurium, 11
Salzmann's nodular dystrophy, 66
Saudi Arabia, 73, 83, 85
Scarring, conjunctival, 64, 65–66,
69, 75, 76, 103, 113–114
Scrapings
cervical, 129
conjunctival, 79, 105
urethral, 124, 128, 132
Serology, 193–205
Serotypes, 72, 99, 179–180
Sex ratio in LGV, 48
Shigellosis, 143
Skin tests (*see* Frei test)
Smears (*see* Scrapings)
Specimen collection, 183
Specimen processing, 206–208
Spleen, 18
Sputum, 206
Stages of trachoma (*see* MacCallan
classification)
Stains (*see* Fluorescent antibody;
Giemsa; Giminez; Iodine;
Macchiavello)

Staphylococcus aureus, 72, 73,
76, 79, 115
Staphylococcus epidermidis, 79
Streptococcus, 73, 115
Streptomycin, 78, 210
Sulfisoxazole, 127
Sulfonamides
genital tract infections, 127, 134
inclusion conjunctivitis, adult,
102–103, 108, 109
inclusion conjunctivitis, neonatal, 116
LGV, 54–55
pneumonia in infants, 118
psittacosis, 26
resistance to, LGV, 55
sensitivity to, taxonomic significance, 4
trachoma, 89, 90, 91, 92–93, 94
Syphilis, 53, 78

T strain mycoplasma, 130, 134, 136
Taiwan
genital tract infections, 131
trachoma, 72, 84
T'ang, F.F., 64
Taxonomy of chlamydiae, 3–7
Tear, antibody, 87, 198
Tears, 82, 198
Tetracyclines, 107, 143
genital tract infections, 130,
132, 133, 134, 135, 138
inclusion conjunctivitis, adult,
108–109
inclusion conjunctivitis, neonatal, 114, 116–117, 118
LGV, 55
NGU, 132–133, 134, 151
pneumonia in infants, 118
psittacosis, 25–26
trachoma, 89–90, 91–92, 93–94,
95
Throat washings, 206
Thygeson, Phillip, 98
Thygeson's superficial punctate
keratitis, 77
Thymidine kinase, 168–169
Tissue culture methods for isolation, 212–216
Tissue culture technique, 216–219

Tissues, 207–208
Toxin, murine, 179
Trachoma, 63–96, 97
  acute, 99
  CF test, 197
  clinical description, 65–70
  cytology, 78–81, 184
  differential diagnosis, 74–78
  dry eye syndrome, 66, 70, 89
  dubium, 67
  epidemiology, 64, 70–74, 95
  "genital," 97, 101
  Herbert's pits, 66
  immunization, 83–88
  intensity, 68, 70, 73
  keratitis, 66, 73, 102, 105, 106,
    109
  laboratory diagnosis, 78–82
  MacCallan classification, 67
  pannus, 66, 70, 75
  paratrachoma, 99
  prototrachoma, 67
  trachome pur, 70
  treatment, 65, 88–96
  trichiasis surgery, 89, 91, 95
Treatment
  genital tract infections, 132–134
  inclusion conjunctivitis, adult,
    108–109
  inclusion conjunctivitis, neo-
    natal, 116–117
  LGV, 54–56
  psittacosis, 25–26
  Reiter's syndrome, 143
  trachoma, 65, 88–96
TRIC agents, 46, 122

Trichiasis surgery, 89, 91, 95
Trichomoniasis, 130
Tunisia, 93
Turkeys, 12, 14, 15, 23, 31, 34
Typhoid fever, 21, 25

Ulceration, corneal, 66, 72, 95
Ureaplasma urealyticum, 134
Ureaplasmas, 127, 134
Urethral scrapings, 124, 128, 132
Urethritis, 122, 124–128
  nongonococcal, 122–123, 124–
    128, 132–133, 134, 135, 138,
    139, 151
  "nonspecific," 133
  postgonococcal, 124, 125, 131–
    132, 134
  in Reiter's syndrome, 142, 151
Urinalysis, 128, 134
Uveitis, 103–104, 109, 143

Vaccination (*see* Immunization)
Venereal bubo, 45
Vernal catarrh, 66, 78, 184
Viral conjunctivitis, 104–107,
  115–116
  cytology, 184
Vomitus, 226

Xerosis bacillus (*see* Diphtheroids)

Yolk sac isolation technique, 122,
  210–212